Internet-Delivered Therapeutic Interventions in Human Services

There has been exponential growth in the use of the Internet to deliver therapeutic and supportive human services. Online interventions are known by a variety of names, including online practice, etherapy, e-therapy, Internet therapy, online (psycho)therapy, Itherapy, Interapy, virtual therapy, online counselling, therap-e, therap-pc and others. All refer to the delivery of services over the Internet through a variety of delivery systems including asynchronous email, chat-based real time communication, video and chat communication, and closed circuit video conferencing. They include services delivered by professionals such as psychiatrists, social workers, psychologists, counsellors and nurses as well as self-help groups with a therapeutic purpose and supportive services provided by trained volunteers.

This book presents the most current research on online practice. Topics include: descriptions of innovative online practice, evaluation studies of online practice with specific disorders, meta-analysis of the effectiveness of online practice, education and training of online practitioners, methods for the delivery of online practice, organizational policy and ethical issues related to online practice, online crisis intervention and hotline services, and considerations for meeting legal and ethical requirements of online practice.

This book was originally published as a special issue of the *Journal of Technology in Human Services*.

Jerry Finn is currently a Professor of Social Work, University of Washington Tacoma teaching research and human behavior. He serves as a reviewer for the *Journal of Information Technology in Human Services* and several other social science journals, and is co-editor of the *Journal of Social Work Values and Ethics*.

Dick Schoech is a Professor teaching administration, community practice, and human services technology at the University of Texas-Arlington (UTA), School of Social Work. He is the chair of HUSITA (www.husita.org), an international organization promoting the ethical and effective use of technology to better serve humanity and is the founding editor (1985) of the *Journal of Technology in Human Services*, published by Taylor & Francis.

Internet-Delivered Therapeutic Interventions in Human Services

Methods, Interventions and Evaluation

Edited by Jerry Finn and Dick Schoech

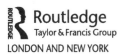

Routledge
Taylor & Francis Group

LONDON AND NEW YORK

First published 2009 by Routledge
2 Park Square, Milton Park, Abingdon, Oxon, OX14 4RN

Simultaneously published in the USA and Canada
by Routledge
711 Third Avenue, New York, NY 10017

Routledge is an imprint of the Taylor & Francis Group, an informa business

© 2009 Edited by Jerry Finn and Dick Schoech

First issued in paperback 2013

Typeset in Times by Value Chain, India

British Library Cataloguing in Publication Data
A catalogue record for this book is available from the British Library

ISBN13: 978-0-415-54888-5 (hbk)
ISBN13: 978-0-415-84531-1 (pbk)

CONTENTS

Introduction

Jerry Finn
Dick Schoech

The growing use of the Internet has made possible a "grapevine society" (Vallee, 1982) through which resources for health, mental health, and supportive services are widely available in industrialized societies through Internet-based professional and self-help services. A variety of terms are used to describe these services, including online practice, etherapy, Internet therapy or counseling, online (psycho) therapy, online counseling, itherapy, interapy, virtual therapy, cybercounseling, telehealth, telepsychiatry, cyberpsychology, e-social work, therap-e, therap-pc, online self-help, and others. All refer to the delivery of therapeutic services over the Internet through a variety of delivery systems, including asynchronous e-mail, chat-based messaging, discussion forums, closed circuit video conferencing, net-guided interventions, virtual reality, games, and Internet-based audio and video communication. The terms include services delivered by professionals such as psychiatrists, social workers, psychologists, counselors, and nurses as well as by therapeutic self-help groups and trained volunteers. Internet-delivered therapeutic interventions include online professional advice, prevention, assessment, intervention, case management, and supportive services for many health and mental health related issues. Fee-based etherapy has been provided by individuals in private practice as early as 1995 (Ainsworth, 2001). The field can no longer be said to be in its "infancy," as evidenced by the tens of thousands of online practitioners that can be found using a simple Google search, the codes of ethics for online practice developed by helping professional organizations, and the growing empirical research that documents the breadth and effectiveness of online practice.

This special issue of the *Journal of Technology and Human Services* goes beyond a discussion of the "potential" of online practice and anecdotal descriptions of services and outcomes; it focuses on the latest empirical evidence that supports etherapy both in the United States and abroad and discusses current issues still confronting the field. Specifically, this issue includes:

Empirical Evidence Regarding Etherapy

- Barak, Hen, Boniel-Nissim, and Shapira provide a meta-analysis of 92 etherapy studies with a total of 9,764 clients that provides strong support for the adoption of online psychological interventions as a legitimate therapeutic activity.
- Andersson and colleagues provide a review of their work in Sweden using cognitive-behavior therapy (CBT) to provide guided self-help over the Internet to intervene in problems such as headache, tinnitus, panic disorder, anxiety disorder, bulimia nervosa, and depression.
- Botella and colleagues present a case study of their approach and provide evidence of the effectiveness of CBT in treating social phobia and fear of public speaking.
- Finn and Hughes describe the evaluation of a new program model for delivering Internet-based sexual assault hotline services. The model includes chat-based interventions by trained volunteers with online supervisors.
- Kernsmith and Kernsmith examine the process and effectiveness of a voluntary online support group for recovering sex offenders facilitated by two nonprofessional recovering sex offenders. The group was found to be a positive therapeutic environment and resulted in significant improvement on several indicators of change for those who were active participants.
- Lintvedt and colleagues provide evidence from one university that suggests many students use the Internet for information about mental health issues. In addition, they found that student need for counseling services for depression is not being met. A substantial proportion of students whose needs were not being met by current services, however, also had positive attitudes about using an online, cognitive-behavior therapy (CBT) self-help program in lieu of face-to-face services.
- Pahwa and Schoech review some of the major online prevention websites and evaluations of their effectiveness. They discuss an evaluation model to evaluate an interactive multimedia anger management exercise that is part of a teen substance abuse prevention website.

The study points to many issues that occur when developing and evaluating online interventions in real-world environments.

- Finn and Bruce describe a case study of the LivePerson website, an etherapy model in which a private company provides the infrastructure for licensed online therapists to provide services using chat or e-mail for service delivery. A content analysis of the website is presented, including policies, number of consumers, consumer ratings, and therapists' degrees, licensure, age, sex, race, fees, and languages offered. In addition, the experiences of one practitioner are presented to highlight methods, processes, and ethical concerns.

Ethical and Legal Issues

- Midkiff and Wyatt discuss specific ethical issues, including boundaries of competence, basis in science, avoidance of harm, confidentiality, avoidance of false or deceptive statements, forums, testimonials, solicitation of clients, fees, and informed consent. In addition, they address interstate issues in online practice and recommend that federal licensing legislation be enacted.
- Zack reviews the current state of practice regarding legal issues related to providing mental health services via the Internet. He discusses jurisdiction, licensure, legal duties, and other legal concerns related to the business of online counseling. He addresses potential criminal and civil liability issues, noting procedural and substantive aspects of the relevant law.

Theoretical Papers and Overviews of Service Delivery

- Abbott, Klein, and Ciechomski highlight important issues in best practices in the delivery of etherapy based on the clinical and research work of members from the Monash University Etherapy Research, Education, and Training Unit and the research literature.
- Peng and Schoech review 10 theories selected from the fields of psychotherapy, social work, health promotion, gaming, and innovation dissemination that can be used for grounding the design, development, implementation, and evaluation of online interventions. Selected studies illustrate how these theories have been used in online human service interventions. An integrated theoretical approach and guidelines for designing online interventions are proposed.
- LaMendola and Krysik examine how current thinking in persuasive technologies may be applied to therapeutic interventions

through a planned and multidisciplinary design process. Design steps identified in the human services and the design sciences are analyzed to generate six design imperatives that provide a framework for optimizing the development of persuasive technology applications in the human services.

- Freddolino and Blaschke discuss online gaming in the twenty-first century as a new tool for human service interventions. They also consider negative and positive aspects of gaming and propose several research, practice, and educational strategies for subsequent development of this genre.

Etherapy Training Programs

- Murphy, MacFadden, and Mitchell describe the development of a university-based cybercounseling certificate program. The web-based program offers experienced face-to-face counselors training in an asynchronous, e-mail form of cybercounseling. Ethical issues such as cross-jurisdictional concerns, client appropriateness, and counselor insurance are discussed.
- Cárdenas, Serrano, Flores, and De la Rosa describe an etherapy teaching program for clinical psychology students by the Virtual Teaching and Cyberpsychology Laboratory of the National Autonomous University of Mexico. The program uses a CBT theoretical base and both asynchronous and synchronous e-mail. Preliminary results indicate that students increase knowledge of clinical interventions and improve in clinical skills.

Taken as a whole, these articles describe an evolving online practice, increasingly grounded in theory and empirical evidence. A number of the articles contain lessons learned for future development of programs and discuss unresolved issues needing further research. They point to the need for practitioners and consumers to be aware of strengths and limitations of online practice and for human service educators to seriously consider the inclusion of online practice in their curriculum.

REFERENCES

Ainsworth, M. (2001). The ABCs of Internet therapy. Retrieved November 27, 2007, from http://www.metanoia.org/imhs/directry.htm.

Vallee, J. (1982). *The network revolution: Confessions of a computer scientist*. Berkeley, CA: And/Or Press.

A Comprehensive Review and a Meta-Analysis of the Effectiveness of Internet-Based Psychotherapeutic Interventions

Azy Barak
Liat Hen
Meyran Boniel-Nissim
Na'ama Shapira

The Internet has been used for psychotherapeutic interventions for more than a decade. Various terms have been used to denote this special professional activity: etherapy (or counseling), online therapy, Internet therapy, and cybertherapy, and sometimes it is referred to as e-health or telehealth, as a part of more general activities. Although attempts have been made to associate specific terms with more focused activities (e.g., cybertherapy for the use of virtual reality software), this terminology has failed in practice, and professionals and laypersons alike normally use different terms interchangeably. There are, however, several major factors that differentiate among the different therapeutic applications conducted by means of the Internet. One of these has to do with the online-intervention method employed—whether it includes human communication (termed here etherapy) or is a self-help, website-based therapy (termed here web-based therapy). A different major factor has to do with another Internet-enabled capacity—whether an intervention is delivered in "real-time" (synchronously) or is delayed (asynchronously). A third important factor has to do with mode of communication—whether conducted textually, by audio only, or by video (webcam). Other important differentiations have to do with individual versus group mode and therapeutic approach, terms normally associated with traditional, face-to-face therapies.

From its start, Internet therapy has been criticized and opposed by both many laypeople (e.g., Skinner & Latchford, 2006) and professionals (e.g., Lester, 2006; Wells, Mitchell, Finkelhor, & Becker-Blease, 2007) on several grounds. First, the lack of face-to-face visibility—which prevents the transmission and detection of a client's nonverbal communication cues, on the one hand, and the use of a therapist's body language, on the other—created massive resistance. This opposition based on the lack of nonverbal communication was considered an essential component of therapeutic relationships. Second, ethical issues—relating to secrecy and confidentiality, identity of patients and therapists, impersonations, handling of emergency situations, and more—became a central problem with the application of computer-mediated, distance therapy. Third, contemporary laws and regulations did not always cover various situations created by online therapy, such as local licensing requirements, legal jurisdiction, professional insurance of negligence, and more, resulting in often unresolved legal issues. Fourth, practical and technical concerns led to arguments related to the training of online therapists, the dependency on electricity and on complicated, fragile technologies, as well as to worries about the digital divide, and more. All of these criticisms, though they still exist, have been answered to a great degree as the field developed, numerous professionals have connected, literally and figuratively, to this new channel of therapy, advanced technologies emerged, ethical codes were developed, training courses and workshops began to be offered, and so on (Chester & Glass, 2006; Grohol, 2004). Not least, many clients seemed to like this innovative therapeutic option (King et al., 2006).

In the attempt to respond to the questions and critiques posed by the opponents of online therapy, quite a few therapeutic *process studies* were conducted that generally tried to examine the special characteristics of the therapeutic dynamics created in distant, invisible, interpersonal circumstances. The findings of those investigations—obviously concentrating in etherapy of different forms—often showed that therapy processes online are, in many ways, similar to the traditional form of therapy, though they possess some unique features as well, which were identified. Cook and Doyle (2002), for example, found that clients of e-mail- or chat-based therapy rated therapeutic working alliance similar and even superior to that of face-to-face therapy. In an analogue study, Mallen, Day, and Green (2003), however, found higher ratings of disclosure, closeness, and satisfaction with the face-to-face therapy experience than with that online, though no difference in emotional understanding was detected between the two interaction modes. Escoffery, McCormick, and Bateman (2004) reported on the process development of goal-setting, consciousness growing, and satisfaction of clients using web-based therapy for smoking cessation. Lewis, Coursol, and Herting (2004) studied client and counselor experiences in videoconferencing-based counseling in a qualitative analysis of a case study. They were able to qualify interesting themes in counselor's and client's experiences, and noted the client's positive feelings. In an analogue study, Rochlen, Land, and Wong (2004) found that men with high emotionality preferred online counseling over face-to-face counseling more than did men with low or restricted emotionality. Bickmore, Gruber, and Picard (2005) showed that bond and working alliance may be achieved even when working with an automated software agent. In an observational analogue study, Rees and Stone (2005) saw that clinicians rated working alliance in videoconferencing-based therapy lower than in traditional, face-to-face sessions. Young (2005) investigated the attitudes of clients treated through online chat groups; although convenience and anonymity were cited as favorable factors, privacy and security concerns were listed against its use. Barak and Bloch (2006) found that session-impact factors in chat-based therapy were related to the perceived helpfulness of sessions. Leibert, Archer, Munson, and York (2006) studied clients' working alliance in, and satisfaction with, e-mail- and chat-based counseling; both were rated inferior to face-to-face experiences. Reynolds, Stiles, and Grohol (2006) found session-impact factors and therapeutic alliance in e-mail-based therapy to be similar to face-to-face therapy for both therapists and clients. According to Ritterband et al. (2006), the use of audio, graphics, and interactivity in website-based treatment of encopresis with children contributed to their elevated knowledge, motivation, and readiness to change. Thus, generally speaking, these studies show that counseling and psychotherapy relationships can effectively take place under the special circumstances enabled by the Internet as far as major therapeutic processes are concerned.

The main questions consistently asked throughout these studies and through numerous other publications have been whether therapy practiced online was effective, whether therapy could be conducted effectively (i.e., achieve its therapeutic goals) through the Internet, whether it was as effective as traditional therapy, and how various methods and variables associated with online therapy affected its effectiveness. Although quite a few individual studies on treating a variety of psychological problems have been conducted to date and numerous case studies have been published and presented, a comprehensive review and examination of these questions are still lacking.

Several attempts were made to provide an inclusive review on the effectiveness of online psychological interventions. These attempts, however, offered a rather limited view of the question at hand, mainly because of their partial inclusion of the published research (e.g., Anthony, 2006; Ritterband et al., 2003; Tate & Zabinski, 2004; Ybarra, Eaton, & Bickman, 2005); stenographic, encyclopedic-style summary (Barak, 2004); emphasis on history and development rather than effectiveness (e.g., Skinner & Zack, 2004); concentration on a specific problem area, such as anxiety (Andersson, Bergström, Carlbring, & Lindefors, 2005), depression (Andersson, 2006), panic disorder (Carlbring & Andersson, 2006), smoking cessation (Etter, 2006; Walters, Wright, & Shegog, 2006), weight loss (Weinstein, 2006), health-related problems (Strecher, 2007), or problem drinking (Walters, Miller, & Chiauzzi, 2005); concentration on web-based interventions only (Andersson, 2006; Griffiths & Christensen, 2006; Pull, 2006); focus on video-based therapy (Simpson, 2003); or their mixing together therapy and support (Mallen, Vogel, Rochlen, & Day, 2005). Although the general conclusion of these reviews, as well as several others, was highly supportive of Internet therapy, it seems that reliance on these resources is insufficient because their surveys of the literature are in effect incomplete or narrow. In addition, none of these reviews made an attempt to examine interactions of relevant moderators (e.g., age of clients, therapeutic approach) with therapy outcome. It should be noted that several books focusing on etherapy and e-counseling (e.g., Derrig-Palumbo & Zeine, 2005; Hsiung, 2002; Kraus, Zack, & Stricker, 2004; Tyler & Sabella, 2003) also provided a general and partial review of research, as well as numerous case examples, but did not provide a thorough and comprehensive view of the area.

Three meta-analytic reviews that are relevant in part to our current research questions were conducted. Wantland, Portillo, Holzemer, Slaughter, and McGhee (2004) conducted a meta-analysis of 22 web-based versus non-web-based psychological interventions intended to educate and create behavioral change in people with chronic illness. They found a large variability in effect size (ES), ranging from -0.01 to $+0.75$, which averaged out to a moderate mean ES.

In another meta-analytic review, Spek et al. (2007) examined 12 studies that tested the effectiveness of web-based cognitive-behavioral therapy (CBT) for depression and anxiety. They found a small-to-moderate *ES* for the treatment of depression and a large *ES* for the treatment of anxiety. Provision of therapist support (provided online) moderated these findings, as therapist support resulted in large effects and no such support resulted in small effects. These two meta-analyses referred only to web-based interventions in specific problem areas. Hirai and Clum (2006b) conducted a meta-analysis of the effectiveness of various self-help venues in helping people with anxiety problems, including computer and Internet self-help interventions among other methods (e.g., printed materials, videotapes). They found that computer- and Internet-based self-help interventions appeared, for the most part, to yield equally effective treatment outcomes as the other self-help interventions.

The aim of the current meta-analytic study was to provide fuller, more comprehensive answers to questions relating to the effectiveness of online psychological interventions. Our research was meant to cover a broad data set that referred to a variety of online technological methods, intervention settings, psychological approaches, problem areas, and other features that exist in the provision of psychotherapy through the Internet. The purpose was to examine the effectiveness of online interventions in general, and specifically in quantitative empirical studies and in the impact of moderators that interact with therapy outcome.

METHOD

Data Collection

We searched and collected all published studies relevant to our meta-analysis. The studies we used met these criteria: (1) they were published in a refereed journal in English at any time until March 2006 (inclusive); (2) they empirically studied the effectiveness of psychological treatments conducted through online channel(s) of communication (that is, Internet-delivered therapy); (3) the intervention was based on the actual implementation of a psychological intervention (rather than just the provision of online support or an online assessment); (4) the study contained more than five participants receiving online treatment; (5) treatment effectiveness was based on at least pre-post quantitative comparisons; (6) effectiveness of treatment was based on at least one actual outcome measure.

The search for studies was conducted by using the PsycINFO and MEDLINE databases as well as the Google Scholar and Scopus online scientific search engines. In addition, we checked the bibliographies of numerous articles to detect possible missing items. Except for a single article, all of the studies included in our research had been published up to and in March 2006; in the single exception, the study was made public by being posted on a publisher's website (it came out in print shortly thereafter).

In total, we collected 69 articles that met the inclusion criteria. Additional 47 articles that examined the effectiveness of online therapy were rejected because they had either insufficient data enabling the calculation of *ES*, used qualitative and descriptive approaches (usually through case studies), were based on mere literature reviews, or lacked major details in regard to the nature of the therapy or the research design employed. In two cases, in which specific information was missing (i.e., unclear treatment for a comparison group, missing information about participants), the authors of the studies were contacted to complete the information. Furthermore, we found that the results reported in 5 of the 69 usable articles had been duplicated and published in other articles in this set; therefore, the information gathered from these studies were included only once in the analysis. The final data set, therefore, contained 64 articles. Most of them reported a single study; several articles, however, described two or more (up to four) studies, each of which differed by gender of patients (e.g., Christensen, Griffiths, Korten, Brittliffe, & Groves, 2004), intervention method (e.g., Carlbring, Ekselius, & Andersson, 2003), or another factor. In sum, the 64 articles reported on 92 independent studies (based on different patients) of various online interventions that were aimed at treating patients who suffered from a psychological problem or distress. This collection, then, contains the final data set for our meta-analysis. (The first author may be contacted for a list of keywords used in searching for articles and for a list of articles rejected from the data set used for the meta-analysis.)

In all, the 92 studies examined 11,922 participants, 9,764 of whom received some form of psychological intervention online. The number of patients in each study ranged from 6 to 2,341 (mean = 106; median = 28). Table 1 presents a summary of the basic characteristics

TABLE 1. Articles Included in the Meta-analysis

Author(s)	Problem Area	Online Channel & Format	N	Therapeutic Approach	Age & Type of Patients	Research Design	Outcome Measures	Findings	ES[1] (CI[2])
Andersson et al. (2005)	Depression	Website and forum	36	CBT	Adults	RCT, compared to WL CG	SR of depression, anxiety, and quality of life	TG improved in all measures while no change in CG. Change maintained in 6-month follow-up	.67 (±43)
Andersson, Lundström, & Ström (2003)	Recurrent headache	1. Website and e-mail	(1) 13	CBT	Adults	RCT, comparison of 2 TGs	Headache diary and SR of stress, anxiety, and depression	No change in headaches in both TGs; improvement in SR outcomes in both TGs	.23 (±.77)
		2. Web-based and telephone support	(2) 17						.18 (±67)
Andersson, Strömgren, Ström, & Lyttkens (2002)	Tinnitus	Website and e-mail support	24	CBT	Adults	RCT, compared to WL CG	SR of tinnitus annoyance, anxiety, and depression	Reduction in tinnitus annoyance and improved psychological measures	.32 (±.49)
Bruning Brown, Winzelberg, Abascal, & Taylor (2004)	Eating disorders	Website and forum	(1) 102 kids	PE	Adolescents and parents	TG vs. no-treatment comparison group	SR of eating disorders-related scales, knowledge test, and parents' attitudes	Improvement in all measures of TG compared to following treatment but not at 1-year follow-up.	.08 (±.34)
			(2) 22 parents					Parents attitudes' positively changed	.57 (±.51)

11

TABLE 1. Articles Included in the Meta-analysis *(continued)*

Author(s)	Problem Area	Online Channel & Format	N	Therapeutic Approach	Age & Type of Patients	Research Design	Outcome Measures	Findings	ES[1] (CI[2])
Buhrman et al. (2004)	Chronic back pain	Website and telephone support	22	CBT	Adults	RCT, compared to WL CG	SR of level of pain, depression, and anxiety	TG improved in some measures, attitudes, and ability to decrease pain but not in others. Some effects maintained at 3-month follow-up	−.04 (±.55)
Carlbring et al. (2003)	Panic disorder	Website and e-mail	(1) 11	(1) CBT	Adults	RCT, compared to applied relaxation treatment	SR of agoraphobia, anxiety, depression, and quality of life; diary of attacks	TG improved in most measures, but was a little inferior to the improvement of the CG	.44 (±.83)
			(2) 11	(2) Applied relaxation					.71 (±.83)
Carlbring, Furmark, Steczkó, Ekselius, & Andersson (2006)	Social phobia	Website and e-mail	26	CBT	Adults	RCT, compared to WL CG	SR of social anxiety, general anxiety, depression, and quality of life	TG improved in all measures at posttreatment, and maintained or further improved at 6-month follow-up	.98 (±.54)
Carlbring et al. (2005)	Panic disorder	Website and e-mail	25	CBT	Adults	RCT, compared to FTF treatment	SR of agoraphobia, anxiety, depression, and quality of life	Both treatment groups improved in all measures. Effects maintained at 1-year follow-up	.81 (±.55)

Carlbring et al. (2001)	Panic disorder	Website and e-mail	20	CBT	Adults	RCT, TG compared to WL CG	SR of panic attacks and anxiety	Positive effects in TG in all outcome measures while no change in CG	.84 (±.61)
Celio et al. (2000)	Body dissatisfaction	Website and forum	24	PE	Female adults	RCT, compared to FTF treatment and to WL CG	SR of body and eating concerns and attitudes	Improvement pre- to posttreatment in all measures. Results maintained and continued to improve at 6-month follow-up	.27 (±.73)
Chiauzzi, Green, Lord, Thum, & Goldstein (2005)	Binge drinking	Website	(1) 42	(1) CBT M	Adults	RCT, TG vs. WL CG (CG instructed to read online articles on consequences of heavy drinking)	SR of attitudes toward drinking, and drinking behaviors	Reduction of drinking and improved attitudes; effects continued and improved in 3-month follow-up	.61 (±.43)
			(2) 63	(2) CBT F					.48 (±.35)
			(3) 50	(3) PE M					.82 (±.39)
			(4) 60	(4) PE F					.51 (±.36)
Christensen, Griffiths, & Jorm (2004)	Depression	Website	(1) 165	(1) PE	Adults	RCT, 2 TGs vs. WL CG	SR of depression and knowledge of treatment	Both treatments effective in reducing depression symptoms	.66 (±.21)
			(2) 182	(2) CBT					.44 (±.21)
Christensen, Griffiths, & Korten (2002)	Depression and anxiety	Website	(1) 30	CBT (1) M	Adults	Pre-post and follow-up comparisons	SR of depression and anxiety	Reduction of depression and anxiety at each measurement point	.30 (±.51)
			(2) 48	(2) F					.45 (±.39)
Christensen et al. (2004)	Depression and anxiety	Website	(1) 102	CBT (1) F	Adults	Compared 2 TGs: experimental trial vs. use of open site	SR of depression and anxiety	Reduction of depression and anxiety of both groups	1.03 (±.27)
			(2) 36	(2) M					.84 (±.46)

(Continued)

TABLE 1. Articles Included in the Meta-analysis (continued)

Author(s)	Problem Area	Online Channel & Format	N	Therapeutic Approach	Age & Type of Patients	Research Design	Outcome Measures	Findings	ES[1] (CI[2])
Clarke et al. (2005)	Depression	Website and phone or postcard reminders	(1) 75	PE and (1) Postcard reminders	Adults	RCT, TG compared to no-treatment CG	SR of depression and utilization of health services	Reduction in depression over therapy period in comparison with CG. No difference in use of health services	.38 (±.31)
			(2) 80	(2) Telephone reminders					.53 (±.31)
Clarke et al. (2002)	Depression	Website	144	PE	Adults	RCT, TG compared to no-treatment CG	SR of depression	No difference between TG and CG in changing over the research period	.04 (±.23)
Cohen & Kerr (1998)	Precounseling anxiety	Chat	12	Unspecified	Adults	TG vs. FTF	SR of anxiety	Anxiety decreased in both groups	.86 (±.80)
Day & Schneider (2002)	Various	1. Audio chat	(1) 26	CBT	Adults	TGs vs. FTF vs. WL CG	SR of complaints and functioning	Audio, video, and FTF were similarly effective	.91 (±.53)
		2. Video chat	(2) 27						1.05 (±.54)
Devineni & Blanchard (2005)	Chronic headache	Website and e-mail	39	CBT	Adults	RCT, TG vs. WL CG	SR of headache symptoms, depression, and anxiety	TG (of 2 versions) effective over CG. Results maintained in 2-month follow-up	.36 (±.43)
Dew et al. (2004)	Heart transplant-related psychological symptoms	Website and forum	(1) 20	PE	Adult (1) patients	RCT, TG vs. CG	SR of depression, anxiety, and social functioning of patients, SR of hostility of caregivers	TG improved in all measures while CG did not change. Greater compliance of TG than CG with medical procedures	.53 (±.57)
			(2) 17		(2) caregivers				.86 (±.58)

Author (year)	Topic	Medium	N	Intervention	Population	Design	Measures	Results	Effect size
Etter (2005)	Smoking cessation	Website	(1) 2341 (2) 1896	PE (1) Emphasis on health risk (2) Emphasis on nicotine replacement	Adults	RCT, comparison of 2 treatments	SR of smoking abstinence	Both treatments produced decrease in smoking, with advantage of 1st over 2nd intervention	.58 (±.06) .49 (±.04)
Farvolden, Denisoff, Selby, Bagby, & Rudy (2005)	Panic disorder and agoraphobia	Website and forum and e-mail	12	CBT	Adults	Pre-post TG	SR of panic attacks	Decrease in panic attacks for each consecutive stage	.60 (±.80)
Gollings & Paxton (2006)	Body image and disordered eating	Chat room and forum	20	CBT group therapy	Female adults	RCT, TG vs. FTF treatment	SR of body image, eating disorders, depression, anxiety, and self-esteem	Both groups improved in all measures with no mode difference	.78 (±.62)
Griffiths, Christensen, Jorm, Evans, & Groves (2004)	Depression	Website	(1) 136 (2) 121	(1) Information (2) CBT	Adults	RCT, TGs vs. CG	SR of depression, stigma, thoughts	Intervention caused slightly reduced stigmatic attitudes of depression	.16 (±.23)
Harvey-Berino et al. (2002)	Overweight	Website and e-mail and chat room	30	Unspecified	Adults	RCT, TG compared to 2 FTF maintenance support	Body weight and adherence to treatment	FTF meetings for maintenance of weight loss treatment more effective than online intervention	.09 (±.24) .45 (±.51)

(Continued)

TABLE 1. Articles Included in the Meta-analysis *(continued)*

Author(s)	Problem Area	Online Channel & Format	N	Therapeutic Approach	Age & Type of Patients	Research Design	Outcome Measures	Findings	ES[1] (CI[2])
Harvey-Berino, Pintauro, Buzzell, & Gold (2004)	Overweight and obese eating	Website and e-mail and chat room	77	Unspecified	Adults	RCT, TG compared to 2 FTF maintenance support	Body weight, adherence to treatment, and energy expense	Online intervention was as effective as 2 FTF support in maintaining treatment effects	.07 (±.31)
Hasson, Anderberg, Theorell, & Arnetz (2005)	Stress	Website and chat	129	CBT	Adults	RCT, TG compared to information-only CG	Physiological markers and self-report of stress management	TG improved over CG in most outcome measures	.29 (±.23)
Hirai & Clum (2006a)	Traumatic event	Website	13	CBT	Adults	RCT, TG compared to WL CG	SR of anxiety, depression, and impact of event	TG improved in all measures relative to CG	.62 (±.75)
Hopps, Pépin, & Boisvert (2003)	Loneliness (for people with disabilities)	Chat rooms, in groups of 2–3 patients	10	CBT	Adults	RCT, TG compared to WL CG	SR of loneliness and acceptance of disability	TG improved in all measures and exceeded CG. Results maintained in 4-month follow-up	1.18 (±.90)
Kenardy, McCafferty, & Rosa (2003)	Anxiety disorders	Website	36	CBT	Adults	RCT, TG compared to WL CG	SR of anxiety, depression, and related cognitions	Some improvement was found, unrelated to treatment	.61 (±.43)
Kenardy, McCafferty, & Rosa (2006)	Anxiety disorders	Website	36	CBT	Adults	RCT, compared to WL CG	SR of anxiety, fear, depression, and related cognitions	Positive effects of treatment in most measures over CG, maintained in 6-month follow-up	.62 (±.45)

Study	Disorder	Intervention	N	Treatment	Age	Design	Outcome measures	Results	Effect size
Kenwright, Marks, Gega, & Mataix (2004)	Phobia or panic disorder	Website and telephone support	10	CBT	Adults	Pre-post evaluation of TG	SR of fear, depression, and social adjustment	Patients improved in all outcome measures. Effects maintained at 1-month follow-up	1.09 (±.88)
Klein & Richards (2001)	Panic disorder	Website	11	CBT	Adults	RCT, TG compared with NT CG	Incidents of panic attacks, SR of anxiety, depression, self-efficacy, and body vigilance	TG improved in most outcome measures while no changes in CG	.26 (±.83)
Klein, Richards, & Austin (2006)	Panic disorder	Website and	19	CBT	Adults	RCT, TG compared CGs of information and written manual	SR of panic attacks, anxiety, depression, body vigilance, and related cognitions	Effective changes to posttherapy and 3-month follow-up of both TG & written manual TC on most outcome measures, but not information TG	1.13 (±.64)
Kypri & McAnally (2005)	Hazardous health behaviors	Site-based assessment and prescriptive feedback	60	PE	Adults	RCT, TG compared to assessment only and minimal contact CGs	SR of behaviors	TG found effective in changing behaviors similar to assessment but better than minimal contact	.30 (±.36)
Kypri et al. (2004)	Hazardous drinking	Site-based assessment and prescriptive feedback	42	PE	Adults	RCT, TG compared to written material CG	SR of behaviors	Reductions in hazardous behaviors in 6 weeks and 6 months following treatment compared to CG	.35 (±.43)
Lange et al. (2003)	Posttraumatic stress	Website	69	CBT	Adults	RCT, TG compared to WL CG	SR of behaviors and relevant emotions	Positive effects of TG on all outcome measures relative to CG; these maintained at 6-month follow-up	.92 (±.42)

(Continued)

17

TABLE 1. Articles Included in the Meta-analysis (continued)

Author(s)	Problem Area	Online Channel & Format	N	Therapeutic Approach	Age & Type of Patients	Research Design	Outcome Measures	Findings	ES[1] (CI[2])
Lange et al. (2000)	Posttraumatic stress	Website	20	CBT	Adults	Pre-post comparisons of TG	Trauma symptoms, anxiety, and depression	Positive effects of the treatment in all outcome measures, sustained 6-week follow-up	.86 (±.62)
Lenert, Muñoz, Perez, & Bansod (2004)	Smoking cessation	1. Website	(1) 70	PE	Adults	Comparisons of several time points between TGs	Percentage of smoke quitting	Higher smoking-quitting rates when e-mail messages sent to site users	.29 (±.33)
		2. Website and e-mail	(2) 74						.40 (±.32)
Lieberman (2003)	Jet lag	Website	20	Prescriptive PE	Adults	Relationship between prescriptive treatment and symptom relief	SR of jet-lag-related symptoms	Negative correlation between compliance with intervention and severity of symptoms	1.06 (±.65)
Lieberman et al. (2005)	Depression in Parkinson's disease patients	Chat room and forum for (1) homogeneous or (2) heterogeneous	(1) 17	PE and general support	Adults	Pre-post comparisons of 2 TGs	SR of depression and quality of life	Reduction in depression in homogeneous but not in heterogeneous groups	−.01 (±.67)
			(2) 14						
Moor et al. (2005)	Binge drinking	E-mail	53	PE	Adults	TG compared with CG receiving written materials	SR of drinking behavior	Effective treatment evident in pre-post comparisons, similar in both groups	.52 (±.74)
									.17 (±.38)

Study	Disorder	Medium	Sessions	Treatment	Population	Design	Outcome measures	Results	Effect size
O'Kearney, Gibson, Christensen, & Griffiths (2006)	Depression	Website	20	CBT	Adolescents	RCT, TG compared with WL CG	SR of depressive symptoms, attribution style, and self-esteem and related cognitions	Some positive moderate effects were found; only change in self-esteem sustained in 16-week follow-up	.19 (±.68)
Owen, Klapow, Roth, Shuster, & Bellis (2005)	Anxiety and mood related to breast cancer	Website and forum	26	CBT	Female adults	RCT, TG compared with WL CG	SR of health-related quality of life, psychological and physical well-being	Weak effects of treatment from pre- to post-intervention and to 12-week follow-up	.19 (±.54)
Patten (2003)	Depression	Website	406	PE	Adults	RCT, TG compared with information-only CG	SR of depression	No effects of the intervention in either group	.04 (±.14)
Richards & Alvarenga (2002)	Panic disorder	Website	9	CBT	Adults	Pre- to 3-month following treatment comparisons	SR of panic and anxiety severity, body vigilance, and body sensations	Improvement in some of the outcome measures	.61 (±1.00)
Richards et al. (2006)	Panic disorder	Website and e-mail	(1) 12 (2) 11 (3) 9 12	(1) CBT (2) CBT and stress management (3) information PE and behavioral	Adults	RCT, 2 TGs compared with information-only CG	SR of panic severity, depression, anxiety, agoraphobic cognitions, body vigilance, and quality of life	Positive improvement in all measures were found equally in both TGs compared to CG; these effects sustained at 3-month follow-up	.78 (±.80) 1.07 (±.83)
Ritterband et al. (2003)	Encopresis	Website	12	PE and behavioral	Children	RCT, TG compared with comparison group that received routine medical care	Relevant knowledge, encopresis incidents, and toilet habits	Effective change in most outcome measures relative to pretreatment and to CG	-.10 (±.92) .65 (±.80)

(Continued)

19

TABLE 1. Articles Included in the Meta-analysis *(continued)*

Author(s)	Problem Area	Online Channel & Format	N	Therapeutic Approach	Age & Type of Patients	Research Design	Outcome Measures	Findings	ES^1 (CI^2)
Robinson & Serfaty (2001)	Eating disorders	E-mail	19	CBT or eclectic	Adults	Pre- to posttreatment comparison	SR of depression, and symptoms and severity of eating disorders	Effective change in all measures from pre- to posttreatment	.37 (±.58)
Rothert et al. (2006)	Weight management	Website	(1) 438 (2) 429	(1) Tailored behavior (2) PE	Adults	RCT, compared TG to information-only CG	Body weight	Reduced body weight in TG more than CG, at both 3- and 6-month follow-up assessment	.19 (±.13) .08 (±.13)
Schneider et al. (2005)	Phobic and panic disorders	Website	(1) 33 (2) 15	(1) CBT, with exposure (2) CBT, self-management without exposure	Adults	RCT, compared 2 TGs	SR of state of problem and evaluation of fear by blind assessor	Both TGs equally improved at posttreatment on most measures, but TG(1) sustained better outcome at 4-week follow-up	1.31 (±.50) 1.28 (±.74)
Strecher et al. (2005)	Smoking cessation	Website and e-mail	(1) 446 (2) 418	(1) Tailored CBT (2) Nontailored CBT	Adults	Compared 2 TGs at 6 and 12 weeks following intervention	SR of smoking abstinence	Over 20 percent abstinence on 28-day continuous rates in both groups, with advantage to tailored intervention	1.68 (±.13) 1.43 (±.14)

Study	Disorder	Medium	N	Treatment	Population	Design	Outcome measures	Results	Effect size
Ström, Pattersson, & Andersson (2000)	Recurrent headache	Website and e-mail	20	CBT	Adults	RCT, TG compared with WL CG	Headache diary and effects and depression	Reduction in headache severity and depression	.41 (±.59)
Ström, Pattersson, & Andersson (2004)	Insomnia	E-mail and web page	30	CBT	Adults	RCT, TG compared with WL CG	Sleep diary, depression, and anxiety	Improved sleeping quality	.32 (±.44)
Swartz, Noell, Schroeder, & Ary (2006)	Smoking cessation	Website	87	PE	Adults	RCT, TG compared with WL CG	Smoking abstinence	Abstinence rate of TG was higher than in CG at 3-month follow-up	.45 (±.28)
Tate, Jackvony, & Wing (2003)	Weight loss	1. Website 2. Website and e-mail	(1) 46 (2) 46	Behavioral	Adults	RCT, 2 TGs compared pre- to posttreatment	Body weight and waist circumference	Both TGs improved in outcome measures; 2nd group was more successful	.25 (±.41) .44 (±.41)
Tate, Wing, & Winett (2001)	Weight loss	1. Website 2. Website and e-mail	(1) 30 (2) 32	(1) PE (2) Behavioral	Adults	RCT, 2 TGs compared pre- to posttreatment	Body weight and waist circumference	Both TGs improved in outcome measures; 2nd group was more successful	.43 (±.49) .46 (±.48)
Wade, Wolfe, Brown, & Pestian (2005)	Traumatic brain injury	Website and webcam	(1) 6 (2) 8	CBT	(1) Parents (2) Children	Pre- to posttreatment comparisons	Child adjustment, parent-child conflicts, family functioning	Small improvement in most outcome measures	.65 (±.98) .44 (±1.13)

(Continued)

TABLE 1. Articles Included in the Meta-analysis *(continued)*

Author(s)	Problem Area	Online Channel & Format	N	Therapeutic Approach	Age & Type of Patients	Research Design	Outcome Measures	Findings	ES[1] (CI[2])
White et al. (2004)	Weight loss	Website or website and e-mail	(1) 29	(1) PE parents	Adolescents and parents	RCT, 2 TGs compared pre- to posttreatment	Body mass index, weight, body fat	TGs improved in all measures over 6 months, both in children and parents, more successful in behavioral TG	−.01 (±.51)
			(2) 28	(2) PE adolescents					−.07 (±.51)
			(3) 29	(3) Behavioral parents					.10 (±.51)
			(4) 28	(4) Behavioral adolescents					.08 (±.51)
Winzelberg et al. (2000)	Body image	Website and forum	24	CBT	Adults	RCT, TG compared with no-treatment CG	SR of body shape, eating disorders, and weight and shape concerns	No differences between groups, but some advantage to TG at 3-month follow-up	.46 (±.60)
Womble et al. (2004)	Weight loss	Website and e-mail and forum	15	Behavioral	Female adults	RCT, TG compared with manual treatment CG	Weight, biochemical data, and SR of quality of life	More changes in CG than in TG	.36 (±.58)

Study	Topic	Medium	N	Therapy	Approach	Population	Design	Outcome measures	Results	ES
Woodruff, Edwards, Conway, & Elliott (2001)	Smoking cessation	Chat room	18	Client-centered		Adolescents	Pre- to posttreatment comparisons	Abstinence rates, amount smoked, and related attitudes	Positive changes occurred, maintained at 1-month follow-up	.51 (±.67)
Zabinski et al. (2001)	Eating pathology and body-image dissatisfaction	Website and forum	27	PE		Female adults	RCT, TG compared with WL CG	Body mass index and SR of body image and eating disorders	Improvement of TG in most outcome measures, sustained at 10-week follow-up	.24 (±.52)
Zabinski, Wilfley, Calfas, Winzelberg, & Taylor (2004)	Eating pathology and body-image dissatisfaction	3 chat rooms	28	PE		Female adults	RCT, TG compared with WL CG	Body mass index, eating disorders, body image	Improvement of TG in most outcome measures, sustained at 10-week follow-up	.53 (±.51)
Zetterqvist, Maanmies, Ström, & Andersson (2003)	Stress	Website	23	CBT		Adults	RCT, TG compared with WL CG	SR of stress, social support, anxiety, and depression	Improvement of TG in most outcome measures, but some improvement in CG too	.70 (±.53)

Note: *ES* = effect size; CBT = cognitive-behavior therapy; PE = psychoeducation; FTF = face-to-face; RCT = randomized controlled trial; SR = self-report; TG = treatment group; CG = control group; WL = waiting list; NT = no treatment. *N* = number of participants receiving online treatment in the statistical analyses.

[1]*ES* = average of effects of outcome measures used in each study.

of the studies included in the analysis. The interventions analyzed were evaluated by a total of 746 measures of effects. Some studies were evaluated by a single outcome measure (e.g., Cohen & Kerr, 1998), whereas others were assessed by several measures, up to as many as 21 (Buhrman, Fältenhag, Ström, & Andersson 2004). On the average, the studies used eight measures to determine the effectiveness of treatment.

Coding of Moderators

Two coders independently coded various study features as possible moderators of effects, based on theoretical or methodological considerations. Interrater consensus between the coders revealed a 95 percent agreement. In cases of disagreement or lack of coherence, a third rater was involved to reach a final, agreed-on rating. The three coders held either masters or doctorate degrees in the behavioral sciences. As mentioned, when the study provided insufficient data with respect to a specific moderator, it was coded as absent and not included in the final analysis. Moderator analyses were performed to examine whether the *ES* of an intervention or a group intervention could be explained by moderating variables. In cases in which a specific moderator resulted in more than two separate groups, it was designated as a moderating variable if the analysis revealed significant heterogeneity between two of the groups, each of which displayed within-group homogeneity (Hedges & Olkin, 1985). A minimum of five cases in a category allowed for a meaningful test of homogeneity (Voyer, Voyer, & Bryden, 1995); however, not all of the coded moderators were used because of the small number of studies in some of the categories.

To avoid sample-size bias, once Hedge's *g* was calculated for a given variable, the corresponding *ES* was weighed according to the number of participants included in the *ES* calculation. These calculations were performed by means of the D-STAT program and according to the formulas developed by Hedges and Olkin (1985).

After the mean weighed *ES* was calculated, tests of homogeneity were performed to determine whether the *ES*s could be considered to share a common population *ES*. If *Q* statistics were significant, homogeneity would be rejected for the *ES*s within the given set and moderator analyses conducted to identify the sources of systematic variations among the *ES*s. In these calculations, the moderator variables represent the independent variables, while the effectiveness of the interventions represents the dependent variables. Moderator analyses were performed as follows: First, the mean effect size and the value of within-group homogeneity (Q_W = within) were calculated for each category of the moderator variables. Next, the degree of homogeneity between the moderator categories (Q_B = between) was calculated. A moderator variable is considered to explain the variance of an effect set if the value of Q_W is not significant while the value of Q_B is significant.

Calculation of Effect Size

The data collected from the 92 studies investigated were converted into a uniform, standardized format to enable a quantitative synthesis by means of meta-analytic calculations, using the fixed-effects method. The studies contained 746 measures of effects of the interventions employed. The intervention *ES* of each of the 746 measures was computed through statistical procedures developed by Hedges and Olkin (1985) and additional mathematical solutions for nonsignificant *ES* (Rosenthal, 1984).

In several cases, some data were missing. We then calculated the *ES* of the effects of individual measures on the available data. When data associated with a specific moderator were missing, we either omitted missing data or included it in the "other" category in presenting the results.

After computing *ES*s for all measures and the average *ES* for each of the studies, we examined as a common procedure in meta-analysis the distribution of effects to detect outliers. Although three of the 92 mean effects were detected as outliers, we decided not to exclude these studies for the following reasons: First, the mean weighted *ES* did not change when outliers were excluded. Second, it became clear when analyzing moderating effects that the outliers' *ES*s significantly associated with moderator interaction, thus excluding the possibility that these studies could actually damage the explanatory value of our review. In other words, the outliers actually contributed to the homogeneity of variance rather than the opposite—the main reason for discarding outliers. Thus, our decision is consistent with statistical requirements and reasoning (Fuller & Hester, 1999; Hedges & Olkin, 1985).

RESULTS

The average weighted *ES* over all 92 studies, across all dependent measures, was 0.53, which is considered to be a medium effect (Cohen, 1988). As can be observed in Table 1, average effects varied greatly from study to study, from a minimum *ES* of –0.10 (Richards, Klein, & Austin, 2006; treating panic disorder through online information alone) to a maximum of 1.68 (Strecher, Shiffman, & West, 2005; treating smoking cessation through tailored CBT). The *ES*s also showed extreme variations along other variables, especially through the 746 dependent measures: from a low of –2.90 (self-report of pain severity in treating chronic back pains; in Buhrman et al., 2004) to 5.10 (self-report of "total phobia" in follow-up versus pretreatment in treating phobic and panic disorders, both with and without exposure in using CBT; in Schneider, Mataix-Cols, Marks, & Bachofen, 2005). Out of the 746 effects calculated, 75 were zero or less (10 percent); out of the 92 mean *ES*s calculated per study, 5 (5.4 percent) were negative.

We then examined the moderation effects on *ES* of the various moderators in searching for meaningful interactions. The following sections present the moderating effects examined.

Type of Outcome Measure of Effectiveness

Effectiveness of treatments was measured in various ways: clients' self-report questionnaires, reports of behaviors and activities, assessments and diagnostics by experts and raters, and physiological measures—all suited to the study and problem in question. Table 2 presents the comparison of *ES*s by type of dependent measure. The differences among *ES* by type of measure were highly significant

TABLE 2. Effect Size by Type of Outcome Measure

Type of Measure	*ES*	*n*	*N*
Evaluation by Expert	0.93	3	140
Behavior	0.61	26	6272
Self-Report	0.43	62	4518
Physical	0.19	26	1892
Other	1.54	8	222

Note: ES = effect size; *n* = number of effects; *N* = number of participants. Number of effects exceeds 92; some of the studies used more than one type of measure.

($Q_B = 226.42$; $p < .001$), varying from 0.93 (evaluation by experts and raters) to 0.19 (physical; e.g., blood pressure, brain waves). The "other" category yielded very high average *ES*, but this seems to be random, as there is no logical common denominator (e.g., number of visits to a general practitioner before and after treatment, therapist satisfaction). It seems that psychological treatments conducted online are less successful in producing problem-related changes that are physical or somatic in nature, such as blood pressure or weight. Without this type of effectiveness outcome measure, however, the average *ES* would apparently have increased significantly and become closer to what is considered high *ES*.

Type of Problem

Patients were treated for a variety of problems and psychological distresses (sometimes associated with medical-considered problems, such as back pains or headaches). We classified most of these problems into several meaningful categories; however, eight specific problems (e.g., insomnia) remained in the "other" category. As may be viewed in Table 3, average *ES* yielded significant variations among the problem categories ($Q_B = 197.98$; $p < .001$). While post-traumatic stress disorder (PTSD) (mean $ES = 0.88$) and panic and anxiety disorders (mean $ES = 0.80$) were treated most effectively, weight loss received the least effective treatment ($ES = 0.17$). Thus, it looks as if Internet-based interventions are better suited to treat problems that are more psychological in nature—that is, problems

TABLE 3. Effect Size by Type of Problem

Type of Problem	ES	n	N
PTSD	0.88	3	148
Panic and Anxiety	0.80	23	498
Smoking Cessation	0.62	8	5460
Drinking	0.48	6	351
Body Image	0.45	5	221
Depression	0.32	16	2500
Physiological	0.27	7	212
Weight Loss	0.17	16	1604
Other	0.55	8	1427

Note: ES = effect size; *n* = number of effects; *N* = number of participants; PTSD = post-traumatic stress disorder dealing with emotions, thoughts, and behaviors—and less suited to treat problems that are primarily physiological or somatic (although these obviously have psychological components, too). If the latter categories were removed from the analysis, the average *ES* would have exceeded 0.6.

We examined possible confounding effects in that differential effectiveness might have been created by different therapeutic approaches, use of certain type of outcome measures, or other factors. We found no support for such confounding effects.

Time of Measuring Effectiveness

Most studies measured effectiveness right at the end of the therapy (i.e., posttreatment) or very close to it; a number of studies measured effectiveness in later follow-up, ranging from four weeks to a year after the end of therapy. The mean *ES* for post-therapy measurement, which involved 85 studies, was 0.52, whereas the mean *ES* of 33 studies that measured effectiveness at follow-up was 0.59. Despite the optical, apparent difference in favor of the follow-up effect, it was not found to be statistically significant ($Q_B = 2.46$; $p > .05$). The lack of difference means that effects of Internet-based interventions last for a longer time than just to the end of therapy, as should be expected of effective treatment intervention.

Therapeutic Theoretical Approach

Three main psychotherapeutic approaches characterized the studies being analyzed: CBT (intervention primarily based on a combination of changing thought patterns and contents, associated with rehearsal of related relevant behaviors), psychoeducational (intervention primarily based on providing information and explanations on a problem area and behaviors and emotions associated with it and prescribed instructions on how to change), and behavioral (intervention primarily based on modification and shaping of target behaviors based on learning principles). Table 4 presents the *ES*s by approach. Significant differences emerged among the therapy categories ($Q_B = 190.22$; $p < .001$), with the CBT (*ES* = 0.83) being found much more effective than the other approaches. The behavioral approach seems to be the least suited for online treatment (*ES* = 0.23). If behavioral approaches were left out of Internet

TABLE 4. Effect Size by Type of Theoretical Approach of Intervention

Type of Intervention	ES	n	N
Cognitive-Behavioral	0.83	51	3960
Psycho-educational	0.46	25	6796
Behavioral	0.23	14	1136
Other	0.65	2	30

Note: ES = effect size; n = number of effects; N = number of participants.

interventions, average *ES* would have increased, it seems, to a much higher level of effectiveness.

Here, too, possible confounding effects were examined to test that differential effectiveness was a result of other factors (e.g., presenting problem). We found no support for such confounding effects.

Age of Patients

We classified the age of clients into five age groups according to the data available from the articles (see Table 5). However, quite a few studies reported only an age range; hence, these data have to be referred to with caution. The effects of the data used for the analysis yielded significant differences among age groups ($Q_B = 181.23$; $p < .001$). An interesting *ES* pattern emerged, as youth and oldest adults seem to be less effectively treated (*ES* = 0.15 and 0.20, respectively), whereas young (19–24) and older (25–39) adults seem to gain more from Internet-based therapy (*ES* = 0.48 and 0.62, respectively).

TABLE 5. Effect Size by Age of Patients

Age Group	ES	n	N
18 and under	0.15	6	287
19–24	0.48	14	840
25–39	0.62	27	6941
40 and above	0.20	31	3172
Age not reported	0.63	14	682

Note: ES = effect size; n = number of effects; N = number of participants.

Form of Online Intervention: Web-based versus Etherapy

Internet-based therapy can be delivered mainly through a website (i.e., web-based therapy, using a number of intervention methods) or online communication (i.e., etherapy, through various communication channels and modalities). Although these two forms of delivering therapy are essentially different, they both use the Internet as a major vehicle for interacting with clients from a distance. Of the 92 studies, the mean *ES* of 65 studies that examined the effectiveness of web-based therapy was 0.54, which is not significantly different from the mean *ES* of 0.46 found for 27 studies that investigated the effectiveness of etherapy ($Q_B = 2.49$; $p > .05$). It is important to note that, generally, web-based and etherapy used similar theoretical approaches with similar patients (in terms of age and gender), with similar presenting problems, and were assessed by similar outcome measures, hence confounding effects are improbable.

Group versus Individual Therapy

The Internet enables delivering therapy in individual or group modes, just as in face-to-face therapy. However, whereas web-based therapy is conducted individually, etherapy in principle (aside from possible supplements of group support offered occasionally in this form of therapy) may be conducted either individually (through various communication channels, such as e-mail and personal chat) or in groups (through a forum or chat room). Table 6 compares the mean *ES* of individual (in web-based therapy and in etherapy) versus group (in etherapy) therapeutic modes. As can be seen in the table, individual therapy—whether delivered through web-based therapy or etherapy—was found to be more effective than group therapy ($Q_B = 7.34$;

TABLE 6. Effect Size of Individual versus Group Modes of Therapy

Mode	d	n	N
Individual—website	0.53	65	10523
Individual—etherapy	0.57	9	490
Group—etherapy	0.36	18	909

Note: d = effect size; *n* = number of effects; *N* = number of participants.

$p < .05$). The individual therapy mode marked 74 of the studies and yielded a mean *ES* of 0.54; group therapy, characterizing the remaining 18 studies, yielded a mean of 0.36, a statistically significant difference ($Q_B = 7.12$; $p < .01$). However, since only a small number of studies included in the analysis used group therapy, and the number of their participants was relatively small compared to the other therapy modes, the impact on the overall *ES* was marginal. Again, it should be noted that, generally, individual and group interventions were provided by similar therapeutic approaches to similar patients with similar problems and were assessed by similar outcome measures, hence the possibility for confounding effects is little.

Web-based Therapy: Interactive versus Static Website

Web-based therapy may be delivered through an interactive website, where users actively interact with the site according to its instructions and applications, or through a static website, where users passively receive information, instructions, and suggestions relating to their area of concern. Interactive sites are characteristic of CBT and the behavioral psychotherapeutic approaches, in which activating patients cognitively and behaviorally is essential. Static sites are more typical of psychoeducational or information-only approaches, which employ didactic and informative techniques. Our analysis found that of the 65 studies that investigated web-based therapy, the *ES* was 0.65 for 51 therapies that used interactive sites, which is significantly higher than the *ES* of 0.52 for the 14 interventions that used static sites ($Q_B = 32.07$; $p < .001$).

It should be noted that problem type were similarly treated by both types of therapies, therefore this factor should not be regarded as a possible confounding variable. However, as mentioned, interactive sites are more typical of CBT, whereas static sites are more typical of psychoeducational approaches, thus confounding might be possible in inferring from the differences reported here.

Web-based Therapy: Open versus Closed Website

Web-based therapy may be delivered through an open-access website, which permits anyone who desires to receive treatment to engage in it, or through a closed-access (filtered) website, for which patients are prescreened (according to various criteria) and the site is accessed only by personal authorization. Among the 65 web-based therapy studies, the *ES* for 51 interventions that used closed sites was 0.68, which is significantly higher than the *ES* of 0.48 for the 14 interventions that used open sites ($Q_B = 50.40; p < .001$). This difference may be interpreted through several possible explanations, such as: web therapy does not fit every patient hence prescreening is essential, professional assessment should precede effective web-based therapy, and/or a closed site creates elevated commitment and motivation for therapy. Future research should look into these hypotheses.

Etherapy: Synchronicity of Communication

Etherapy can use either the synchronous communication mode—through chat, audio, or webcam—or asynchronous communication, via e-mail and forum. Of the 27 studies that investigated the effectiveness of etherapy, the mean *ES* of the 12 studies that studied the use of the synchronous communication modality for therapy was 0.49, whereas the mean *ES* of the 15 studies that investigated asynchronous therapeutic communication tools was 0.44. This difference was not found to be statistically significant ($Q_B = 0.20; p > .05$).

Etherapy: Type of Modality

The 27 studies that investigated the effectiveness of etherapy examined chat (nine studies), forum (eight studies), e-mail (seven studies), audio (two studies), and webcam (one study) as means of communication between therapists and clients. Table 7 presents the mean *ES* of each modality. The differences among the mean *ES* values were found to be significant ($Q_B = 55.16; p < .001$). It appears that chat and e-mail (both in the 0.50 s) were more effective than forum and

TABLE 7. Effect Size of Etherapy by Communication Modality (27 Studies)

Communication Modality	ES	n	N
Audio	0.91	1	54
Chat	0.53	9	231
Webcam	0.31	2	208
E-mail	0.51	7	383
Forum	0.34	8	523

Note: ES = effect size; *n* = number of effects; *N* = number of participants.

webcam (both in the 0.30 s). As the number of studies for this analysis is small and the common denominator between webcam and forum, unlike the other communication modalities, is not obvious, various speculations may be offered to account for these differences, such as reduced sense of privacy.

It should be noted that, generally, no systematic difference was present between the various modalities in terms of problem type, theoretical approach, or type of clients, hence confounding effects seem to be improbable. The small number of studies in each modality, however, does not allow further examination of this effect.

Contribution of Online Supplements to Main Treatment Mode

Several Internet-based treatment methods tried online supplements to accompany the main treatment modality, whether it involved the use of web-based therapy or any etherapy modality. In some studies, clients were offered the supplemental (and sporadic) use of e-mail (e.g., Carlbring, Westling, Ljungstrand, Ekselius, & Andersson, 2001) or a forum (e.g., Dew et al., 2004) in addition to the use of web-based therapy as the primary therapeutic method. In other studies, a complementary website to etherapy was offered that used e-mail (e.g., Moore, Soderquist, & Werch, 2005) or a forum supplement where chat was used as primary therapeutic communication channel (e.g., Gollings & Paxton, 2006).

In a comparison of studies that used a *website as a supplement* to other modes of treatment and those that did not, the supplementary websites were revealed in fact to have the possibility of *reducing* the effectiveness of the treatment (mean *ES* of 0.41 versus 0.54, respectively; $Q_B = 4.26$; $p < .05$). A further analysis showed no differences between supplementary-site types, open or closed, static or interactive.

Use of *e-mail as a supplement* to the main treatment modality, too, was found to be noncontributing, as mean *ES* of studies that used this method was 0.53, identical to the studies that did not e-mail as a supplement. Nor did the use of a *forum as a supplement* contribute to therapy effectiveness: the mean *ES* of the 15 studies that used this method was 0.44, the result of which was not different from the studies that did not use a forum supplement (mean $ES = 0.54$; $Q_B = 1.74$; $p > .05$).

Furthermore, the use of an online *audio feature as a supplement* did not contribute to therapy; in fact, it actually *decreased* the value of *ES*. The mean *ES* of the eight studies that used this feature was 0.32, versus a mean *ES* of 0.54 for the studies that did not ($Q_B = 7.65$; $p < .01$). The use of *chat as a supplement* to the main treatment modality, too, had a *diminishing* effect: the six studies that used chat as a complementary channel of communication had a mean *ES* of 0.15, as opposed to a mean *ES* of 0.54 for the rest of the studies ($Q_B = 25.32$; $p < .001$). The use of a *webcam as a supplementary* channel revealed that this method *hindered* effectiveness, as the six studies that used it had a mean *ES* of 0.35, compared to a mean *ES* of 0.54 for the studies that did not ($Q_B = 3.74$; $p < .05$).

It should be noted that this finding does not necessarily pertain to causality, as various variables might moderate and be responsible for this difference. Several explanations may be provided as to why supplementary features seem not to significantly contribute to the effectiveness of therapy, such as: multichanneling of communication with clients may distract their focus and attention, and/or communication channels that reduce level personal sense of anonymity harm Internet-delivered therapy effectiveness. These (or other) hypotheses should be tested in future research.

Internet-Based versus Face-to-Face Therapy

Among the 92 studies included in the analysis, there were 14 that directly compared the Internet-based ($n = 940$) with the face-to-face ($n = 593$), traditional treatment of the same problem, with participants being assigned randomly to each treatment mode. While the average weighted *ES* of the Internet-based interventions was 0.39, the weighted *ES* of the face-to-face interventions was 0.34. This difference is not statistically significant ($Q_B = 0.32$; $p > .05$). It should be mentioned that there was no systematic factor or obvious reason why these particular studies yielded effects lower than the average of the rest of the studies; we thus assume there were no confounding effects involved in this analysis.

DISCUSSION

Overall Effectiveness of Internet-Based Interventions

The meta-analysis performed on 92 studies that investigated the effectiveness of Internet-based psychological interventions revealed that, on the average, such an intervention has an *ES* of 0.53, or a medium effect. This average *ES* was found across different intervention methods and approaches, types of measure of effectiveness, problem areas, Internet channels and modalities, age of patients, and other variables. Our analysis of the interaction effects of moderators showed that the average *ES* could have been much higher if, for example, specific types of outcome measures (e.g., physical and physiological) were not employed. Actually, our examination showed that if studies used only the best (i.e., most improved) measures of effectiveness, the average weighted *ES* would have increased to 1.05, which is considered a very high *ES*. However, despite the poor effects on some of the outcome measures, despite that some psychological methods were found to be less appropriate for online application than others (e.g., behavioral), and despite that some problems are apparently less psychologically treatable through the Internet (e.g., weight loss), the average *ES* that we found, 0.53, is quite impressive. Incidentally, it should be mentioned that—generally parallel to our findings—some problems (e.g., weight loss) are less effectively treated by quite a few traditional, face-to-face therapeutic approaches too (Hardeman, Griffin, Johnston, Kinmonth, & Wareham, 2000; Shaw, O'Rourke, Del Mar, & Kenardy, 2007), hence these differences might not have to be attributed to the Internet as the mode of delivery of the intervention.

Our conclusion concerning the impressive nature of the level of effectiveness found is based on three foundations. First, on the average, face-to-face psychotherapeutic interventions are not significantly more effective in producing change in clients. Although quite a few studies showed that in-person therapy could attain a relatively high *ES* in treating certain problems in a specific population by using specific methods, the average effectiveness—parallel to the average *ES* of 0.53 found in our meta-analysis—was found to be of medium size, too. This finding is based on quite a few comprehensive reviews of the efficacy of psychotherapy, such as the Consumer Report study (see Seligman, 1995) and the comprehensive meta-analyses conducted by Smith and Glass (1977), Wampold and colleauges (1997), and Luborsky and colleagues (1999). Actually, if one summarizes all of the meta-analytic study results included in Lambert's and Ogles' (2004) comprehensive review of meta-analyses of the effectiveness of psychotherapy, one would find that the average of a medium-size effect best represents the results of the numerous studies. The conclusion, then, is that Internet-based therapy, on the average, is as effective, or nearly as efficacious, as face-to-face therapy. In this context, Wampold's (2001) summation in regard to the effectiveness of traditional, face-to-face psychological interventions, "Simply stated, *psychotherapy is remarkably efficacious*" (p. 71; emphasis in original), would seem to apply, as well, to Internet-based psychological interventions.

Second, the data collected for our meta-analytic review revealed no difference in *ES* between Internet and face-to-face interventions when compared in the same study. In fact, the average *ES* of the Internet intervention in the 14 studies that made such a comparison was only 0.39—for some unknown reason, a lower than average *ES* of all the studies included in our meta-analysis—but the average *ES* of face-to-face interventions included in this data set was 0.34. This difference was not found to be statistically significant, thus supporting the contention that Internet interventions are as effective as parallel face-to-face psychological interventions.

Third, despite the common myth (Fenichel et al., 2002) that therapy cannot or should not be delivered through the Internet—especially because of the lack of visibility and of nonverbal communication cues and the absence of evidence for its effectiveness (e.g., Clinical Social Work Federation, 2001)—our findings clearly show that, in most cases, online therapy can be delivered effectively, by using various Internet applications and exploiting several online communication options. If we take into consideration that the use of modern computers and the Internet for therapeutic purposes is a relatively new professional pursuit, and if we add to this that computer and communication technologies have continuously and significantly developed over the past decade, and if we also pay attention to the fact that, generally, therapy professionals are relative novices to and lack advanced education and training in this area—the findings of the current meta-analysis are not only impressive but surprisingly, actually stand high.

Moderating Effects of Theoretical Approaches

The analysis of moderators revealed that several important variables significantly moderate the effectiveness of Internet therapy. Some of these findings are not surprising and were actually anticipated. For instance, it can reasonably be expected that the type of outcome measures is associated with the degree of effectiveness, as this association is quite common in psychotherapy-outcome research (Hill & Lambert, 2004). In this context, it should be noted that expert ratings were found to be associated the most with effectiveness of interventions in the current meta-analysis. However, although "blind" raters were used in most studies, it makes sense that an expert's evaluation might be the most sensitive (even if in principle biased) to therapeutic effects—a speculation that directly corresponds to the well-documented problem of reactivity of outcome measures (Smith, Glass, & Miller, 1980). The obvious, and simple, possibility that interviewers could become aware of a patient's method of intervention and of his or her experiences in the process somewhat invalidates this type of outcome criterion or, at least, imparts to it a substantial bias. In this respect, therapist and/or researcher allegiance (Luborsky et al., 2002) might significantly affect any examination of effectiveness and influence ratings.

Our findings showed that CBT was more effective than other therapeutic approaches applied online, while behavioral techniques were much inferior. This finding—despite its saliency—is far from being simple. If we take into account that computer and Internet technology are advancing rapidly, we must consider that approaches having less of a text basis might not only become more attractive, they might even *elevate* effectiveness. For instance, Dallery and his associates (Dallery & Glenn, 2005; Dallery, Glenn, & Raiff, 2007; Glenn & Dallery, 2007) showed that behavioral treatment—using Skinnerian behavior-modification techniques and advanced remote technologies to bring about smoking cessation—can effectively be delivered through the Internet with exceptional success. (The first study cited was excluded from the meta-analysis for too few participants.) Additional examples are studies by Gold, Burke, Pintauro, Buzzell, and Harvey-Berino (2007) and Polzien, Jakicic, Tate, and Otto (2007), which recently presented highly effective behaviorally oriented web-therapy technique assisting in reducing clients' body weight—both an approach and a problem area that were relatively inferior in our meta-analysis. In other words, it might be a question of time, skill, and method-development before a variety of clinical approaches is implemented online with a degree of effectiveness similar to CBT. For instance, Ritterband and colleagues (2006) showed that adding unique online tools (audio, graphics, interactivity) to previously developed, mainly textual interventions indeed contributed an added value to therapeutic efficacy.

Web-Based Therapy, Etherapy, and Additional Internet-Delivered Interventions

The number of studies that investigated the effectiveness of web-based therapy ($n = 65$) included in our review significantly exceeded those that studied etherapy ($n = 27$). Apparently, the reason for this difference has to do with the relative ease with which research can be conducted on web-based interventions than on etherapy. In web-based therapy, clients enter a site and follow instructions, including filling out online questionnaires at various points in time, whereas etherapy more resembles face-to-face therapy in that a client meets a therapist for a therapeutic dialogue; hence, in the latter practice, forms and questionnaires are perceived as irrelevant and a nuisance, and contacting patients for questionnaires and other measurements is usually troublesome and involves ethical and methodological difficulties in addition to practical problems. This difference between the two modes of Internet-based interventions, however, is in reversed direction to that of process research reviewed earlier. It is also interesting to note that the efficacy of etherapy—perhaps because of its basic, more natural therapeutic nature—has been in the subject of numerous nonquantitative studies, including illustrative descriptive case studies (e.g., Chechele & Stofle, 2003; Luce, Winzelberg, Zabinski, & Osborne, 2003) and advanced qualitative analyses (e.g., Stofle, 2002). These publications could not be included in our quantitatively based meta-analytic review; however, their existence should not be overlooked, especially as they provide much evidence in support of the application of etherapy in various online communication modalities and for numerous problem areas. These problem areas include individual therapy in treating such issues as marital difficulties (Jedlicka & Jennings, 2001), sex problems (Hall, 2004), addictive behaviors (Stofle, 2002), anxiety and social phobia (Przeworski & Newman, 2004), and eating disorders (Grunwald & Busse, 2003); and group therapy in treating diverse problems (e.g., Barak & Wander-Schwartz, 2000; Colòn, 1996; Przeworski & Newman, 2004; Sander, 1999). Perhaps this type of methodology better suits etherapy-type intervention, especially since experiential-oriented therapy is commonly applied (Suler, 2008). It seems that with the development and improved training in this emerging area (Coursol & Lewis, 2004; Mallen, Vogel, & Rochlen, 2005; Trepal, Haberstroh, Duffey, & Evans, 2007) therapeutic process and outcome will elevate.

Our findings showed that, on the average, web-based intervention provides as effective therapy as etherapy. This finding does not mean that both approaches are as effective in treating similar individuals and/or similar problems. Web-based therapy is focused on self-help; that is, individual people make use of therapeutic resources—be it online information, psychoeducation interventions, or a tailored, clinical protocol based on CBT principles—to change their condition. The essential role and responsibility of a therapist lie in preparing the materials and providing them online in a way that is attractive, friendly, and optimally effective. In etherapy, however, a therapist is actively engaged in therapeutic communication with clients and in exploiting the Internet for a channel of communication of choice (Suler, 2000, 2004, 2008). It is possible, therefore, that clients characterized by different preferences, needs, or habits would benefit differentially from each of these two approaches in interaction with the problem area. The absence of a meaningful difference in average effectiveness that we found between the two approaches might reflect the self-selection of patients and/or therapists; the available data cannot as yet provide answers to these questions. Future research should focus on these interesting hypotheses.

Very little research has been published on two other uses of the Internet to deliver therapy: Internet component(s) that may complement face-to-face therapy (e.g., use of e-mail in between face-to-face sessions, ask in-person clients to publish posts on a personal blog, use of a website to prepare clients for face-to-face therapy) and Internet-operated software (a programmed robot that simulates a therapist based on principles of artificial intelligence or prescribed protocols, such as ELIZA). These two category uses, in addition to web-based therapy and etherapy, create a comprehensive toolkit for therapists who wish to exploit Internet capabilities in their clinical work. However, only very limited outcome research has been published to date on the growing use of Internet-assisted therapy as a complementary therapeutic vehicle, such as using e-mail, blogs, online information, or an online support group in parallel with traditional, face-to-face therapy (Baily, Yager, & Jensen, 2002; Castelnuovo, Gaggioli, Mantovani, & Riva, 2003; Suler, 2008; Tate & Zabinski, 2004; Zuckerman, 2003). Findings published on such therapeutic use have been promising, however. For example, Baily and colleagues (2002) described the use of e-mail as an adjunctive treatment tool for an adolescent with anorexia nervosa and the use of a chat room for the enhancement of social life for a patient with social phobia. Likewise, Peterson and Beck (2003) presented a model, and several illustrative cases, of the use of e-mail as an adjunctive tool in psychotherapy. Golkaramnay, Bauer, Haug, Wolf, and Kordy (2007) recently presented the use of group therapy, conducted through a chat room, following the termination of a patient's in-person therapy in order to reduce the risk of relapse. In regard to the category of more robotic, therapeutic online software (Marks, Cavanagh, & Gega, 2007), empirical outcome research is rare; however, descriptions of such applications exist, such as in helping the treatment of problem drinkers (Squires & Hester, 2004) or the more general use of ELIZA (Epstein & Klinkenberg, 2001).

Considerations of Age as a Moderating Factor

The differential effects of age group on Internet-based therapy outcome require special attention. The findings of the meta-analysis showed that clients' age made a difference in terms of their ability to gain from the therapy. Specifically, among four age-group categories employed, the findings showed that the *ES* of Internet-based therapy provided to mid-age adults (19–39) was higher than either to older or younger clients. This finding, however, might be a temporal result of a vanishing factor: that of pervasiveness, acceptance, and usage skills associated with the Internet. In other words, we believe that nowadays—after the general penetration of computers and the Internet into homes, schools, and workplaces—these differences might have disappeared. Actually, recent studies of Internet-based therapy for older adults and children—published after the end of the data collection for the current analysis (March, 2006)—showed strong therapeutic effects. For instance, using web-based CBT, Spence, Holmes, March, and Lipp (2006) showed highly effective results on anxious children, while Nelson, Barnard, and Cain (2006) gained similar results on depressive children. Hicks, von Baeyer, and McGrath (2006) presented highly effective online intervention for children's recurrent pains. Similarly, at the other end of the age continuum, Brattberg (2006) presented a highly effective, Internet-delivered, psychoeducation intervention in treating the chronic pains of older adults; Hill, Weinert, and Cudney (2006) showed highly effective web-based intervention of psychological symptoms of chronically ill older women. Lorig, Ritter, Laurent, and Plant (2006) presented a highly effective online intervention program for developing the self-management skills of older adults suffering from chronic diseases; Marziali and Donahue (2006) very effectively treated older caregivers (mean age 68) through video-conferencing. Thus, it seems that an age gap interacting with online-intervention effectiveness is indeed vanishing.

Since cyberspace has become a major social environment for children and adolescents (Fox & Madden, 2006; Hall, 2006; Valkenburg & Peter, 2007), it is not surprising to learn that Internet-based therapeutic and support applications operating online are highly useful for youngsters (Barak, 2007; Hoffmann, 2006; Mangunkusumo, Brug, Duisterhout, de Koning, & Raat, 2007), in contrast to what our review seemingly found. Likewise, the use nowadays of computers and the Internet by older people is quickly growing (Carpenter & Buday, 2007); indeed, this age group may gain much mental support through computer use (Shapira, Barak, & Gal, 2007).

Limitations of the Meta-Analytic Review

Meta-analysis—although becoming a common procedure in reviewing quantitative empirical findings of various phenomena—is far from being a flawless procedure. It has been criticized on statistical and methodological grounds in the context of evaluating the effectiveness of psychotherapy (e.g., Wampold, 2001) and other, more general issues (e.g., Field, 2003). One of the main criticisms has to do with publication bias and "file-drawer effect," created either by researchers themselves or by scientific journals, which results in an overestimation of effects. Although this point might be true, no doubt it affects face-to-face and Internet-based outcome research similarly; hence, a comparison of the two methods is not erroneous. In addition, it seems that the results of the moderator analyses that we conducted add to the validity of our conclusions. We considered using the "fail-safe N" (FSN) statistics in order to examine how many unpublished studies would have been needed to jeopardize our conclusions; we have avoided this step because of the clear nature of the results, on the one hand, and the problematic assumptions related to calculating FSN, on the other.

Another issue worth mentioning has to do with the statistical methods employed here. Since we used the fixed-effects method for our analysis, different results might be derived from those of the random- or mixed-effects methods, throwing into question the accuracy of our results. However, if we compare our results with those of previous meta-analyses of Internet interventions—though these are more limited in scope and content (Hirai & Clum, 2006b; Spek et al., 2007; Wantland et al., 2004) but employ alternative statistical models and assumptions—we find that the general nature of our findings is highly consistent with those others, thus supporting the validity of our conclusions from this aspect, as well. Future research should utilize different statistical models to replicate our analysis.

Also, our data set for performing the meta-analysis included all eligible articles according to the inclusion criteria determined; quality of research, however, was not one of them. Using this criterion—suggested by some meta-analysis experts—might be problematic, especially as the objective and professional ability to assess quality of published research is limited and might be erroneous or biased. After close consideration and actual trials we decided to avoid this selection criterion and base research quality merely on acceptance for publication in a peer-reviewed journal. Our approach, however, might have introduced some error variance into the results. Future meta-analyses in this area should attempt to evaluate research quality of studies and either select those meeting a minimal level of this additional criterion or, perhaps in using a more informative approach, using research quality level as an additional moderator and examine its effects.

SUMMARY AND CONCLUSIONS

The findings presented in this meta-analytic review provide much support for the application of psychotherapeutic interventions through the Internet, using various approaches, methods, and online modalities, to treat various problems differentially but effectively; online therapy is especially effective for treating anxiety and stress—effects that last after therapy ends—and, on the average, is as effective as face-to-face intervention. The effectiveness of interventions can be detected by a variety of outcome measures, but less so when using physiological or physical measures. When web-based, self-help therapy is applied on an interactive website that may be accessed only by prescreened, authorized patients, it should increase therapy success. E-mail reminders for patients who use web-based therapy are expected to contribute to the success of the therapeutic intervention, too. When etherapy is applied, it seems that textual are preferred to nontextual modes (e.g., use of audio and webcam), though this should be regarded cautiously due to the small number of studies reviewed using these features. Furthermore, it seems that individual Internet therapy is more effective than group intervention online.

The use of computers and the Internet is rapidly increasing and becoming a common personal and social phenomenon (Barak & Suler, 2008; Bargh & McKenna, 2004; Haythornthwaite & Hagar, 2004; Madden, 2006). Moreover, the Internet-connected computer is turning into a highly influential social tool (Sassenberg & Jonas, 2007) all while innovative and advanced technology is introduced frequently and is rapidly changing the culture. Psychotherapy and counseling should adjust to this changing world and adopt new, innovative tools accordingly to fit into the world of today and tomorrow so as to better meet clients' expectations and needs. The current review shows that this is not only theoretically possible but actually a developing professional reality.

REFERENCES

Note: References marked with an asterisk indicate studies included in the meta-analysis

Andersson, G. (2006). Internet-based cognitive-behavioral self help for depression. *Expert Review of Neurotherapeutics, 6,* 1637–1642.
Andersson, G., Bergström, J., Carlbring, P., & Lindefors, N. (2005). The use of the Internet in the treatment of anxiety disorders. *Current Opinion in Psychiatry, 18,* 73–77.
*Andersson, G., Bergström, J., Hollandäre, F., Carlbring, P., Kaldo V., & Ekselius, L. (2005). Internet-based self-help for depression: Randomised controlled trial. *British Journal of Psychiatry, 187,* 456–461.
*Andersson, G., Lundström, P., & Ström, L. (2003). Internet-based treatment of headache: Does telephone contact add anything? *Headache, 43,* 353–361.
*Andersson, G., Strömgren, T., Ström, L., & Lyttkens, L. (2002). Randomized controlled trial of Internet-based cognitive behavior therapy for distress associated with tinnitus. *Psychosomatic Medicine, 64,* 810–816.
Anthony, K. (2006). Electronically delivered therapies. In C. Feltham & I. Horton (Eds.), *The SAGE handbook of counselling and psychotherapy* (pp. 518–523). London, UK: Sage.

Baily, R., Yager, J., & Jensen, J. (2002). The psychiatrist as clinical computerologist in the treatment of adolescents: Old barks in new bytes. *American Journal of Psychiatry, 159*, 1298–1304.

Barak, A. (2004). Internet counseling. In C. E. Spielberger (Ed.), *Encyclopedia of applied psychology* (pp. 369–378). San Diego, CA: Academic Press.

Barak, A. (2007). Emotional support and suicide prevention through the Internet: A field project report. *Computers in Human Behavior, 23*, 971–984.

Barak, A., & Bloch, N. (2006). Factors related to perceived helpfulness in supporting highly distressed individuals through an online support chat. *CyberPsychology & Behavior, 9*, 60–68.

Barak, A., & Suler, J. (2008). Reflections on the psychology and social science of cyberspace. In A. Barak (Ed.), *Psychological aspects of cyberspace: Theory, research, applications*, 1–12. Cambridge, UK: Cambridge University Press.

Barak, A., & Wander-Schwartz, M. (2000). Empirical evaluation of brief group therapy conducted in an Internet chat room. *Journal of Virtual Environments, 5*(1) [online]. Retrieved August 1, 2007, from http://www.brandeis.edu/pubs/jove/HTML/v5/cherapy3.htm.

Bargh, J. A., & McKenna, K. Y. A. (2004). The Internet and social life. *Annual Review of Psychology, 55*, 573–590.

Bickmore, T., Gruber, A., & Picard, R. (2005). Establishing the computer-patient working alliance in automated health behavior change interventions. *Patient Education and Counseling, 59*, 21–30.

Brattberg, G. (2006). Internet-based rehabilitation for individuals with chronic pain and burnout: A randomized trial. *International Journal of Rehabilitation Research, 29*, 221–227.

*Bruning Brown, J, Winzelberg, A. J., Abascal, L. B., & Taylor, C. B. (2004). An evaluation of an Internet-delivered eating disorder prevention program for adolescents and their parents. *Journal of Adolescent Health, 35*, 290–296.

*Buhrman, M., Fältenhag, S., Ström, L., & Andersson, G. (2004). Controlled trial of Internet-based treatment with telephone support for chronic back pain. *Pain, 111*, 368–377.

Carlbring, P., & Andersson, G. (2006). Internet and psychological treatment: How well can they be combined? *Computers in Human Behavior, 22*, 545–553.

*Carlbring, P., Ekselius, L., & Andersson, G. (2003). Treatment of panic disorder via the Internet: A randomized trial of CBT vs. applied relaxation. *Journal of Behavior Therapy and Experimental Psychiatry, 34*, 129–140.

*Carlbring, P., Furmark, T., Steczkó, J., Ekselius, L., & Andersson, G. (2006). An open study of Internet-based bibliotherapy with minimal therapist contact via e-mail for social phobia. *Clinical Psychologist, 10*, 30–38.

*Carlbring, P., Nilsson-Ihrfelt, E., Waara, J., Kollenstam, C., Buhrman, M., Kaldo, V., et al. (2005). Treatment of panic disorder: Live therapy vs. self-help via the Internet. *Behaviour Research and Therapy, 43*, 1321–1333.

*Carlbring, P., Westling, B. E., Ljungstrand, P., Ekselius, L., & Andersson, G. (2001). Treatment of panic disorder via the Internet: A randomized trial of a self-help program. *Behavior Therapy, 32*, 751–764.

Carpenter, B. D., & Buday, S. (2007). Computer use among older adults in a naturally occurring retirement community. *Computers in Human Behavior, 23,* 3012–3024.

Castelnuovo, G., Gaggioli, A., Mantovani, F., & Riva, G. (2003). New and old tools in psychotherapy: The use of technology for the integration of the traditional clinical treatments. *Psychotherapy: Theory, Research, Practice, Training, 40,* 33–44.

*Celio, A. A., Winzelberg, A. J., Wilfley, D. E., Eppstein-Herald, D., Springer, E. A., Dev, P., et al. (2000). Reducing risk factors for eating disorders: Comparison of an Internet and a classroom-delivered psychoeducational program. *Journal of Consulting & Clinical Psychology, 68,* 650–657.

Chechele, P. J., & Stofle, G. (2003). Individual therapy online via email and internet relay chat. In S. Goss & K. Anthony (Eds.), *Technology in counselling and psychotherapy: A practitioner's guide* (pp. 39–58). Houndmills, UK: Palgrave Macmillan.

Chester, A., & Glass, C. A. (2006). Online counseling: A descriptive analysis of therapy services on the Internet. *British Journal of Guidance and Counselling, 34,* 145–160.

*Chiauzzi, E., Green, T. C., Lord, S., Thum, C., & Goldstein, M. (2005). My student body: A high-risk drinking prevention Web site for college students. *Journal of American College Health, 53,* 263–274.

*Christensen, H., Griffiths, K. M., & Jorm, A. F. (2004). Delivering interventions for depression by using the Internet: Randomised controlled trial. *British Medical Journal, 328*(7), 265–268. [this article provides findings also reported in Griffiths, K. M., Christensen, H., Clarke, G., Eubanks, D., Reid, E., Kelleher, C., et al. (2005). Overcoming depression on the Internet (ODIN) (2): A randomized trial of a self-help depression skills program with reminders. *Journal of Medical Internet Research, 7*(2), e16 [online]. Retrieved August 1, 2007, from: http://www.jmir.org/2005/2/e16.

*Christensen, H., Griffiths, K. M., & Korten, A. (2002). Web-based cognitive behavior therapy: Analysis of site usage and changes in depression and anxiety scores. *Journal of Medical Internet Research, 4*(1), e3 [online]. Retrieved August 1, 2007, from http://www.jmir.org/2002/1/e3.

*Christensen, H., Griffiths, K. M., Korten, A. E., Brittliffe, K., & Groves, C. (2004). A comparison of changes in anxiety and depression symptoms of spontaneous users and trial participants of a cognitive behavior therapy website. *Journal of Medical Internet Research, 6*(4), e46 [online]. Retrieved August 1, 2007, from http://www.jmir.org/2004/4/e46.

*Clarke, G., Eubanks, D., Reid, E., Kelleher, C., O'Connor, E., DeBar, L. L., et al. (2005). Overcoming depression on the Internet (ODIN) (2): A randomized trial of a self-help depression skills program with reminders. *Journal of Medical Internet Research, 7*(2), e16 [online]. Retrieved August 1, 2007, from http://www.jmir.org/2005/2/e16.

*Clarke, G., Reid, E., Eubanks, D., O'Connor, E., DeBar, L. L., Kelleher, C. et al. (2002). Overcoming depression on the Internet (ODIN): A randomized controlled trial of an Internet depression skills intervention program. *Journal of Medical Internet Research, 4*(3), e14 [online]. Retrieved August 1, 2007, from: http://www.jmir.org/2002/3/e14.

Clinical Social Work Federation (2001). CSWF position paper on internet text-based therapy [online]. Retrieved August 1, 2007, from http://www.associationsites.com/page.cfm?usr=cswa&pageid=3670.

*Cohen, G. E., & Kerr, A. B. (1998). Computer-mediated counseling: An empirical study of a new mental health treatment. *Computers in Human Services, 15*(4), 13–27.

Cohen, J. (1988). *Statistical power analysis for the behavioral sciences* (2nd ed.). Hillsdale, NJ: Erlbaum.

Colòn, Y. (1996). Chatt(er)ing through the fingertips: Doing group therapy online. *Woman & Performance: A Journal of Feminist Theory, 17*, 205–215.

Cook, J. E., & Doyle, C. (2002). Working alliance in online therapy as compared to face-to-face therapy: Preliminary results. *CyberPsychology & Behavior, 5*, 95–105.

Coursol, D., & Lewis, J. (2004). Counselor preparation for a cyber world: Curriculum design and development. In J. W. Bloom & G. R. Walz (Eds.), *Cybercounseling & cyberlearning: An encore* (pp. 19–34). Alexandria, VA: American Counseling Association.

Dallery, J., & Glenn, I. M. (2005). Effects of an Internet-based voucher reinforcement program for smoking abstinence: A feasibility study. *Journal of Applied Behavior Analysis, 38*, 349–357.

Dallery, J., Glenn, I. M., & Raiff, B. R. (2007). An Internet-based abstinence reinforcement treatment for cigarette smoking. *Drug and Alcohol Dependence, 86*, 230–238.

*Day, S. X., & Schneider, P. L. (2002). Psychotherapy using distance technology: A comparison of face-to-face, video and audio treatment. *Journal of Counseling Psychology, 49*, 499–503.

Derrig-Palumbo, K., & Zeine, F., (2005). *Online therapy: A therapist's guide to expanding your practice.* New York: Norton.

*Devineni, T., & Blanchard, E. B. (2005). A randomized controlled trial of an Internet-based treatment for chronic headache. *Behaviour Research & Therapy, 43*, 277–292.

*Dew, M. A., Goycoolea, J. M., Harris, R. C., Lee, A., Zomak, R., Dunbar-Jacob, J., et al. (2004). An Internet-based intervention to improve psychosocial outcomes in heart transplant recipients and family caregivers: Development and evaluation. *Journal of Heart and Lung Transplantation, 23*, 745–758.

Epstein, J., & Klinkenberg, W. D. (2001). From Eliza to Internet: A brief history of computerized assessment. *Computers in Human Behavior, 17*, 295–314.

Escoffery, C., McCormick, L., & Bateman, K. (2004). Development and process evaluation of a Web-based smoking cessation program for college smokers: Innovative tool for education. *Patient Education & Counseling, 53*, 217–225.

*Etter, J.-F. (2005). Comparing the efficacy of two Internet-based, computer-tailored smoking cessation programs: A randomized trial. *Journal of Medical Internet Research, 7*(1), *e2* [online]. Retrieved August 1, 2007, from http://www.jmir.org/2005/1/e2.

Etter, J. (2006). The Internet and the industrial revolution in smoking cessation counselling. *Drug and Alcohol Review, 25*, 79–84.

*Farvolden, P., Denisoff, E., Selby, P., Bagby, M. R., & Rudy, L. (2005). Usage and longitudinal effectiveness of a Web-based self-help cognitive behavioral therapy program for panic disorder. *Journal of Medical Internet Research, 7*(1), e7 [online]. Retrieved August 1, 2007, from http://www.jmir.org/2005/1/e7.

Fenichel, M., Suler, J., Barak, A., Zelvin, E., Jones, G., Munro, K., et al. (2002). Myths and realities of online clinical work. *CyberPsychology & Behavior, 5,* 481–497.

Field, A. P. (2003). Can meta-analysis be trusted? *The Psychologist, 16,* 642–645.

Fox, S., & Madden, M. (2006). *Generations online.* Pew Internet and American Life Project [online]. Retrieved August 1, 2007, from http://www.pewinternet.org/pdfs/PIP_Generations_Memo.pdf.

Fuller, J. B., & Hester, K. (1999). Comparing the sample-weighted and unweighted meta-analysis: An applied perspective. *Journal of Management, 25,* 803–828.

Glenn, I. M., & Dallery, J. (2007). Effects of Internet-based voucher reinforcement and a transdermal nicotine patch on cigarette smoking. *Journal of Applied Behavior Analysis, 40,* 1–13.

Gold, B. C., Burke, S., Pintauro, S., Buzzell, P., & Harvey-Berino, J. (2007). Weight loss on the web: A pilot study comparing a structured behavioral intervention to a commercial program. *Obesity, 15,* 155–164.

Golkaramnay, V., Bauer, S., Haug, S., Wolf, M., & Kordy, H. (2007). The exploration of the effectiveness of group therapy through an Internet chat as aftercare: A controlled naturalistic study. *Psychotherapy & Psychosomatics, 76,* 219–225.

*Gollings, E. K., & Paxton, S. J. (2006). Comparison of Internet and face-to-face delivery of a group body image and disordered eating intervention for women: A pilot study. *Eating Disorders: The Journal of Treatment & Prevention, 14,* 1–15.

Griffiths, K. M., & Christensen, H. (2006). Review of randomised controlled trials of Internet interventions for mental disorders and related conditions. *Clinical Psychologist, 10,* 16–29.

*Griffiths, K. M., Christensen, H., Jorm, A. F., Evans, K., & Groves, C. (2004). Effect of web-based depression literacy and cognitive-behavioural therapy interventions on stigmatising attitudes to depression: Randomised controlled trial. *British Journal of Psychiatry, 185,* 342–349.

Grohol, J. M. (2004). Online counseling: A historical perspective. In R. Kraus, J. Zack, & G. Stricker (Eds.), *Online counseling: A handbook for mental health professionals* (pp. 51–68). San Diego, CA: Elsevier Academic Press.

Grunwald, M., & Busse, J. C. (2003). Online consulting service for eating disorders— Analysis and perspectives. *Computers in Human Behavior, 19,* 469–477.

Hall, G. (2006). Teens and technology: Preparing for the future. *New Directions for Youth Development, 111,* 41–52.

Hall, P. (2004). Online psychosexual therapy: A summary of pilot study findings. *Sexual and Relationship Therapy, 19,* 167–178.

Hardeman, W., Griffin, S., Johnston, M., Kinmonth, A. L., & Wareham, N. J. (2000). Interventions to prevent weight gain: A systematic review of psychological models and behaviour change methods. *International Journal of Obesity, 24,* 131–143.

*Harvey-Berino, J., Pintauro, S., Buzzell, P., DiGiulio, M., Gold, B. C, Moldovan, C., et al. (2002). Does using the Internet facilitate the maintenance of weight loss? *International Journal of Obesity, 26,* 1254–1260.

*Harvey-Berino, J., Pintauro, S., Buzzell, P., & Gold, E. C. (2004). Effect of Internet support on the long-term maintenance of weight loss. *Obesity Research, 12,* 320–329.

*Hasson, D., Anderberg, U. M., Theorell, T., & Arnetz, B. B. (2005). Psychophysiological effects of a web-based stress management system: A prospective, randomized controlled intervention study of IT and media workers. *BMC Public Health, 5,* 78 [online]. Retrieved August 1, 2007, from http://www.biomedcentral.com/1471-2458/5/78.

Haythornthwaite, C., & Hagar, C. (2004). The social worlds of the web. *Annual Review of Information Science and Technology, 39,* 311–346.

Hedges, L. V., & Olkin, I. (1985). *Statistical methods for meta-analysis.* Orlando, FL: Academic Press.

Hicks, C. L., von Baeyer, C. L., & McGrath, P. J. (2006). Online psychological treatment for pediatric recurrent pain: A randomized evaluation. *Journal of Pediatric Psychology, 31,* 724–736.

Hill, C. E., & Lambert, M. J. (2004). Methodological issues in studying psychotherapy processes and outcomes. In M. J. Lambert (Ed.), *Bergin and Garfield handbook of psychotherapy and behavior change* (5th ed.; pp. 84–135). New York: Wiley.

Hill, W., Weinert, C., & Cudney, S. (2006). Influence of a computer intervention on the psychological status of chronically ill rural women: Preliminary results. *Nursing Research, 55,* 34–42.

*Hirai, M., & Clum, G. A. (2006a). An Internet-based self-change program for traumatic event related fear, distress, and maladaptive coping. *Journal of Traumatic Stress, 18,* 631–636.

Hirai, M., & Clum, G. A. (2006b). A meta-analytic study of self-help interventions for anxiety problems. *Behavior Therapy, 37,* 99–111.

Hoffmann, W. A. (2006). Telematic technologies in mental health caring: A web-based psychoeducational program for adolescent suicide survivors. *Issues in Mental Health Nursing, 27,* 461–474.

*Hopps, S. L., Pépin, M., & Boisvert, J. M. (2003). The effectiveness of cognitive-behavioral group therapy for loneliness via inter-relay-chat among people with physical disabilities. *Psychotherapy: Theory, Research, Practice, Training, 40,* 136–147.

Hsiung, R. C. (Ed.) (2002). *Etherapy: Case studies, guiding principles, and the clinical potential of the Internet.* New York: Norton.

Jedlicka, D., & Jennings, G. (2001). Marital therapy on the Internet. *Journal of Technology in Counseling, 2*(1) [online]. Retrieved August 1, 2007, from http://jtc.colstate.edu/vol2_1/Marital.htm.

*Kenardy, J., McCafferty, K., & Rosa, V. (2003). Internet-delivered indicated prevention for anxiety disorders: A randomized controlled trial. *Behavioural & Cognitive Psychotherapy, 31,* 279–289.

*Kenardy, J., McCafferty, K., & Rosa, V. (2006). Internet-delivered indicated prevention for anxiety disorders: Six-month follow-up. *Clinical Psychologist, 10*, 39–42.

*Kenwright, M., Marks, I. M., Gega, L., & Mataix, D. (2004). Computer-aided self-help for phobia/panic via Internet at home study. *British Journal of Psychiatry, 184*, 448–449.

King, R., Bambling, M., Lloyd, C., Gomurra, R., Smith, S., Reid, W., et al. (2006). Online counselling: The motives and experiences of young people who choose the Internet instead of face to face or telephone counselling. *Counselling and Psychotherapy Research, 6*, 169–174.

*Klein, B., & Richards, J. C. (2001). A brief Internet-based treatment for panic disorder. *Behavioural & Cognitive Psychotherapy, 29*, 113–117.

*Klein, B., Richards, J. C., & Austin, D. W. (2006). Efficacy of Internet therapy for panic disorder. *Journal of Behavior Therapy and Experimental Psychiatry, 37*, 213–238.

Kraus, R., Zack, J., & Stricker, G. (Eds.) (2004). *Online counseling: A handbook for mental health professionals.* San Diego, CA: Elsevier Academic Press.

*Kypri, K., & McAnally, H. M. (2005). Randomized controlled trial of a web-based primary care intervention for multiple health risk behaviors. *Preventive Medicine, 41*, 761–766.

*Kypri, K., Saunders, J. B., Williams, S. M., McGee, R. O., Langley, J. D., Cashell-Smith, M. L., et al. (2004). Web-based screening and brief intervention for hazardous drinking: A double-blind randomized controlled trial. *Addiction, 99*, 1410–1417.

Lambert, M. J., & Ogles, B. M. (2004). The efficacy and effectiveness of psycho-therapy. In M. J. Lambert (Ed.), *Bergin and Garfield handbook of psychotherapy and behavior change* (5th ed.; pp. 139–193). New York: Wiley.

*Lange, A., Rietdijk, D., Hudcovicova, M., van de Ven, J.-P., Schrieken, B., & Emmelkamp, P. M. G. (2003). Interapy: A controlled randomized trial of the standardized treatment of posttraumatic stress through the Internet. *Journal of Consulting & Clinical Psychology, 71*, 901–909.

*Lange, A., Schieken, B., van de Ven, J., Bredeweg, B., Emmelkamp, P. M. G., van der Kolk, J., et al. (2000). "Interapy": The effects of a short protocolled treatment of posttraumatic stress and pathological grief through the Internet. *Behavioural and Cognitive Psychotherapy, 28*, 175–192. [this article provides findings also reported in Lange, A., van de Ven, J-P. Q. R., Schrieken, B. A. L., Bredeweg, B., & Emmelkamp, P. M. G. (2000). Internet-mediated, protocol-driven treatment of psychological dysfunction. *Journal of Telemedicine and Telecare, 6*, 15–21.]

Leibert, T., Archer, J. Jr., Munson, J., & York, G. (2006). An exploratory study of client perceptions of Internet counseling and the therapeutic alliance. *Journal of Mental Health Counseling, 28*, 69–83.

*Lenert, L., Muñoz, R. F., Perez, J. E., & Bansod, A. (2004). Automated e-mail messaging as a tool for improving quit rates in an Internet smoking cessation intervention. *Journal of the American Medical Informatics Association, 11*, 235–240.

Lester, D. (2006). Etherapy: Caveats from experiences with telephone therapy. *Psychological Reports, 99*, 894–896.

Lewis, J., Coursol, D., & Herting, W. (2004). Researching the cybercounseling process: A study of the client and counselor experience. In J. W. Bloom & G. R. Walz (Eds.), *Cybercounseling & cyberlearning: An encore* (pp. 307–325). Alexandria, VA: American Counseling Association.

*Lieberman, D. Z. (2003). An automated treatment for jet lag delivered through the Internet. *Psychiatric Services, 54*, 394–396.

*Lieberman, M. A., Winzelberg, A., Golant, M., Wakahiro, M., DiMinno, M., Aminoff, M., et al. (2005). Online support groups for Parkinson's patients: A pilot study of effectiveness. *Social Work in Health Care, 42*(2), 23–38.

Lorig, K. R., Ritter, P. L., Laurent, D. D., & Plant, K. (2006). Internet-based chronic disease self-management: A randomized trial. *Medical Care, 44*, 964–971.

Luborsky, L., Diguer, L., Seligman, D. A., Rosenthal, R., Krause, E. D., Johnson, S., et al. (1999). The Researcher's Own Therapy Allegiances: A "Wild Card" in Comparisons of Treatment Efficacy. *Clinical Psychology: Science & Practice, 6*, 95–106.

Luborsky, L., Rosenthal, R., Diguer, L., Andrusyna, T. P., Berman, J. S., Levitt, J. T., et al. (2002). The dodo bird verdict is alive and well—Mostly. *Clinical Psychology: Science & Practice, 9*, 2–12.

Luce, K. H., Winzelberg, A. J., Zabinski, M. F., & Osborne, M. I. (2003). Internet-delivered psychological interventions for body image dissatisfaction and disordered eating. *Psychotherapy: Theory, Research, Practice, Training, 40*, 148–154.

Madden, M. (2006). *Internet penetration and impact.* Pew Internet & American Life Project [online]. Retrieved September 20, 2007, from http://www.pewinternet. org/pdfs/PIP_Internet_Impact.pdf.

Mallen, M. J., Day, S. X., & Green, M. A. (2003). Online versus face-to-face conversation: An examination of relational and discourse variables. *Psychotherapy: Theory, Research, Practice, Training, 40*, 155–163.

Mallen, M. J., Vogel, D. L., & Rochlen, A. B. (2005). The practical aspects of online counseling: Ethics, training, technology, and competency. *The Counseling Psychologist, 33*, 776–818.

Mallen, M. J., Vogel, D. L., Rochlen, A. B., & Day, S. X. (2005). Online counseling: Reviewing the literature from a counseling psychology framework. *The Counseling Psychologist, 33*, 819–871.

Mangunkusumo, R. T., Brug, J., Duisterhout, J. S., de Koning, H. J., & Raat, H. (2007). Feasibility, acceptability, and quality of Internet-administered adolescent health promotion in a preventive-care setting. *Health Education Research, 22*, 1–13.

Marks, I. M., Cavanagh, K., & Gega, L. (2007). *Hands-on help: Computer-aided psychotherapy.* Florence, NY: Taylor & Francis.

Marziali, E., & Donahue, P. (2006). Caring for others: Internet video-conferencing group intervention for family caregivers of older adults with neurodegenerative disease. *The Gerontologist, 46*, 398–403.

*Moore, M. J., Soderquist, J., & Werch, C. F. (2005). Feasibility and efficacy of a binge drinking prevention intervention for college students delivered via the Internet versus postal mail. *Journal of American College Health, 54,* 38–44.

Nelson, E., Barnard, M., & Cain, S. (2006). Feasibility of telemedicine intervention for childhood depression. *Counselling and Psychotherapy Research, 6,* 191–195.

*O'Kearney, R., Gibson, M., Christensen, H., & Griffiths, K. M. (2006). Effects of a cognitive-behavioural Internet program on depression, vulnerability to depression and stigma in adolescent males: A school-based controlled trial. *Cognitive Behaviour Therapy, 35,* 43–54.

*Owen, J. E., Klapow, J. C., Roth, D. L., Shuster, J. L., & Bellis, J. (2005). Randomized pilot of a self-guided Internet coping group for women with early-stage breast cancer. *Annals of Behavioral Medicine, 30,* 54–64.

*Patten, S. B. (2003). Prevention of depressive symptoms through the use of distance technologies. *Psychiatric Services, 54,* 396–398.

Peterson, M. R., & Beck, R. L. (2003). E-mail as an adjunctive tool in psychotherapy: Response and responsibility. *American Journal of Psychotherapy, 57,* 167–181.

Polzien, K. M., Jakicic, J. M., Tate, D. F., & Otto, A. D. (2007). The efficacy of a technology-based system in a short-term behavioral weight loss intervention. *Obesity, 15,* 825–830.

Przeworski, A., & Newman, M. G. (2004). Palmtop computer-assisted group therapy for social phobia. *Journal of Clinical Psychology, 60,* 179–188.

Pull, C. B. (2006). Self-help Internet interventions for mental disorders. *Current Opinion in Psychiatry, 19,* 50–53.

Rees, C. S., & Stone, S. (2005). Therapeutic alliance in face-to-face versus videoconferenced psychotherapy. *Professional Psychology: Research and Practice, 36,* 649–653.

Reynolds, D. J., Jr., Stiles, W. B., & Grohol, J. M. (2006). An investigation of session impact and alliance in Internet based psychotherapy: Preliminary results. *Counseling and Psychotherapy Research, 6,* 164–168.

*Richards, J. C., & Alvarenga, M. E. (2002). Extension and replication of an Internet-based treatment program for panic disorder. *Cognitive Behaviour Therapy, 31*(5), 41–47.

*Richards, J. C., Klein, B., & Austin, D. W. (2006). Internet cognitive behavioural therapy for panic disorder: Does the inclusion of stress management information improve end-state functioning? *Clinical Psychologist, 10,* 2–15.

Ritterband, L. M., Cox, D. J., Gordon, T. L., Borowitz, S. M., Kovatchev, B. P., Walker, L. S., et al. (2006). Examining the added value of audio, graphics, and interactivity in an Internet intervention for pediatric encopresis. *Children's Health Care, 35,* 47–59.

*Ritterband, L. M., Cox, D. J., Walker, L. S., Kovatchev, B., McKnight, L., Patel, K., et al. (2003). An Internet intervention as adjunctive therapy for pediatric encopresis. *Journal of Consulting & Clinical Psychology, 71,* 910–917.

Ritterband, L. M., Gonder-Frederick, L. A., Cox, D. J., Clifton, A. D., West, R. W., & Borowitz, S. M. (2003). Internet interventions: In review, in use, and into the future. *Professional Psychology: Research and Practice, 34,* 527–534.

*Robinson, P. H., & Serfaty, M. A. (2001). The use of e-mail in the identification bulimia nervosa and its treatment. *European Eating Disorders Review, 9*, 182–193. [Adjunct analyses reported in part also at: Robinson, P., & Serfaty, M. (2003). Computers, e-mail and therapy in eating disorders. *European Eating Disorders Review, 11*, 210–221.]

Rochlen, A. B., Land, L. N., & Wong, Y. J. (2004). Male restrictive emotionality and evaluations of online versus face-to-face counseling. *Psychology of Men & Masculinity, 5*, 190–200.

Rosenthal, R. (1984). *Meta-analytic procedures for social research.* London, UK: Sage.

*Rothert, K., Strecher, V. J., Doyle, L. A., Caplan, W. M., Joyce, J. S., Jimison, H. B., et al. (2006). Web-based weight management programs in an integrated health care setting: A randomized, controlled trial. *Obesity Research, 14*, 266–272.

Sander, F. M. (1999). Couples group therapy conducted via computer-mediated communication: A preliminary case study. *Computers in Human Behavior, 12*, 301–312.

Sassenberg, K., & Jonas, K. J. (2007). Attitude change and social influence on the net. In A. Joinson, K. McKenna, T. Postmes, & U. Reips (Eds.), *The Oxford handbook of Internet psychology* (pp. 273–289). Oxford, UK: Oxford University Press.

*Schneider, A. J., Mataix-Cols, D., Marks, I. M., & Bachofen, M. (2005). Internet-guided self-help with or without exposure therapy for phobic and panic disorders—A randomised controlled trial. *Psychotherapy and Psychosomatics, 74*, 154–164.

Seligman, M. E. P. (1995). The effectiveness of psychotherapy: The Consumer Reports study. *American Psychologist, 50*, 965–974.

Shapira, N., Barak, A., & Gal, I. (2007). Promoting older adults' well-being through Internet training and use. *Aging & Mental Health, 11*, 477–484.

Shaw, K., O'Rourke, P., Del Mar, C., & Kenardy, J. (2007). Psychological interventions for overweight or obesity. *Cochrane Database of Systematic Reviews*, Issue 3. Art. No.: CD003818. DOI: 10.1002/14651858.CD003818.pub2.

Simpson, S. (2003). Video counselling and psychotherapy in practice. In S. Goss & K. Anthony (Eds.), *Technology in counselling and psychotherapy: A practitioner's guide* (pp. 109–128). Houndmills, UK: Palgrave Macmillan.

Skinner, A. E. G., & Latchford, G. (2006). Attitudes to counselling via the Internet: A comparison between in-person counselling clients and Internet support group users. *Counselling and Psychotherapy Research, 6*, 158–163.

Skinner, A., & Zack, J. S. (2004). Counseling and the Internet. *American Behavioral Scientist, 48*, 434–446.

Smith, M. L., & Glass, G. V. (1977). Meta-analysis of psychotherapy outcome studies. *American Psychologist, 32*, 752–760.

Smith, M. L., Glass, G. V., & Miller, T. I. (1980). *The benefits of psychotherapy.* Baltimore, MD: John Hopkins University Press.

Spek, V., Cuijpers, P., Nyklícek, I., Riper, H., Keyzer, J., & Pop, V. (2007). Internet-based cognitive behaviour therapy for symptoms of depression and anxiety: A meta-analysis. *Psychological Medicine, 37*, 319–328.

Spence, S. H., Holmes, J. M., March, S., & Lipp, O. V. (2006). The feasibility and outcome of clinic plus Internet delivery of cognitive-behavior therapy for childhood anxiety. *Journal of Consulting and Clinical Psychology, 74,* 614–621.

Squires, D. D., & Hester, R. K. (2004). Using technical innovations in clinical practice: The Drinker's Check-Up software program. *Journal of Clinical Psychology, 60,* 159–169.

Stofle, G. S. (2002). Chat room therapy. In R. C. Hsiung (Ed.), *eTherapy: Case studies, guiding principles and the clinical potential of the Internet* (pp. 92–135). New York: Norton.

Strecher, V. (2007). Internet methods for delivering behavioral and health-related interventions (eHealth). *Annual Review of Clinical Psychology, 3,* 53–76.

*Strecher, V. J., Shiffman, S., & West, R. (2005). Randomized controlled trial of a Web-based computer-tailored smoking cessation program as a supplement to nicotine patch therapy. *Addiction, 100,* 682–688.

*Ström, L., Pattersson, R., & Andersson, G. (2000). A controlled trial of recurrent headache conducted via the Internet. *Journal of Consulting and Clinical Psychology, 68,* 722–727.

*Ström, L., Pattersson, R., & Andersson, G. (2004). Internet-based treatment for insomnia: A controlled evaluation. *Journal of Consulting and Clinical Psychology, 72,* 113–120.

Suler, J. (2000). Psychotherapy in cyberspace: A 5-dimensional model of online and computer-mediated psychotherapy. *CyberPsychology & Behavior, 3,* 151–159.

Suler, J. (2004). The psychology of text relationships. In R. Kraus, J. Zack & G. Stricker (Eds.), *Online counseling: A handbook for mental health professionals* (pp. 19–50). San Diego, CA: Elsevier Academic Press.

Suler, J. (2008). Cybertherapeutic theory and techniques. In A. Barak (Ed.), *Psychological aspects of cyberspace: Theory, research, applications,* 102–128. Cambridge, UK: Cambridge University Press.

*Swartz, L. H. G., Noell, J. W., Schroeder, S. W., & Ary, D. V. (2006). A randomised control study of a fully automated Internet based smoking cessation programme. *Tobacco Control, 15,* 7–12.

*Tate, D. F., Jackvony, E. H., & Wing, R. R. (2003). Effects of Internet behavioral counseling on weight loss in adults at risk for type 2 diabetes. *Journal of the American Medical Association, 289,* 1833–1836.

*Tate, D. F., Wing, R. R., & Winett, R. A. (2001). Using Internet technology to deliver a behavioral weight loss program. *Journal of the American Medical Association, 285,* 1172–1177.

Tate, D. F., & Zabinski, M. F. (2004). Computer and Internet applications for psychological treatment: Update for clinicians. *Journal of Clinical Psychology, 60,* 209–220.

Trepal, H., Haberstroh, S., Duffey, T., & Evans, M. (2007). Considerations and strategies for teaching online counseling skills: Establishing relationships in cyberspace. *Counselor Education & Supervision, 46,* 266–279.

Tyler, J. M., & Sabella, R. A. (2003). *Using technology to improve counseling practice: A primer for the 21st century.* Alexandria, VA: American Counseling Association.

Valkenburg, P. M., & Peter, J. (2007). Preadolescents' and adolescents' online communication and their closeness to friends. *Developmental Psychology, 43,* 267–277.

Voyer, D., Voyer, S., & Bryden, M. P. (1995). Magnitude of sex differences in spatial abilities: A meta-analysis and consideration of critical variables. *Psychological Bulletin, 117,* 250–270.

*Wade, S. L., Wolfe, C., Brown, T. M., & Pestian, J. P. (2005). Putting the pieces together: Preliminary efficacy of a web-based family intervention for children with traumatic brain injury. *Journal of Pediatric Psychology, 30,* 437–442. (60) [This article reports of findings published also in Wade, S. L., Wolfe, C. R., Maines Brown, T., & Pestian, J. P. (2005). Can a web-based family problem-solving intervention work for children with traumatic brain injury? *Rehabilitation Psychology, 50,* 337–345.]

Walters, S. T., Miller, E., & Chiauzzi, E. (2005). Wired for wellness: e-Interventions for addressing college drinking. *Journal of Substance Abuse Treatment, 29,* 139–145.

Walters, S. T., Wright, J. A., & Shegog, R. (2006). A review of computer and Internet-based interventions for smoking behavior. *Addictive Behaviors, 31,* 264–277.

Wampold, B. E. (2001). *The great psychotherapy debate: Models, methods, and findings.* Mahwah, NJ: Erlbaum.

Wampold, B. E., Mondin, G. W., Moody, M., Stich, F., Benson, K., & Ahn, H.-N. (1997). A meta-analysis of outcome studies comparing bona fide psychotherapies: Empirically, "all must have prizes." *Psychological Bulletin, 122,* 203–215.

Wantland, D. J., Portillo, C. J., Holzemer, W. L., Slaughter, R., & McGhee, E. M. (2004). The effectiveness of web-based vs. non-web-based interventions: A meta-analysis of behavioral change outcomes. *Journal of Medical Internet Research, 6*(4:e40) [online]. Retrieved December 15, 2006, from http://www.jmir.org/2004/4/e40/.

Weinstein, P. K. (2006). A review of weight loss programs delivered via the Internet. *Journal of Cardiovascular Nursing, 21,* 251–258.

Wells, M., Mitchell, K. J., Finkelhor, D., & Becker-Blease, K. A. (2007). Online mental health treatment: Concerns and considerations. *CyberPsychology & Behavior, 10,* 453–459.

*White, M. A., Martin, P. D., Newton, R. L., Walden, H. M., York-Crowe, E. E., Gordon, S. T., et al. (2004). Mediators of weight loss in a family-based intervention presented over the Internet. *Obesity Research, 12,* 1050–1059. [This article provides findings published also in Williamson, D. A., Davis Martin, P., Whito, M. A., Newton, R., Walden, H., York Crowe, E., et al. (2005). Efficacy of an Internet-based behavioral weight loss program for overweight adolescent African-American girls. *Eating and Weight Disorders, 10,* 193–203.]

*Winzelberg, A. J., Eppstein, D., Eldredge, K. L., Wilfley, D., Dasmahapatra, R., Dev, P., et al. (2000). Effectiveness of an Internet-based program for reducing risk factors for eating disorders. *Journal of Consulting and Clinical Psychology, 68,* 346–350.

*Womble, L. G., Wadden, T. A., McGuckin, B. G., Sargent, S. L., Rothman, R. A., & Krauthamer-Ewing, E. S. (2004). A randomized controlled trial of a commercial Internet weight loss program. *Obesity Research, 12,* 1011–1018.

*Woodruff, S. I., Edwards, C. C., Conway, T. L., & Elliott, S. P. (2001). Pilot test of an Internet virtual chat room for rural teen smokers. *Journal of Adolescent Health, 29,* 239–243.

Ybarra, M. L., Eaton, W. W., & Bickman, L. (2005). Internet-based mental health interventions. *Mental Health Services Research, 7,* 75–87.

Young, K. S. (2005). An empirical examination of client attitudes toward online counseling. *CyberPsychology & Behavior, 8,* 172–177.

*Zabinski, M. F., Pung, M. A., Wilfley, D. E., Eppstein, D. L., Winzellberg, A. J., Celio, A., et al. (2001). Reducing risk factors for eating disorders: Targeting at-risk women with computerized psychoeducational program. *International Journal of Eating Disorders, 29,* 401–408.

*Zabinski, M. F., Wilfley, D. E., Calfas, K. J., Winzelberg, A. J., & Taylor, C. B. (2004). An interactive psychoeducational intervention for women at risk of developing an eating disorder. *Journal of Consulting & Clinical Psychology, 72,* 914–919.

*Zetterqvist, K., Maanmies, J., Ström, L., & Andersson, G. (2003). Randomized controlled trial of Internet-based stress management. *Cognitive Behaviour Therapy, 32,* 151–160.

Zuckerman, E. (2003). Finding, evaluating, and incorporating Internet self-help resources into psychotherapy practice. *Journal of Clinical Psychology, 59,* 217–225.

Development of a New Approach to Guided Self-Help via the Internet: The Swedish Experience

Gerhard Andersson
Jan Bergström
Monica Buhrman
Per Carlbring
Fredrik Holländare
Viktor Kaldo
Elisabeth Nilsson-Ihrfelt
Björn Paxling
Lars Ström
Johan Waara

Across the world the Internet is rapidly spreading and helping humans communicate as well as obtain and exchange information. It is therefore highly anticipated that Internet-mediated communication and information gathering already has had implications for the provision of psychological services. A growing literature exists on the social implications of the Internet (Bargh & McKenna, 2004), and the Internet has had a large impact on health care systems (Umefjord, Petersson, & Hamberg, 2003). A related literature has focused on Internet support groups (Houston, Cooper, & Ford, 2002), with conflicting findings regarding benefits and possible harm in a few cases (such as instructions on how to harm oneself) (Bessell et al., 2002). In this article we will give an overview of another use of the Internet, namely the provision of minimal contact psychological treatment (guided self-help) for various health conditions. The focus will be on cognitive behavior therapy (CBT), as this is the psychological treatment approach that has often been translated to self-help format with good empirical support (den Boer, Wiersma, & Van den Bosch, 2004). It is also increasingly the most widely disseminated form of psychological treatment (Norcross, Karpiak, & Santoro, 2005).

It is important at this early stage to briefly comment on the concept of guided self-help. In contrast to self-help groups and what is normally regarded as self-help, guided self-help is often based on a structured protocol, most commonly a text such as the widely spread and empirically validated book, *Feeling Good: The New Mood Therapy* (Burns, 1999). Guided self-help also often involves minimal contact with a responsible clinician, but this contact can vary in form and in amount of time. It is also the case that guided self-help most often involves professionals in the helping professions in either the design or delivery of the treatment. Clinician input is, however, often markedly reduced compared to traditional psychological treatments. In many studies on guided self-help the support has been in the form of telephone contact, but there are also examples of other forms of support, for example by having group meetings (den Boer et al., 2004; Hirai & Clum, 2006; Marrs, 1995). With the advent of the Internet, another common way to communicate is via e-mail.

Often the time spent by the therapist is markedly reduced in guided self-help, regardless of format. In computerized self-help it is also common that at least some of the treatment decisions (such as getting access to the next step of treatment after completing an online test) are delegated to the computer (Marks, Cavanagh, & Gega, 2007). However, the time spent *by the client/patient* is not less, which can be a source of misunderstanding of the treatment approach. In fact, guided self-help can under some circumstances be even more time consuming for the client, as texts are used in homework assignments and the client can continuously report on progress and get faster feedback if exercises fail. In contrast to virtual reality approaches, in which exercises such as exposure to feared objects is conducted via the computer program, guided self-help in the form outlined here almost exclusively focuses on real-life exposure and behavioral and emotional change not mediated by the computer per se.

The focus in this review will be on Internet-delivered CBT that is assisted by a live therapist either by e-mail only or by e-mail and telephone support. We will begin by defining the approach and then move on to a selective review of the Swedish trials conducted by our research group. We will next cover strengths and problems of the approach and comment on what we believe is needed for Internet-delivered CBT to work effectively.

DEFINING GUIDED INTERNET-DELIVERED SELF-HELP

There are several varieties of computerized treatments, some of which have been transferred to the Internet, and others that are outside of the scope of the present paper. For example, computerized CBT (CCBT) has been tested in several studies (Marks et al., 2007) but is a broader concept than the more specific application of Internet for psychological treatment. For example, in several CCBT studies the Internet has not been involved at all and instead standalone computers have been used (Proudfoot et al., 2004).

Another application of the Internet is so called e-mail therapy, which does not require a written text or self-help material but can be handled on a one-to-one basis between a client and a therapist (Manhal-Baugus, 2001; Murphy & Mitchell, 1998). Yet another format is video counseling, which can be conducted via the Internet (Ruskin et al., 2004), and there are also treatment applications using chat forums (Rassau & Arco, 2003).

A common approach to online therapy in Sweden and in some other countries (e.g., Australia) is best described as a mixture between bibliotherapy and e-mail therapy, but with relatively little use of e-mail correspondence. In fact, therapist contact ranges between below 100 minutes for a 8–10 week program in most Swedish studies to extensive therapist interaction in a therapy form called Interapy (Lange, van de Ven, & Schrieken, 2003), in which almost no reduction in therapist time is achieved compared with face-to-face treatment.

Thus for the present purpose, we define guided Internet-delivered self-help as a therapy that is based on self-help books, guided by an identified therapist who gives feedback and answers to questions, with a scheduling that mirrors face-to-face treatment, and which also can include interactive online features such as queries to obtain passwords in order to get access to treatment modules. In practice, this means that guided Internet-delivered self-help falls somewhere between face-to-face treatments (with extensive therapist contact) and purely computerized treatments with no therapist contact. While some treatment decisions and tasks can be delegated to the computer in guided Internet-delivered self-help, in some respects this treatment form is similar to guided self-help using a book and support via telephone (den Boer et al., 2004; Hirai & Clum, 2006; Newman, Erickson, Preworski, & Dzus, 2003).

One additional qualification is that most studies and clinical applications of guided Internet-delivered self-help have relied on principles and treatment techniques derived from CBT. This does not by definition mean that other therapeutic orientations cannot be transferred to the Internet, but it does suggest that CBT has been dominant in the psychological treatment literature on self-help.

SERVICE DELIVERY CONSIDERATIONS

Three issues are relevant to discuss when outlining the treatment approach. First, there is the role and skills of the guiding therapist. Many aspects of this role could possibly be handled by a layperson, such as encouragement and emotional support via e-mail. Other parts of the therapist role are harder to handle without at least basic training in the treatment modality presented and the presenting complaint (for example, knowledge about anxiety). Expertise can also be required for monitoring and planning of follow-up visits. Unfortunately, there is no research on the qualifications of those who use the treatment approach, but we believe that basic knowledge of the CBT principles is required.

The client is the second issue. To date, there have been no systematic reviews of characteristics of clients suitable for guided Internet-delivered self-help or even of the participants who have been included in the studies, albeit this has been mentioned in some reviews (Spek et al., 2007). While the early Swedish studies had a higher proportion of well-educated participants than in the Swedish population in general, later studies do not clearly show this pattern, which might reflect the spread of the Internet. However, certain requirements are worth mentioning. Language skills is one aspect, as much of the information is presented in text form. Sound files and use of translated texts could possibly handle this restriction partly, but in common with bibliotherapy (e.g., text-based treatment) guided Internet-delivered self-help as it stands now requires that the client can read, follow instructions, and communicate via text (often e-mail). This implies that the actual texts used in guided Internet-delivered self-help need to be well-written and comprehensive, but also that clients with neurological and/or reading deficits for various other reasons might benefit less from treatment. Being able to handle the basics of computers and also basic typing skills are needed as well.

The third possible concern has to do with the technological requirements from both the provider and client perspective. The web has expanded rapidly, and yesterday's high tech is today's old fashion. A guiding principle in many studies conducted in Sweden has been to stay alongside the public at large and keep the web inter-action technically as simple as possible while still retaining the useful part of the expanding Internet and computer technology. For example, this means staying away from most plug-in programs. Instead we mostly rely on plain text, simple pictures, and download-able PDF files. The therapeutic utility of a number of technical advances that has become easily accessible to the public during recent years is not evident either. For instance, the therapeutic use of web-cams is yet to be studied thoroughly, although the technique has been available to the public during the past years. Client expectations regarding the level of technology will most likely play a role in future applications of Internet-delivered self-help.

OVERVIEW OF OUTCOME IN THE SWEDISH TRIALS

In the following we will focus on the Internet studies we have been involved in as researchers and clinicians. There are a few other Swed-ish studies not covered here, including a few unpublished papers. We will not provide a detailed analysis of effect sizes, which has been done in previous reviews and meta-analyses (Andersson, Cuijpers, Carlbring, & Lindefors, 2007; Cuijpers, van Straten, & Andersson, 2008; Spek et al., 2007).

The first Swedish randomized trial targeted headache (Ström, Pettersson, & Andersson, 2000). Participants were recruited via mass media, and the immediate result of treatment was promising, with 50 percent of the Internet treatment group showing an improvement of 50 percent on an index of headache severity. However, the dropout rate was substantial (56 percent). A later replication trial concerned the role of structured telephone support in addition to the Internet program (Andersson, Lundström, & Ström, 2003). Somewhat different results were obtained, with a statistical significant improvement on a broad measure relating to disability caused by the headache (Jacobson, Ramadan, Aggrawal, & Newman, 1994), but less clear effects on headache activity (an index of headache intensity divided by the number of days with headache), with only a fourth reporting clinical significant improvement. The promising effects of Internet-delivered CBT for headache have been replicated in an independent trial (Devineni & Blanchard, 2005).

A second early project concerned tinnitus (ringing or buzzing in the ear), which is a common condition that can cause irritation, insomnia, and concentration problems in addition to the auditory intrusiveness of the tinnitus sound (Andersson, Baguley, McKenna, & McFerran, 2005). Tinnitus is often impossible to cure, and CBT has been found to help sufferers cope with their tinnitus (Martinez Devesa, Waddell, Perera, & Theodoulou, 2007). One randomized controlled trial showed promising effects of an Internet-delivered, therapist-guided CBT program for tinnitus distress (Andersson, Strömgren, Ström, & Lyttkens, 2002), and in a later effectiveness study, the results were even better (Kaldo-Sandström, Larsen, & Andersson, 2004). Effectiveness studies examine whether a treatment works in real-world settings and in situations that clinicians encounter in their practices. They often constitute the next level of obtaining evidence that a treatment works after it has been investigated under more ideal circumstances; for example, in a research university clinic with participants recruited via advertisements (so called efficacy trials). In the most recent trial, Internet-delivered guided self-help using CBT for tinnitus distress was found to yield similar outcome as live-group treatment (Kaldo et al., in press). A case report on this treatment has also been published (Andersson & Kaldo, 2004). This program was rapidly implemented in clinical practice and has been running as a regular clinical service at Uppsala Academic Hospital in Sweden since 1999. This is part of the National Health Service and not funded by external funds.

In the area of psychiatric disorders, the first project concerned panic disorder. Several studies have been conducted in Sweden following the first randomized trial showing very promising results in terms of symptom reduction (Carlbring, Westling, Ljungstrand, Ekselius, & Andersson, 2001). In the second study the guided self-help

CBT program was compared with applied relaxation in a small study (Carlbring, Ekselius, & Andersson, 2003), showing relatively minor differences but good results for both treatment conditions. The third study on panic disorder from our group compared live treatment against the effects of Internet-delivered self-help (Carlbring et al., 2005). Results showed that the two treatment formats were largely equivalent in terms of outcome, with a vast majority in both groups receiving substantial symptom reduction. A later study by our group explored the effects of combining the Internet treatment with weekly brief telephone calls. The calls focused on providing support but were also structured and covered progress in the program. Results were similar to the previous studies, but in contrast to the previously mentioned headache trial (Andersson, Lundström, et al., 2003) we noticed that the telephone calls improved adherence to the treatment protocol (Carlbring, Bohman, et al., 2006). The most recent panic study was an effectiveness trial that showed that the treatment format could be transferred to a regular psychiatric outpatient setting (Bergström et al., 2007). We are not alone in conducting research on panic disorder, with promising results also seen in trials conducted in Australia (Klein, Richards, & Austin, 2006).

In the area of behavioral medicine, apart from tinnitus, we have also conducted a study on chronic pain patients (Buhrman, Fältenhag, Ström, & Andersson, 2004). In a randomized controlled trial we had very good adherence to the protocol (i.e., few dropouts), possibly because of the addition of brief telephone calls. Outcome was good compared to a waiting-list control condition, with significant reductions of catastrophizing regarding pain. A later unpublished study largely replicates these findings, but did not include the telephone calls (Buhrman et al., unpublished data). An interesting feature of the Buhrman and colleagues (2004) trial was an indication of improvement in the wait-list control group. A similar observation was seen in a trial we conducted on stress management (Zetterqvist, Maanmies, Ström, & Andersson, 2003). In that study positive effects were found, but we also noticed improvements in the waiting-list control group, which might be attributed to easily available information on stress management on the Internet.

Insomnia is another problem that we believe is very suitable for Internet treatment. In one controlled trial we found positive effects using Internet-delivered guided self-help (Ström, Pettersson, & Andersson, 2004).

In another study of Internet-administered treatment, we conducted an analog study of computer versus live administration of applied relaxation (Carlbring, Björnstjerna, Norkrans, Waara, & Andersson, 2007). In the study we included both physiological and self-report measures. Overall, using a randomized controlled design, that also included a nonrelaxation control condition (surfing on the web), we found that computers can be used to administer relaxation.

At an early stage in the late 1990 s we conducted a trial on major depression, which lead to a research program. The first trial used a chat forum as a control condition, which was compared to a guided self-help CBT program with standard ingredients (e.g., behavioral activation and cognitive restructuring) (Andersson, Bergström et al., 2005; Andersson, Bergström, Holländare, Ekselius, & Carlbring, 2004). No telephone support was given in that study. An interesting observation in that trial was that the discussion group proved ineffective in contrast to a previous trial from the United States (Houston et al., 2002) that found some improvements in a trial of Internet support groups. Since the first study we have conducted two randomized control trials (RCTs) on depression that are yet unpublished. This is an area in which many other researchers are active (Christensen, Griffiths, & Jorm, 2004), and many studies are in progress or have already been conducted (Andersson, 2006).

Moving on to another anxiety disorder, we began doing research on social phobia. In the first trial we hesitated to rely on Internet-mediated treatment only and included two live exposure sessions in addition to a nine-week guided self-help program (Andersson et al., 2006). Results from that first trial were very promising, and in a later randomized trial telephone support in addition to the treatment program was found to yield equally good outcome even without the live exposure sessions (Carlbring, Gunnarsdóttir, et al., 2007). An open trial with less therapist input also resulted in good outcome (Carlbring, Furmark, Steczkó, Ekselius, & Andersson, 2006). Other studies on psychiatric disorders, including bulimia nervosa and binge eating disorder (Ljotsson et al., 2007), have been conducted. Studies on specific phobia, generalized anxiety disorder, and pathological gambling represent work in progress.

In total we have now conducted several controlled trials, a few open trials, and one effectiveness study that all used the same treatment format with minor modifications. The work summarized in meta-analyses mentioned earlier (Andersson et al., 2007; Cuijpers et al.,

2007; Spek et al., 2007) suggests that our Swedish trials generate large effect sizes (often in the range of d = .80, which is equal to face-to-face therapy). In fact, in many cases we have larger effects than found in Internet studies conducted in other countries. In several of these studies follow-ups have been included, ranging between three months to one year posttreatment. This leads us to a discussion of the important lesson we have learned thus far from our research program.

LESSONS LEARNED

Since the first headache trial we have made several observations, and in fact our experiences have "shaped" the way we conduct studies and constructed our programs. As already commented on, we decided early on to refrain from technologically advanced technological web solutions, as most clients were not prepared for this when we began. This can be posed as a limitation to our approach as more advanced programs (relying more on automated interactive features than "manual" e-mail contact) save therapist time and can also be attractive for the user. In fact, when comparing approaches to computerized CBT, Marks and coworkers referred to our approach as "net biblioCBT" (Marks et al., 2007), and also characterized a series of Australian trials under the same heading (Richards, Klein, & Carlbring, 2003). The advantage with using mainly text, downloadable as PDF files, is that new programs can easily be constructed and updates of texts can be made without much effort. However, as web solutions are becoming increasingly user-friendly and require less expertise in terms of programming, we expect to use more interactive features (for example, feedback on questionnaire ratings and a decision tree guiding the feedback depending on the score obtained), which also will be more easily done when clients have broadband Internet access. Obviously, in some of our programs (e.g., the tinnitus program which is situated within a hospital IT environment and runs within a regular clinical service), more advanced web solutions have been constructed, not least because of security issues; for example, using a server located within the hospital firewalls. Another reason for having clients interact more with the web page is that we can get important data from the clients (e.g., online behavior).

Among the lessons learned are our experiences of recruiting participants to our trials. A general web page in Swedish is available in which potential research participants can sign up for interest in participating in upcoming trials. To date, all of our studies have been conducted in the Swedish language, and while there have been a few distant participants living overseas, they have been too few to draw any conclusions regarding differential effects. Visitors can also read summaries of previous trials and link to registration if a trial is running. Having a general web page facilitates contacts with mass media, and in effect we can at any moment have hundreds of potential study participants when recruiting for an upcoming trial on, for instance, social phobia. Overall, we have used different channels to recruit participants for trials, including leaflets and posters (mainly in general practice waiting rooms and other health care settings), regular articles in newspapers (which will generate many interested persons), radio and television appearances, and occasionally advertisements in local press, although the latter is rarely needed and seldom very effective. In effectiveness trials, patients are obviously not recruited in this way, but rather via referrals within a psychiatric clinical setting (Bergström et al., in press), since the aim is to maximize external validity. Here one faces other challenges, often related to difficulties in implementing completely novel treatment formats in traditional clinical settings, as well as issues concerning assessment, screening, and responsibility for patients. One lesson worth commenting on is that participants with different diagnoses differ even at the stage of recruitment. For instance, panic disorder patients tend to be very motivated, whereas persons with major depression tend to be slower to report interest in the trials. For the somatic conditions, recruitment differs depending on how well psychological treatment is accepted as a treatment option, experience with previous treatment, and how difficult it is to get referral to CBT practitioners.

The next lesson concerns selection of participants for inclusion in trials. Persons with very minor or too severe problems will report interest in participating in the study. When the person has only very mild or inversely very severe problems, guided Internet-delivered self-help might be unsuitable. This is an empirical question that can be resolved only by systematic research efforts, but for many of the psychiatric conditions we have studied, such as panic disorder and social phobia, the diagnostic criteria are strict (American Psychiatric Association, 2000), and people who suffer from some degree of anxiety (e.g., panic attacks) often do not fulfill the criteria for a diagnosis. On the other side of this dilemma we find the severe clients, who might be in acute need for psychiatric/medical consultations and for whom Internet treatment is not safe enough as a single intervention. However, concerning the patients we do include, we suspect that our effort to include "real patients" with diagnosis (e.g., as defined in the DSM-IV) is a contributing factor for the strong effects we have found. In other trials within the field, researchers have often used less strict diagnostic criteria, which sometimes result in lower effects, at least judging from the meta-analysis recently published by Spek et al. (2007). However, some people do have very severe problems and are therefore excluded. This is a group we have not yet studied. Targeting more severe and even suicidal clients could possibly be done if a combined treatment format were developed, including telephone monitoring, live sessions, and Internet self-help. Indeed, cognitive therapy appears to be a promising treatment approach to the prevention of suicide (Brown et al., 2005), which could be extended to the Internet, and studies are currently conducted in that field. When selecting participants for a study, it is important to find a balance between the information collected in web-based screening formulas (which should be as brief as possible while still proving a reliable likelihood of getting a diagnosis), the need for confirmation in a telephone or even live diagnostic interview, and the need to inform people as rapidly as possible in cases when they are not suitable for the treatment. Indeed, a few rare people get irritated when they are not accepted for participation, but a vast majority appreciates the feedback they get (which must be personalized, and present alternatives such as suggestions about where to seek help). Effectiveness trials in traditional clinical settings raises other questions mentioned earlier related to specificity of referrals, assessment practices, and patient security issues when professional feedback to patients might not be as fast as in efficacy studies.

With regard to the task of developing treatment protocols, we have the experience of consulting all available sources, but the lesson learned has been to mainly rely on self-help books that have been tested in controlled trials. As CBT is rapidly progressing, there may be shifts in focus on which treatment components to emphasize. For example, in the treatment of major depression, recent evidence suggest that behavioral activation is not only important to include, but perhaps sufficient (Dimidjian et al., 2006), and when developing our treatment program for social phobia we paid attention to recent concepts such as safety behaviors (misdirected coping that increases rather than decreases the social anxiety) and other recent developments (Clark et al., 2006). Marks et al. (2007), among others, has commented on the potential to conduct dismantling studies online, and a few examples of such studies have been published (Christensen, Griffiths, Mackinnon, & Brittliffe, 2006). In a dismantling study, ingredients in a treatment protocol can be deleted in order to "dismantle" what the effective ingredients are. For example, in the case of depression an important question is whether behavioral activation really is needed or if it is enough to work on beliefs and cognitions. Our focus has rather been on finding ways to increase the effects of Internet treatment, which has included varying the amount of therapist contact instead of removing treatment ingredients (such as removing cognitive restructuring from the depression program). However, once effective programs have been developed, by which we mean as effective as possible with the potential of generating equal outcome as in live, face-to-face treatment (Carlbring et al., 2005) and in regular clinical settings (Bergström et al., in press), a focus on dismantling studies could be called for. We should, however, consider using combined treatment formats (i.e., live sessions and Internet treatment in combination) to generate even better outcome than in live-only treatment.

Treatment design issues cannot be discussed without considering costs. While some work has been published on the cost-effectiveness of computerized CBT (Kaltenthaler et al., 2006), much more work needs to be done regarding Internet delivered treatment (Palmqvist, Carlbring, & Andersson, 2007). Another unexplored issue concerns the environment and how Internet treatment might be justified from an environmental perspective. For example, traveling to a specialist clinic for live treatment can involve hours by car or train. On the other hand, printing PDF files has the disadvantage of just printing on one side of the paper (in comparison with books that print on both sides). Pending better reader-friendly computer screens and/or digital paper, it is possible that this will change in the future. Another possibility we consider is using published books and to have only supplementary material and interaction online. To our knowledge the environmental implications of "remote" treatment has not yet been considered in the literature.

When we began doing Internet studies we did not consider the implications of using online questionnaires (Buchanan, 2003), and for a while we decided to use paper and pencil tests until we had evaluated the psychometric properties of online questionnaires and tests. We now believe we have robust support for the use of online question-naires (e.g., Austin, Carlbring, Richards, & Andersson, 2006), but are less convinced regarding diagnostic issues (Carlbring et al., 2002). The lesson learned is that we usually rely on web-administrated questionnaires, but that we check their characteristics (Andersson, Kaldo-Sandström, Ström, & Strömgren, 2003). When it comes to diagnoses of psychiatric conditions, we prefer live or at least telephone interviews to supplement the online screening. As we work in many areas, we regularly consult physicians for accuracy of our judgments in screening conferences, or we use physicians to directly make a diagnosis when conducting effectiveness trials. For example, in a recent ongoing trial on generalized anxiety disorder, all persons who passed the first screening test online were then interviewed using a structured psychiatric interview over the telephone by a psychologist (recorded on audiotape), and the diagnoses were later presented to and confirmed by a psychiatrist. Obviously, this will add to the costs of delivering the treatment, but we benefit from the safety and accuracy when making clinical decisions.

While the main part of the treatment lies in the text material, we do see the need for support by a trained professional during the treatment period. In our trials we have mostly used supervised clinical psychologists near the end of the master's degree in clinical psychology, but we have also had more experienced therapists. In an ongoing analysis of therapist effects we see some indications that therapist factors (e.g., different outcome depending on who is the therapist) do make a difference even in this treatment approach. What is yet to be structured and evaluated is the need for training of therapists to act as e-therapists. In our experience, the therapist should be knowledgeable about the principles behind the treatment (i.e., CBT), but as the interaction is via text (e-mail) they also need to be good communicators and have sufficient writing skills. Supervision of the therapist who is in touch with the client is another aspect we increasingly focus on to boost the effects in our trials. While the supervision differs from regular psychotherapy supervision, important advice can be given to the therapist, either in live supervision sessions, telephone consultations, or via e-mail. Since clients can present with various problems and issues during the treatment process, there can be many issues to focus on during supervision.

From a research point of view we found early that the risk of dropping out of treatment was high (Eysenbach, 2005). To handle this we scheduled follow-up calls at the beginning of the treatment, and as a result we now have a much lower dropout rate, even similar to regular treatment studies. However, other researchers have more problems with this (Christensen, Griffiths, Groves, & Korten, 2006; Christensen, Griffiths, Mackinnon et al., 2006), which can be regarded as a major limitation to the treatment approach. Our lesson learned is that there should be some human interaction and the participant in a trial must know early what we expect in terms of completing follow-up assessments. This does not, however, mean that all participants complete all modules (chapters); for example, in a 10-week program. However since we can keep track of the modules completed, we can ascertain if there are correlations between modules completed and outcome. We know from experience that one of the most common reasons for not completing all treatment modules in time is that the participants lack time. Giving access to the rest of the modules give them an opportunity to complete the treatment after the follow-up interview and assessment. It is not obvious how to handle this problem, as a decreased number of modules can still lead to the same problem or be equally effective, perhaps depending on what modules are included (Christensen, Griffiths, Mackinnon et al., 2006). In fact, in the tinnitus program mentioned earlier we demanded more instead of less of the participants in the second treatment study, which resulted in better outcome and less dropout. Using Internet for research opens up new possibilities since follow-up studies of research trials can be easier than in regular face-to-face follow-ups. On the other hand, in long-term follow-ups former clients might have changed their contact address (e.g., e-mail), and researchers are therefore advised to obtain alternative ways to contact research participants for long-term follow-ups (provided that ethical permission has been obtained).

FUTURE IMPLICATIONS

It is hard, if not impossible, to predict the future of the Internet, and this also holds true for Internet-delivered treatment. From a research point of view, we can foresee effectiveness and dissemination trials, and also treatment studies that take more advantage of the medium. For example, we have a study in progress in which we plan to tailor treatment according to the problems the patient has. This was partly done in the tinnitus program. With other diagnoses, for example, anxiety disorders in which there is high comorbidity between different anxiety disorders and mood disorders, it could be feasible to accept clients who do not have a clear diagnosis. We believe that our clinical colleagues will welcome this approach, which would necessitate clinical judgment and most likely fit better with the kinds of clients that clinicians see. Issues surrounding dissemination of Internet treatment would require a separate review. In Sweden we have recently had the treatment approach evaluated by the Swedish Council on Technology Assessment in Health Care (Statens Beredning för Medicinsk Utvärdering, 2007), a Cochrane-type of organization. This review gave preliminary support for dissemination of Internet-based interventions into health care. There are, however, both private and governmental (tax financed) providers of health care in Sweden. Dissemination issues by both types of providers will need to be addressed in the future.

CONCLUSION

In this review we presented the development of our approach to Internet delivered CBT. It may strike some readers as more different than what they expect when thinking about computerized and Internet-delivered treatment. In fact, we must conclude that our approach is somewhere in between more standard provision of therapy, bibliotherapy, and computerized treatment. In effect, we do save therapist time (between 50 to 80 percent), but not as much as in a purely computerized treatment or in bibliotherapy without any guidance. We have strong reasons to believe that at this phase of online treatment development we cannot replace the clinician with a computer, but it might increasingly be the case that more decisions and routine tasks such as generating feedback on submitted registrations/homework will be handled automatically. While we have used automated replies for some time, we have retained the "manual" interactive features with a live therapist. In particular in sensitive cases the clinical judgment cannot be replaced. In the future we are confident that Internet treatment will find its place as a natural complement and assistance in the practice of CBT.

ACKNOWLEDGEMENT

The preparation of this manuscript was sponsored in part from grants from the from the Swedish Research Council, the Swedish Cancer Foundation, Swedish Council for Working and Life Research, and the Hard of Hearing Research Fund.

REFERENCES

American Psychiatric Association. (2000). *Diagnostic and statistical manual of mental disorders* (4th ed., text revision ed.). Washington, DC: American Psychiatric Press.

Andersson, G. (2006). Internet based cognitive behavioral self-help for depression. *Expert Review of Neurotherapeutics, 6,* 1637–1642.

Andersson, G., Baguley, D. M., McKenna, L., & McFerran, D. J. (2005). *Tinnitus: A multidisciplinary approach.* London: Whurr.

Andersson, G., Bergström, J., Holländare, F., Carlbring, P., Kaldo, V., & Ekselius, L. (2005). Internet-based self-help for depression: A randomised controlled trial. *British Journal of Psychiatry, 187,* 456–461.

Andersson, G., Bergström, J., Holländare, F., Ekselius, L., & Carlbring, P. (2004). Delivering CBT for mild to moderate depression via the Internet. Predicting outcome at 6-months follow-up. *Verhaltenstherapie, 14,* 185–189.

Andersson, G., Carlbring, P., Holmström, A., Sparthan, E., Furmark, T., Nilsson-Ihrfelt, E., et al. (2006). Internet-based self-help with therapist feedback and in-vivo group exposure for social phobia: A randomized controlled trial. *Journal of Consulting and Clinical Psychology, 74,* 677–686.

Andersson, G., Cuijpers, P., Carlbring, P., & Lindefors, N. (2007). Effects of Internet delivered cognitive behaviour therapy for anxiety and mood disorders. *Review Series: Psychiatry, 9,* 9–14.

Andersson, G., & Kaldo, V. (2004). Internet-based cognitive behavioral therapy for tinnitus. *Journal of Clinical Psychology, 60,* 171–178.

Andersson, G., Kaldo-Sandström, V., Ström, L., & Strömgren, T. (2003). Internet administration of the hospital anxiety and depression scale (HADS) in a sample of tinnitus patients. *Journal of Psychosomatic Research, 55,* 259–262.

Andersson, G., Lundström, P., & Ström, L. (2003). Internet-based treatment of headache. Does telephone contact add anything? *Headache, 43,* 353–361.

Andersson, G., Strömgren, T., Ström, L., & Lyttkens, L. (2002). Randomised controlled trial of Internet based cognitive behavior therapy for distress associated with tinnitus. *Psychosomatic Medicine, 64,* 810–816.

Austin, D. W., Carlbring, P., Richards, J. C., & Andersson, G. (2006). Internet administration of three commonly used questionnaires in panic research: Equivalence to paper administration in Australian and Swedish samples of people with panic disorder. *International Journal of Testing, 6,* 25–39.

Bargh, J. A., & McKenna, K. Y. A. (2004). Internet and social life. *Annual Review of Psychology, 2004,* 573–590.

Bergström, J., Andersson, G., Karlsson, A., Andreewitch, S., Rück, C., Carlbring, P., et al. (in press). An open study of the effectiveness of Internet treatment for panic disorder delivered in a psychiatric setting. *Nordic Journal of Psychiatry.*

Bessell, T. L., McDonald, S., Silagy, C. A., Anderson, J. N., Hiller, J. E., & Sansom, L. N. (2002). Do Internet interventions for consumers cause more harm than good? A systematic review. *Health Expectations, 5,* 28–37.

Brown, G. K., Ten Have, T., Henriques, G. R., Xie, S. X., Hollander, J. E., & Beck, A. T. (2005). Cognitive therapy for the prevention of suicide attempts: A randomized controlled trial. *Journal of the American Medical Association, 294,* 563–570.

Buchanan, T. (2003). Internet-based questionnaire assessment: Appropriate use in clinical contexts. *Cognitive Behaviour Therapy, 32,* 100–109.

Buhrman, M., Fältenhag, S., Ström, L., & Andersson, G. (2004). Controlled trial of Internet-based treatment with telephone support for chronic back pain. *Pain, 111,* 368–377.

Burns, D. D. (1999). *Feeling good: The new mood therapy.* New York: Avon Books.

Carlbring, P., Björnstjerna, E., Norkrans, A., Waara, J., & Andersson, G. (2007). Applied relaxation: An analog study of therapist vs. computer administration. *Computers in Human Behavior, 23,* 2–10.

Carlbring, P., Bohman, S., Brunt, S., Buhrman, M., Westling, B. E., Ekselius, L., et al. (2006). Remote treatment of panic disorder: A randomized trial of Internet-based cognitive behavioral therapy supplemented with telephone calls. *American Journal of Psychiatry, 163,* 21.

Carlbring, P., Ekselius, L., & Andersson, G. (2003). Treatment of panic disorder via the Internet: A randomized trial of CBT vs. applied relaxation. *Journal of Behavior Therapy and Experimental Psychiatry, 34,* 129–140.

Carlbring, P., Forslin, P., Ljungstrand, P., Willebrand, M., Strandlund, C., Ekselius, L., et al. (2002). Is the Internet-administered CIDI-SF equivalent to a human SCID-interview? *Cognitive Behaviour Therapy, 31,* 183–189.

Carlbring, P., Furmark, T., Steczkó, J., Ekselius, L., & Andersson, G. (2006). An open study of Internet-based bibliotherapy with minimal therapist contact via e-mail for social phobia. *Clinical Psychologist, 10,* 30–38.

Carlbring, P., Gunnarsdóttir, M., Hedensjö, L., Andersson, G., Ekselius, L., & Furmark, T. (2007). Treatment of social phobia: Randomized trial of internet delivered cognitive behaviour therapy and telephone support. *British Journal of Psychiatry, 190,* 123–128.

Carlbring, P., Nilsson-Ihrfelt, E., Waara, J., Kollenstam, C., Buhrman, M., Kaldo, V., et al. (2005). Treatment of panic disorder: Live therapy vs. self-help via Internet. *Behaviour Research and Therapy, 43,* 1321–1333.

Carlbring, P., Westling, B. E., Ljungstrand, P., Ekselius, L., & Andersson, G. (2001). Treatment of panic disorder via the Internet—A randomized trial of a self-help program. *Behavior Therapy, 32,* 751–764.

Christensen, H., Griffiths, K., Groves, C., & Korten, A. (2006). Free range users and one hit wonders: Community users of an Internet-based cognitive behaviour therapy program. *Australian and New Zealand Journal of Psychiatry, 40,* 59–62.

Christensen, H., Griffiths, K. M., & Jorm, A. (2004). Delivering interventions for depression by using the Internet: Randomised controlled trial. *British Medical Journal, 328*, 265–268.

Christensen, H., Griffiths, K. M., Mackinnon, A. J., & Brittliffe, K. (2006). Online randomized trial of brief and full cognitive behaviour therapy for depression. *Psychological Medicine, 36*, 1737–1746.

Clark, D. M., Ehlers, A., Hackmann, A., McManus, F., Fennell, M., Grey, N., et al. (2006). Cognitive therapy versus exposure and applied relaxation in social phobia: A randomized controlled trial. *Journal of Consulting and Clinical Psychology, 74*, 568–578.

Cuijpers, P., van Straten, A.-M., & Andersson, G. (2008). Internet-administered cognitive behavior therapy for health problems: A systematic review. *Journal of Behavioral Medicine, 31*, 169–177.

den Boer, P. C., Wiersma, D., & Van den Bosch, R. J. (2004). Why is self-help neglected in the treatment of emotional disorders? A meta-analysis. *Psychological Medicine, 34*, 959–971.

Devineni, T., & Blanchard, E. B. (2005). A randomized controlled trial of an internet-based treatment for chronic headache. *Behaviour Research and Therapy, 43*, 277–292.

Dimidjian, S., Hollon, S. D., Dobson, K. S., Schmaling, K. B., Kohlenberg, R. J., & Addis, M. E., et al. (2006). Randomized trial of behavioral activation, cognitive therapy, and antidepressant medication in the acute treatment of adults with major depression. *Journal of Consulting and Clinical Psychology, 74*, 658–670.

Eysenbach, G. (2005). The law of attrition. *Journal of Medical Internet Research, 7*(1), e11.

Hirai, M., & Clum, G. A. (2006). A meta-analytic study of self-help interventions for anxiety problems. *Behavior Therapy, 37*, 99–111.

Houston, T. K., Cooper, L. A., & Ford, D. E. (2002). Internet support groups for depression: A 1-year prospective cohort study. *American Journal of Psychiatry, 159*, 2062–2068.

Jacobson, G. P., Ramadan, N. M., Aggrawal, S. K., & Newman, C. W. (1994). The Henry Ford Hospital headache disability inventory (HDI). *Neurology, 44*, 837–842.

Kaldo, V., Levin, S., Widarsson, J., Buhrman, M., Larsen, H. C., & Andersson, G. (in press). Internet versus group cognitive-behavioural treatment of distress associated with tinnitus. A randomised controlled trial. *Behavior Therapy.*

Kaldo-Sandström, V., Larsen, H. C., & Andersson, G. (2004). Internet-based cognitive-behavioral self-help treatment of tinnitus: Clinical effectiveness and predictors of outcome. *American Journal of Audiology, 13*, 185–192.

Kaltenthaler, E., Brazier, J., De Nigris, E., Tumur, I., Ferriter, M., Beverley, C., et al. (2006). Computerised cognitive behaviour therapy for depression and anxiety update: a systematic review and economic evaluation. *Health Technology Assessment (Winchester, England), 10*(33), iii, xi-xiv, 1–168.

Klein, B., Richards, J. C., & Austin, D. W. (2006). Efficacy of Internet therapy for panic disorder. *Journal of Behavior Therapy and Experimental Psychiatry, 37*, 213–238.

Lange, A., van de Ven, J.-P., & Schrieken, B. (2003). Interapy: Treatment of post-traumatic stress through the Internet. *Cognitive Behaviour Therapy, 32,* 110–124.

Ljotsson, B., Lundin, C., Mitsell, K., Carlbring, P., Ramklint, M., & Ghaderi, A. (2007). Remote treatment of bulimia nervosa and binge eating disorder: A randomized trial of Internet-assisted cognitive behavioural therapy. *Behaviour Research and Therapy, 45*(4), 649–661.

Manhal-Baugus, M. (2001). Etherapy: Practical, ethical, and legal issues. *Cyberpsychology & Behavior, 4,* 551–563.

Marks, I. M., Cavanagh, K., & Gega, L. (2007). *Hands-on help. Maudsley monograph no. 49.* Hove: Psychology Press.

Marrs, R. W. (1995). A meta-analysis of bibliotherapy studies. *American Journal of Community Psychology, 23,* 843–870.

Martinez Devesa, P., Waddell, A., Perera, R., & Theodoulou, M. (2007). Cognitive behavioural therapy for tinnitus. *Cochrane database of systematic reviews (Online)*(1), CD005233.

Murphy, L. J., & Mitchell, D. L. (1998). When writing helps to heal: E-mail as therapy. *British Journal of Guidance and Counselling, 26,* 21–32.

Newman, M. G., Erickson, T., Preworski, A., & Dzus, E. (2003). Self-help and minimal-contact therapies for anxiety disorders: Is human contact necessary for therapeutic efficacy? *Journal of Clinical Psychology, 59,* 251–274.

Norcross, J. C., Karpiak, C. P., & Santoro, S. O. (2005). Clinical psychologists across the years: The division of clinical psychology from 1960 to 2003. *Journal of Clinical Psychology, 61,* 1467–1483.

Palmqvist, B., Carlbring, P., & Andersson, G. (2007). Internet-delivered treatments with or without therapist input: Does the therapist factor have implications for efficacy and cost? *Expert Review of Pharmacoeconomics & Outcomes Research, 7,* 291–297.

Proudfoot, J., Ryden, C., Everitt, B., Shapiro, D. A., Goldberg, D., Mann, A., et al. (2004). Clinical efficacy of computerised cognitive-behavioural therapy for anxiety and depression in primary care: Randomised controlled trial. *British Journal of Psychiatry, 185,* 46–54.

Rassau, A., & Arco, L. (2003). Effects of chat-based on-line cognitive behavior therapy on study related behavior and anxiety. *Behavioural and Cognitive Psychotherapy, 31,* 377–381.

Richards, J., Klein, B., & Carlbring, P. (2003). Internet-based treatment for panic disorder. *Cognitive Behaviour Therapy, 32,* 125–135.

Ruskin, P. E., Silver-Aylaian, M., Kling, M. A., Reed, S. A., Bradham, D. D., & Hebel, J. R., et al. (2004). Treatment outcomes in depression: Comparison of remote treatment through telepsychiatry to in-person treatment. *American Journal of Psychiatry, 161,* 1471–1476.

Spek, V., Cuijpers, P., Nyklicek, I., Riper, H., Keyzer, J., & Pop, V. (2007). Internet-based cognitive behaviour therapy for symptoms of depression and anxiety: A meta-analysis. *Psychological Medicine, 37,* 319–328.

Statens Beredning för Medicinsk Utvärdering. (2007). *Datorbaserad kognitiv beteendeterapi vid ångestsyndrom eller depression [Computerized cognitive behavior therapy for anxiety syndromes and depression]* (No. 2007–03). Stockholm: SBU.

Ström, L., Pettersson, R., & Andersson, G. (2000). A controlled trial of self-help treatment of recurrent headache conducted via the internet. *Journal of Consulting and Clinical Psychology, 68*, 722–727.

Ström, L., Pettersson, R., & Andersson, G. (2004). Internet-based treatment for insomnia: A controlled evaluation. *Journal of Consulting and Clinical Psychology, 72*, 113–120.

Umefjord, G., Petersson, G., & Hamberg, K. (2003). Reasons for consulting a doctor on the Internet: Web survey of users of an Ask the Doctor service. *Journal of Medical Internet Research, 5*, e26.

Zetterqvist, K., Maanmies, J., Ström, L., & Andersson, G. (2003). Randomized controlled trial of Internet-based stress management. *Cognitive Behaviour Therapy, 3*, 151–160.

An Internet-Based Self-Help Program for the Treatment of Fear of Public Speaking: A Case Study

C. Botella

M. J. Gallego

A. Garcia-Palacios

R. M. Baños

S. Quero

V. Guillen

Social phobia is the third most prevalent mental disorder, after major depressive disorder and alcohol dependence (Kessler et al., 1994). An estimated 13.3 percent of the population in United States experiences social phobia at some point in their lives (Magee, Eaton, Wittchen, McGonagle, & Kessler, 1996). The essential feature of social phobia is persistent and intense fear of one or more social situations in which the person is exposed to the observation of others (APA, 2000). DSM-IV-TR specified a generalized subtype of social phobia, which is diagnosed when someone fears all or almost all social situations. However, the variability of social situations feared by social phobics has opened up a discussion on the necessity of distinguishing among different social phobia subtypes. Heimberg, Holt, Scheneier, Spitzer, and Liebowitz (1993) distinguished three social phobia subtypes: *generalized social phobia*, which includes fear across almost all social situations; *nongeneralized social phobia*, which includes fear of multiple social situations, but no problems in at least one social domain; and finally, *discrete (or specific) social phobia*, which includes fear in only one or two circumscribed social situations (e.g., public speaking or eating in public). In this article we have centered our attention on fear of public speaking. This is the most feared situation among the general population. Its prevalence ranges from 20 percent (Cho & Won, 1997; Pollard & Henderson, 1988) to 34 percent (Stein, Walter, & Forde, 1996).

Cognitive behavioural therapy (CBT) including exposure, specifically in vivo exposure, is considered the treatment of choice for social phobia and specific phobias. Regarding social phobia this intervention has received wide empirical support from numerous clinical trials (e.g., Butler, Cullington, Munby, Amies, & Gelder, 1984; Mattick, Peters, & Clarke, 1989; Turner, Beidel, & Jacob, 1994). The APA report on empirically supported treatments (Task Force on Promotion and Dissemination of Psychological Procedures, 1995, last updated by Woody Barlow, 1997; Heimberg, 1991; Marks, 1978b; Turner, Beidel, & Cooley, 1997).

In vivo exposure consists of confronting the feared situation in a gradual and systematic way. It begins with lower-ranked situations and moves up to more highly feared situations. In a typical exposure session the therapist encourages the patient to confront the feared situation. The therapist asks the patient about the degree of fear from 0 to 10 (or 0 to 100) using the subjective units of discomfort (SUDs; Wolpe, 1969) every few minutes. When fear goes down significantly the patient can move on to confront a more difficult situation. Exposure therapy is based on the notion that individuals are able to adjust to anxiety-provoking stimuli through a process known as habituation (Marks, 1987). Foa and Kozak (1986) used the concept of emotional processing to explain fear reduction during exposure. They support the hypothesis that exposure to feared stimuli allows the activation of the fear structure and the presentation of corrective information incompatible with the pathological elements of the fear structure.

In vivo exposure is an effective therapy technique, although it is not free of limitations. Some patients (approximately 25 percent of those who start an exposure program) refuse exposure therapy or drop out of therapy (Marks, 1978a, 1992). One reason for this percentage of refusal could be that the main feature of exposure is confronting the feared stimuli; some people may find this too frightening. Furthermore, the vast majority (approximately 60 to 85 percent) of those afflicted with specific or social phobias never seek treatment for their problem (Boyd et. al., 1990; Magee et al., 1996). In the case of social phobics, they may abstain from seeking treatment because of the embarrassment associated with meeting an unknown person, the psychologist. Finally, in vivo exposure programs and other CBT programs entail an important amount of therapy time. This means an important financial cost for patients and public mental health institutions. Also, it is difficult for some patients living in remote areas (i.e., rural areas) to get CBT treatment. An important goal in clinical psychology is reducing cost of treatment without decreasing effectiveness. The main factor to minimize economic issues is reducing contact with the therapist (Al-Kubaiy et al., 1992; Marks, 1987; Öst, Salkovskis, & Hellström, 1991). The length of the therapist contact has varied from one visit per week to structure new exposure tasks (Mathews, Gelder, & Johnston, 1981) to no contact at all during the treatment (Ghosh & Marks, 1987; Hellström & Üst, 1995; Öst et al., 1991). Self-directed exposure has shown to be as successful as standard therapist-directed treatment (Ghosh & Marks, 1987). In another study the improvement achieved by self-directed exposure was maintained at two-year follow-up (Park et al., 2001).

One way of reducing therapy contact time and overcoming some of these limitations is telepsychology. Telepsychology has been defined as "the use of telecommunication technologies to put patients in contact with the mental health practitioners with the aim of providing a suitable diagnosis, education, treatment, consultations, communication and storage of the patients' records, research data, and other activities" (Brown, 1998, p. 963). One way to deliver telepsychology is though the Internet (online therapy). Recently, Schneider, Mataix-Cols, Marks, and Bachofen (2005) compared two Internet-guided self-help treatments for phobic and panic disorders, one included exposure instructions and the other did not. They found that at posttest both were equally effective, however at one-month follow-up the Internet-guided self-help treatment with exposure instructions was more effective than the other.

In the field of social phobia there are some studies that reported data on the use of online telepsychology programs to treat this disorder. These studies could be classified in two groups according to the classification of Glasgow and Rosen (1978): (1) Internet-based self-help programs with therapist contact, and (2) Internet-based self-help programs without therapist contact.

Regarding the first group, Andersson et al. (2006) combined an Internet-based self-help program with therapist contact via e-mail with two group exposure sessions. This treatment showed its efficacy in a controlled randomized study. The same Internet program plus weekly therapist contact via e-mail without the group exposure sessions was administered to 26 social phobics (Carlbring, Furmark, Stezkó, Ekselius, & Andersson, 2006). The participants improved significantly from pre- to posttest and the results were maintained at six-month follow-up. Carlbring et al. (2007) compared in a controlled randomized study their Internet program plus weekly phone calls with a waiting-list group. They also found this treatment effective to treat social phobia, and it improved program adherence. This improvement was maintained after one year.

There is only one telepsychology treatment program completely delivered over the Internet to treat social phobia (Botella et al., 2000). It is an Internet-based self-help program for the treatment of fear of public speaking called Talk to Me, designed by our team. This treatment has shown preliminary efficacy in a case study (Botella, Hofmann, & Moscovitch, 2004), and two single case series (Gallego et al., 2007; Guillen, 2001). In these studies there are no data of within-exposure sessions.

The aim of the present study is to describe the Talk to Me program and its application to a person with social phobia, with the most important contribution being presenting data of within-exposure sessions in order to show how the program is able to activate anxiety and promote habituation.

METHOD

Participant

The patient is a 30-year-old Caucasian woman. She is an undergraduate student. She lives with her husband in a Spanish town. An important issue in the history of the problem is that she did not need to confront a public speaking situation until she began her studies at the university. The problem appeared three years ago when she had to present a project in class. She remembers that it was a very bad experience because she was very nervous and noticed that her heart beat very fast, her hands sweat, and her face got red. At that moment the patient was concerned about her anxiety symptoms, and she thought that she was acting in a humiliating way. Furthermore, she found it difficult to center her attention on the project because thoughts such as "they are evaluating me negatively" or "I am doing it badly" were crossing her mind. After this situation the patient feared and avoided public speaking situations. The patient looked for help when she realized that the problem impaired her studies. At the time she was afraid of attending some classes because she knew that speaking in public was possible. In one class, students were assigned to perform a role-play simulating a therapist-patient interaction. The patient felt very nervous during these classes and she avoided performing the role-play. Another feared situation was when the professor asked questions in class; then she felt very nervous thinking of the possibility of having to speak.

In the initial assessment she met DSM-IV-TR (APA, 2000) criteria for social phobia. Two experienced clinicians performed two independent interviews using a structured interview (see the measures section), and both of them confirmed the diagnosis. Taking into account Heimberg and colleagues' (1993) classification, both therapists agreed on the diagnosis of discrete social phobia. The patient did not present comorbidity with any other diagnosis. Regarding the scores in some measures of fear of public speaking (self-statements during public speaking [SSPS], personal report of confidence as a speaker [PRCS], and public speaking self-efficacy questionnaire [PSSEQ]; see measures in the following section), the patient's scores were similar to the scores found in clinical population suffering social phobia. Finally, patient and therapist selected two target behaviors. The first one was presenting a project in class and the second one was giving a talk to high school students or their parents. The main catastrophic thought associated to each of them was "People will think I'm stupid."

Measures

We used several instruments in order to have a thorough assessment of the patient's problem. In this section we describe those instruments. The key assessment instruments of Talk to Me are marked with an asterisk.

Consent Form. The participant read and signed a consent form.

Diagnosis: Anxiety disorders interview schedule IV (ADIS-IV; Di Nardo, Brown, & Barlow, 1994). We used an adapted version of this semistructured interview that assesses the DSM-IV-TR (APA, 2000) criteria for social phobia and the degree of severity of the problem.

Brief version of the fear of negative evaluation scale (BFNE) (Leary, 1983). This scale assesses apprehension at the prospect of being negatively evaluated by others. It is comprised of 12 items that are rated on a scale of 1–5, where 1 is "not at all characteristic of me" and 5 is "extremely characteristic of me." This instrument has shown good psychometric properties in a clinical Spanish population (Botella & Gallego, 2007).

Self-statements during public speaking (SSPS) (Hofmann & DiBartolo, 2000). This scale is composed of 10 items that are rated in 1–5 scales, where 1 is "I completely disagree" and 5 is "I completely agree." It measures self-statements and levels of discomfort while someone is speaking in public. This instrument is comprised of two subscales: positive self-statements subscale (SSPS-P) and negative self-statements subscale (SSPS-N). Both subscales have excellent internal consistency (SSPS-P $\alpha = .80$; SSPS-N $\alpha = .86$) and test-retest reliability (SSPS-P $r = .78$; SSPS-N $r = .80$) (Hofmann & DiBartolo, 2000).

Personal report of confidence as a speaker (PRCS) (Paul, 1966). This measure was developed by Gilkinson (1942) as a 104-item self-report measure of fear of public speaking. Paul (1966) shortened this instrument to 30 true-false items. In Spain, Bados (1986) changed the true-false items format for a six-point scale (1 is "not at all characteristic of me," and 10 is "extremely characteristic of me"). This instrument is validated in Spanish populations by Méndez, Inglés, and Hidalgo (1999), and they found good psychometric properties.

*Public speaking self-efficacy questionnaire (PSSEQ) (adapted from Bados, 1986). This instrument has been adapted from the questionnaire "self-efficacy for speaking in public" (Bados, 1986). This measure was validated in Spanish populations and showed good psychometric properties. It assesses the degree of self-efficacy for speaking in public on a 0–10 scale (0 being "I can't do that at all," and 10 being "I can definitely do that").

*Target behaviors (adapted from Marks & Mathews, 1979). The therapist and the patient established two target behaviors. She had to rate the level of fear and avoidance she had in several social situations on a scale of 0–10 (0 being "no fear at all; I never avoid," and 10 being "severe fear; I always avoid"). Each social situation is a different scenario of the program.

Subjective units of discomfort (adapted from wolpe, 1969). During the exposure sessions the patient reports the level of fear regarding confronting the feared situation on a scale from 0 to 10.

Impairment questionnaire (adapted from echeburúa, Corral, & Fernández-Montalvo, 2000). This measure was adapted from Echeburúa and colleagues (2000). This questionnaire measures the level of impairment of the problem caused in different areas of the patient's life, although we centered our attention on work impairment. A five-point Likert scale from 0 ("no impairment") to 4 ("great impairment") was used.

Attitudes Toward the Treatment Programs Measures

Confidence in the internet and computer expertise (CICE) (Botella et al., 2007). We created a four-item questionnaire to assess confidence in the following: Internet as a medium for finding information to solve personal problems, computers as an instrument that can help solve psychological problems, treatment program, and ability to self-apply this treatment. The items were rated on a scale of 0 (total disagreement) to 10 (total agreement). The maximum score on this measure was 40.

Satisfaction with treatment (adapted from Borkovec & Nau, 1972). Our research group developed a questionnaire to assess satisfaction with the treatment. The content of the items covered how logical the treatment is, to what extend it satisfies the patient, if it is useful to treat other problems, its usefulness for the patient's problem, and to what extent it could be aversive. An 11-point Likert scale from 0 to 10 was used.

Apparatus and Software

The hardware used was a Pentium II personal computer (400 Hz, 256 MB of RAM, and graphics card of 64 MB). The peripherals the patient used were a monitor, a mouse, a keyboard, and speakers. A modem was used for the Internet access. The software used to develop the treatment was Microsoft Windows 98, Windows Media Player, and Internet Explorer 5 or 6. An important technical aspect of the Talk to Me is video streaming. This technology makes it possible to watch and hear videos in real-time through the Internet.

Procedure

After a first screening, two diagnostic sessions were conducted in which the diagnosis of social phobia was established by one experienced psychologist and confirmed by an independent assessor. After that the patient was asked if she agreed to use an Internet-based self-help program for the treatment of her problem. She was very pleased to use Talk to Me and signed a consent form. At pretest the patient completed the self-report measures previously described. After that the psychologist explained in detail to the patient how to use the Talk to Me program. The patient self-applied the program at home without any difficulty. She finished the program in two months. During this time she received four education sessions, eight exposure sessions, and one prevention relapse session. After the treatment and at one year follow-up she completed the same measures.

Treatment

Talk to Me is an Internet-based self-help program created to guide the patient through the whole therapeutic process. This program is composed of an assessment protocol and a structured treatment protocol. Both components are comprised of separate blocks through which users must progress in a specified order, which ensures that the patient does not skip any steps in the treatment. Furthermore, Talk to Me assesses the patient periodically during the treatment and makes subsequent treatment recommendations.

Initially the system provides the patient information about the program to ensure ethical issues are addressed: information about the research and the clinical team that developed the program, description of the problem that the system addresses (fear of public speaking), rationale about the treatment, safety measures to ensure confidentiality, and finally how to use the system.

Assessment. The assessment protocol presents a number of self-report instruments for evaluating the problem. The program uses the outcomes of these measures to establish the patient diagnosis and to obtain detailed information about the problem. Talk to Me creates an individualized treatment for each user based on pretreatment assessment. Depending on the initial scores, the program informs the patient that he or she can benefit from the program or it recommends looking for another kind of mental health help. This decision is made taking into account the criteria established by the standardized self-reports included in the assessment protocol. The next step is to construct a hierarchy of targeted behaviors for the exposure task. As previously stated, in the measures section the key assessment instruments of Talk to Me are marked with an asterisk.

Scenarios. This program offers six scenarios consisting of videos of real videotaped audiences that simulate different public speaking situations. Every patient confronts some of the scenarios depending on the pretreatment assessment. The reader can see a sample of each scenario at the following website: www.internetmeayuda.com/inicio_en.htm.

- *The class:* The program has two class scenarios; one is comprised of 7 to 8 students and the other of 20 to 30 students. The public is seated, and the students are looking at the user situated in front of the class.
- *The conference:* The scenario depicts a formal situation; the user must give a talk at a conference. The audience is composed of 50 people wearing formal clothes, who are gazing toward the user.
- *The oral exam:* There are different scenarios depending on the number of professors (2, 3, or 5) and the gender (all women, all men, and mixed tribunals). The user must perform an oral exam.
- *The work meeting:* The patient must present a project in front of 9 colleagues and the boss. All of them are seated around a conference table.
- *Job interview:* There are two scenarios, in one of them the interviewer is a woman and in the other a man. The interviewer asks some questions of the patient.
- *The wedding:* The patient and other people are seated around a restaurant table, and they talk to one another.

The treatment. After the assessment, the treatment starts. It is a cognitive-behavioral treatment for fear of public speaking comprised of three components: education, cognitive-therapy, and exposure. Exposure and cognitive therapy are included in the list of empirically supported treatments (Task Force of Promotion and Dissemination of Psychological procedures, 1995, last updated Woody & Sanderson, 1998).

The educational component of the program gives information about the rationale of the treatment and its components. After presenting this information, Talk to Me asks some questions that the user must answer correctly to progress to a new step. If the user answers incorrectly, he or she has to read the information again. The cognitive therapy component involves teaching users to identify and challenge automatic thoughts. The program teaches the patient to develop rational responses in public speaking situations by using questions. During the exposure the user is instructed to use the learned skills.

A very important treatment component is exposure. Talk to Me puts into order several scenarios depending on the scores obtained in the assessment phase regarding the target behaviors. Therefore, it presents a hierarchy of scenarios that the user must confront. Each scenario has several modulators to make the hierarchy: number of people, gender, difficulty of speech, and level of audience attention. The system selects the scenarios that the user fears more than 4 in a 0 to 10 scale.

At the beginnig of the exposure sessions Talk to Me instructs the user via text about what he or she has to do. Before confronting the scenario the program asks the degree of fear, avoidance, and belief on an automatic thought. Next the program has a narrative to introduce the user to the situation. This narrative explains the situation that the patient is going to confront. The next step is to give a speech in front of a virtual audience. The system asks the user's degree of fear every five minutes. In the case that the patient wants to give up the exposure before a fear decrease Talk to Me advises him or her to continue in the situation. The length of the exposure is not limited because there are individual differences regarding habituation. After the exposure session the program presents the user with graphs about the progress of anxiety during the task. Furthermore, Talk to Me reinforces the patient for the effort and success achieved. Each exposure session follows the same procedure. The treatment concludes when the user has overcome all of the target behaviors.

Another relevant point is that the program does not give real-world self-exposure instructions because our purpose is to find out the telepsychology program efficacy. An exposure program usually includes self-exposure instructions in order to carry out in vivo exposure between sessions. In this case we did not ask the patient to carry out in vivo self-exposure tasks because then it would have been very difficult to distinguish the contribution of the self-applied telepsychology program from the contribution of the in vivo exposure tasks in the treatment success.

RESULTS

Progress Within Sessions

Before and after every video exposure session, the program asks the degree of fear and avoidance related to the social situation that the patient was going to confront. Figure 1 shows the evolution of those measures along the eight exposure sessions. After each exposure session a reduction in fear was observed. Furthermore, Talk to Me asked the degree of fear (SUDs) every five minutes during each exposure session. We can see in Figure 2 the degree of fear during the first and the last exposure session. We observe a decrease of fear along both sessions.

Other Efficacy Measures

After the treatment, as can be seen in Table 1, there was an important reduction in the measures related to social phobia. This reduction was so pronounced in specific measures of fear of public speaking that patient's scores were similar to the scores of normal samples. This improvement was maintained at one-year follow-up.

Attitudes Toward the Internet-Based Treatment Program

The patient accepted the program before and after the treatment in the same rate. She reported high motivation toward Talk to Me before starting this program. Furthermore, the patient reported high confidence in the Internet to find information to solve personal problems, she trusted computers to solve her problem and she trusted the treatment and herself to self-apply Talk to Me. As we can see in Table 2 the confidence results were maintained at posttest and at one-year follow-up.

At the end of the treatment the patient thought that the program was logical, useful for her problem, and useful for other problems.

FIGURE 1. Ratings Regarding the Target Behaviors Taken in Session Before and After Each Exposure Session *Note:* Degree of fear and avoidance measured by the fear and avoidance scale adapted from Marks & Mathews (1979). We also included the maximum degree of fear during the session. The diamond line represents the ratings before exposure at the beginning of the session, the triangle represents the ratings during the exposure session, and the asterick line represents the ratings after the exposure task at the end of the session.

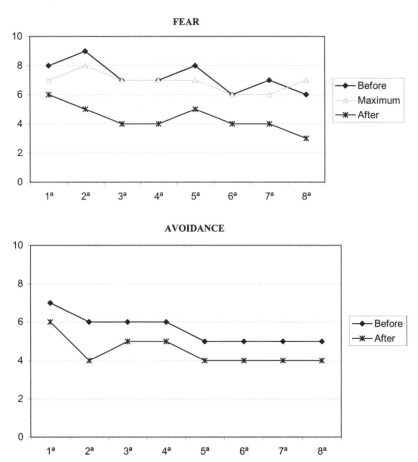

She also was satisfied with the treatment and would recommend the program to others with the same problem. With regard to components and scenarios, the patient found them very useful.

Botella et al.

FIGURE 2. Degree of Fear (SUDs from 0 to 10) During the First Session (Exposure to a Class) and the Last Session (Oral Exam)

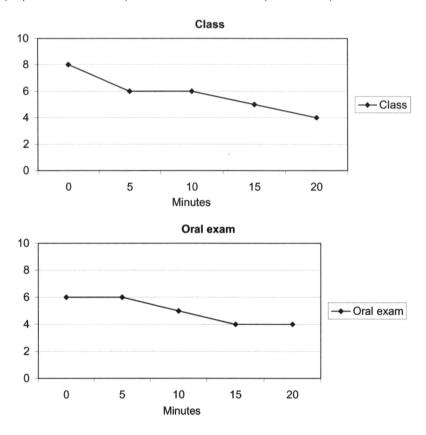

DISCUSSION

This work provides preliminary data about the utility of an Internet-based self-help program for the fear of public speaking and presents data on the degree of fear within exposure sessions. We saw a reduction in the clinical measures of social phobia from pretest to posttest, and this improvement was maintained at one-year follow-up. Although not the only component, video exposure was the main component of the program. As we see in Figure 2, the degree of fear decreased across the exposure session. Furthermore, the fear and avoidance degree related to the target behavior was reduced from the beginning to the end of each session and across the sessions (see Figure 1). With regard

TABLE 1. Measures of Efficacy at Pretest, Posttest and One-Year Follow-up

Target Behaviors		Pre	Post	FU	
To present a project in class/"People will think I'm stupid."	Fear	6	2	2	Clinical sample
	Avoidance	10	0	0	
To give a talk/"People will think I'm stupid."	Fear	6	3	3	Gallego (2006)
	Avoidance	10	0	0	
Social Phobia Measures					Mean (SD)
BFNE		32	22	20	43.03 (9.15)
SSPS-P		14	21	22	12.38 (5.78)
SSPS-N		4	0	0	9.90 (6.68)
PRCS		121	79	99	135.25 (19.48)
PSSEQ		29	56	50	23.86 (11.56)
Severity		3	1	1	2.60 (.85)
Impairment					
Work impairment		2	0	0	2.82 (1.30)

Note: FU: one year follow-up; BFNE: brief version of the fear of negative evaluation scale; SSPS-P: self-statements during public speaking–positive subscale; SSPS-N: self-statements during public speaking–negative subscale; PRCS: personal report of confidence as a speaker; PSSEQ: public speaking self-efficacy questionnaire.

TABLE 2. Variables of the Talk to Me Acceptance

	Pretest	Posttest	Follow-up
Measure			
Motivation	10		
Internet solves problems	9	6	9
Trust computers	9	10	9
Trust treatment	10	10	10
Trust myself	10	10	10
Logic		10	10
Satisfaction		10	10
Recommendation to others		10	10
Utility for other problems		10	10
Utility for the patient		10	10
Aversiveness		0	0
Components utility			
Education		10	10
Cognitive		10	10
Exposure		10	8
Scenarios utility			
Class		10	9
Oral exam		10	8
Conference		10	10

to the results in the fear of public speaking measures at pretest, the patient's scores could be considered as belonging to a clinical population. After the treatment, the reduction of the scores was so dramatic that they were similar to a normal sample (see Table 1). The patient found the treatment program useful in overcoming her problem. In addition, she trusted Talk to Me and was satified.

We would like to highlight a relevant result: the maintenance of the therapeutic gains at one-year follow-up. The patient did not receive any other psychological or pharmacological treatment for social phobia during the follow-up period. In general, she maintained the goals achieved, and in some measures such as the PSSEQ (a self-efficacy questionnaire) she even improved, although in others such as the PRCS (personal report of confidence as a public speaker) she did not. In the last follow-up assessment we saw that the follow-up score was lower than the pretest score. Internet-based self-help efficacy is a recent line of research, and although there are some empirical reports of the efficacy of these treatments, none of them used exposure to videos for the treatment of social phobia. Our work presents preliminary data about the degree of fear within exposure session. These data showed that Talk to Me was able to activate fear and promote habituation, key elements for the success of exposure.

Another important point is that changes observed in relevant measures were clinically significant. On the one hand, the patient achieved the therapeutic goals established at pretest. On the other hand, her scores in fear of public speaking measures were similar to the scores of a clinical sample at pretest and they were reduced at posttest.

Furthermore, the patient reported at follow-up that she had presented a project in class without too much anxiety and she performed it very well, in fact the vote she got in the project was very good. This is a crucial issue in etherapy. The patient habituated to videotaped audiences and the outcomes generalized to real public speaking situations. This is a promising result, but this is only a case study and further research is needed in this particular matter.

The acceptance of this treatment by the patient is crucial for its administration. Before the treatment she was very motivated to begin the program and she had confidence in Talk to Me. After the treatment she also trusted the program, probably because this program met patient expectations. In addition, she thought that the treatment was logical and useful for her and for other problems. Regarding the components utility, she reported high utility for all of them (education, cognitive, and exposure) and for the three scenarios that she had confronted.

We can conclude that this study offers preliminary data about the efficacy and effectiveness (or clinical utility) of an Internet-based self-help program. Also, we have seen the importance of the video exposure component. Internet-based treatments can help patients overcome some limitations of the cognitive-behavioral treatments for this disorder.

This study is not free of limitations. We have to take into account that it is a case study and the data are preliminary, so we cannot draw strong conclusions. Because of this we have conducted a controlled study that compare Talk to Me with the same treatment administered by a therapist and a waiting-list control group (Gallego, 2006). Talk to Me was equally effective as a therapist-administered treatment and more effective than a waiting-list condition.

Talk to Me involves an intensive assessment throughout all of the treatment process. This could be seen as a limitation because we are asking more effort of the patient. On the other hand, we think the assessment during the treatment is important because it is self-administered. The patient has not the expertise to determine if he or she can go a step forward in the difficulty of the exposure tasks. Because of this we set the criteria using expert clinical judgment and used the system to make the decisions. Decision making based on the assessment during the treatment is needed for optimal levels of exposure to the feared situation.

Internet-based self-help programs offer some advantatges. Patients need less therapist time because they can self-administer the program at home. Another issue related to time is that they can enter the program at any time during the week, on holidays, and day or night. Confidentiality is also important. Receiving treatment at home assures a high degree of privacy. Some of these points and not having therapist contact reduces treatment costs. Regarding exposure tasks, Talk to Me offers a safe environment where the patient can explore the problem and practice the therapeutic tools.

Our work offers preliminary data that support the use of online therapy completely delivered by the user through an Internet-based program. The program was a useful and effective alternative to conducting exposure therapy in the treatment of anxiety disorders. We understand, however, that any case study involves considerable risk in drawing conclusions about the causes of the outcome. The patient may have been particularly motivated or may be different from others with social phobia in innumerable ways. The novelty of the program and the extensive evaluation may also have influenced the results. Further research with larger samples and controlled studies are needed.

ACKNOWLEDGEMENT

The research presented in this paper was funded in part by Ministerio de Educación y Ciencia, Spain. PROYECTOS CON-SOLIDER-C (SEJ2006-14301/PSIC). CIBER Fisiopatologia de la Obesidad y Nutricion is an initiative of ISCIII.

REFERENCES

Al-Kubaiy, T., Marks, I. M., Logsdail, S., Marks, M. P., Lovell, K., Sungur, M. et al. (1992). Role of exposure home work in phobia reduction a controlled study. *Behavior Therapy, 23,* 599–621.

American Psychiatric Association (APA) (2000). *Diagnostic and statistical manual of mental disorder* (5th ed.) Washington, DC: APA (Barcelona, Masson, 2000).

Andersson, G., Carlbring, P., Holmström, A., Spartan, L., Furmark, T., Nilsson-Ihrfelt, E., et al. (2006). Internet-based self-help with therapist feedback and in-vivo group exposure for social phobia: A behaviour controlled trial. *Journal of Consulting and Clinical Psychology, 74,* 677–686.

Bados, A. (1986). *Análisis de componentes de un tratamiento cognitivo-somático-conductual del miedo a hablar en público.* Doctoral Dissertation, Universidad de Barcelona.

Borkovec, T. D., & Nau, S. D. (1972). Credibility of analogue therapy rationales. *Journal of Behaviour Therapy and Experimental Psychiatry, 3,* 257–260.

Botella, C., Baños, R. M., Guillén, V., Perpiña, C., Alcañiz, M., & Pons, A. (2000). Telepsychology: Public speaking fear treatment on the Internet. *CyberPsychology & Behavior, 3,* 959–968.

Botella, C., Guillen, V., Baños, R. M., Garcia-Palacios, A., Gallego, M. J. & Alcañiz, M. (2007). Telepsychology and self-help: The treatment of fear of public speaking. *Cognitive and Behavioral Practice, 14,* 46–57.

Botella, C., Hofmann, S. G., & Moscovitz, D. A. (2004). A self-applied Internet-based intervention for fear of public speaking. *Journal of Clinical Psychology, 60,* 1–10.

Boyd, J. H., Rae, D. S., Thompson, J.W., Burns, B. J., Bourdon, K., Locke, B. Z., et al. (1990). Phobia: Prevalence and risk factors. *Social Psychiatry and Psychiatric Epidemiology*, *25*, 314–323.

Brown, F. W. (1998). Rural telepsychiatry. *Psychiatric Services*, *49*, 963–964.

Butler, C., Cullington, A., Munby, M., Amies, P., & Gelder, M. (1984). Exposure and anxiety management in the treatment of social phobia. *Journal of Consulting and Clinical Psychology*, *52*, 642–650.

Carlbring, P., Furmark, T., Steczkó, J., Ekselius, L., & Andersson, G. (2006). An open study of Internet-based bibliotherapy with minimal therapist contact via e-mail for social phobia. *Clinical Psychology*, *10*, 30–38.

Carlbring, P., Gunnarsdóttir, M., Hedensjö, L., Andersson, G., Ekselius, L., & Furmark, T. (2007). Treatment of social phobia: Randomized trial of Internet-delivered cognitive-behavioural therapy with telephone support. *The British Journal of Psychiatry*, *190*, 123–128.

Cho, Y., & Won, H. (1997). Cognitive assessment of social anxiety: a study on the development and validation of the social interaction self-efficacy scale. *Issues in Psychological Research*, *4*, 397–434.

Craske, M. G., Antony, M. M., & Barlow, D. H. (1997). *Mastery of your specific phobia, therapist guide*. San Antonio, TX: The Psychological Corporation.

Di Nardo, P. A., Brown, E. L., & Barlow, D. H. (1994). *Anxiety disorders interview schedule for DSM-IV: Lifetime version (ADIS-IV-L)*. Albany, NY: Gaywind Publications Incorporated.

Echeburúa, E., Corral, P., & Fernández-Montalvo, J. (2000). Escala de inadaptación: Propiedades psicométricas en contextos clínicos. Análisis en contextos clínicos. *Análisis y modificación de conducta*, *26*, 325–338.

Foa, E. B., & Kozak, M. J. (1986). Emotional processing of fear: Exposure to corrective information. *Psychological Bulletin*, *99*, 20–35.

Gallego, M. J. (2006). *An Internet-delivered program for the treatment of fear of public speaking*. Doctoral Dissertation, Universitat Jaume I.

Gallego, M. J., Botella, C., Quero, S., Baños, R. M., & Garcia-Palacios, A. (2007). Psychometric properties of the brief version of the Fear of Negative Evaluation Scale (BFNE) in a clinical sample. *Revista de Psicopatología y Psicología Clínico*, *12*, 163–176.

Garcia-Palacios, A., Botella, C., Hoffman, H., & Fabregat, S. (2007, October). Comparing acceptance and refusal rates of Virtual Reality exposure vs. in vivo exposure by patients with specific phobias. *Cyberpsychology and Behavior*, *10*(5), 722–724.

Ghosh, A., & Marks, I. M. (1987). Self-treatment of agoraphobia by exposure. *Behavior Therapy*, *18*, 3–16.

Gilkinson, H. (1942). Social fears as reported by students in collage speech classes. *Speech Monoghraphy*, *9*, 141–160.

Glasgow, R., & Rosen, G. (1978). Behavioral bibliotherapy: A review of self-help behavior therapy manuals. *Psychological Bulletin*, *85*, 1–23.

Guillen, V. (2001). *Miedo a hablar en público: Un tratamiento autoaplicado en internet*. Tesis de licenciatura no publicada, Universidad de Valencia.

Heimberg, R. G. (1991). *A manual for conducting cognitive-behavioral group therapy for social phobia.* Unpublished manuscript, State University of New York at Albany, Center for Stress and Anxiety Disorders, Albany, NY.

Heimberg, R. G., Dodge, C. S., Hope, D. A., Kennedy, C. R., Zollo, L., & Becker, R. E. (1990). Cognitive behavioral group treatment of social phobia: Comparison to a credible placebo control. *Cognitive Therapy and Research, 14,* 1–23.

Heimberg, R. G., Holt, C. S., Schneier, F. R., Spitzer, R. L., & Liebowitz, M. R. (1993). The issue of subtypes in the diagnosis of social phobia. *Journal of Anxiety Disorders, 7,* 249–269.

Hellström, K., & Öst, L. G. (1995). One-session therapist directed exposure vs. two forms of manual directed self-exposure in the treatment of spider phobia. *Behavior Research and Therapy, 33,* 959–965.

Hofmann, S. G., & DiBartolo, P. M. (2000). An instrument to assess self-statements during public speaking: Scale development and preliminary psychometric properties. *Behavior Therapy, 31,* 499–515.

Kessler, R. C., McGonagle, K. A., Zhao, S., Nelson, C. B., Hughes, M., Eshleman, S., et al. (1994). Lifetime and 12-month prevalence of DSM-III-R psychiatric disorders in the United States. *Archives of General Psychiatry, 51,* 8–19.

Leary, M. R. (1983). A brief version of the fear of negative evaluation scale. *Personality and Social Psychology Bulletin, 9,* 371–375.

Magee, W. J., Eaton, W. W., Wittchen, H.U., McGonagle, K. A., & Kessler, R. C. (1996). Agoraphobia, simple phobia, and social phobia in the National Comorbidity Survey. *Archives of General Psychiatry, 53,* 159–168.

Marks, I. M. (1978a). Behavioral psychotherapy of adult neurosis. In S. L. Gardfield & a. E. Bergin (Eds.), *Handbook of psychotherapy and behavior change* (2nd ed.). New York: Wiley.

Marks, I. M. (1978b). *Living with fear.* New York: McGraw Hill.

Marks, I. M. (1992). Tratamiento de exposición en la agorafobia y el pánico. In Echeburua, E. (Ed.), *Avances en el tratamiento psicológico de los trastornos de ansiedad.* Madrid: Piramide.

Marks, I. M. (1987). *Fear, phobias, and rituals: Panic, anxiety, and their disorders.* New York: Oxford University Press.

Marks, I. M. & Matthews, A. M. (1979). Brief standard self-rating for phobic patients. *Behaviour Research and Therapy, 17,* 263–267.

Mathews, A. M., Gelder, G., & Johnston, D. W. (1981). *Agoraphobia: Nature and Treatment.* New Cork: Guilford.

Mattick, R. P., Peters, L., & Clarke, J. (1989). Exposure and cognitive restructuring for social phobia: A controlled study. *Behavior Therapy, 20,* 3–23.

Méndez, F. J., Inglés, C. J., & Hidalgo, M. D. (1999). Propiedades psicométricas del cuestionario de confianza para hablar en público: estudio con una muestra de alumnos de enseñanzas medias. *Psicothema, 1,* 65–74.

Park, J. M., Mataix-Cols, D., Marks, I. M., Ngamthipwatthna, T., Marks, M., Araya, R. et al. (2001). Two-year follow-up after a randomized controlled trial of self- and clinician-accompanied exposure for phobia/panic disorders. *The British Journal of Psychiatry: The Journal of Mental Science, 178,* 543–548.

Paul, G. L. (1966). *Insight vs. desensitization in psychotherapy.* Standford, CA: Standford University Press.

Pollard, C. A., & Henderson, J. F. (1988). Four types of social phobia in a community sample. *Journal of Nervous and Mental Disease, 176,* 440–445.

Roy, S., Kingler, E., Légeron, P., Lauer, F., Chemin, I. & Nugues, P. (2003). Definition of a VR-based protocol to treat social phobia. *CyberPsychology & Behavior, 6,* 411–420.

Schneider, A. J., Mataix-Cols, D., Marks, I. M., & Bachofen, M. (2005). Internet-guided self-help with or without exposure therapy for phobic and panic disorders. *Psychotherapy and Psychosomatics, 74,* 154–164.

Stein, M. B., Walter, J. R., & Forde, D. R., (1996). Public speaking fears in a community sample: prevalence, impact on functioning, and diagnostic classification. *Archives of General Psychiatry, 53,* 169–174.

Turner, S. M., Beidel, D. C., & Cooley, M. (1997). *Social effectiveness therapy: A program for overcoming social anxiety and phobia.* Toronto: Multi-Health Systems.

Turner, S. M., Beidel, D. C., & Jacob, R. G. (1994). Social phobia: A comparison of behavior therapy and atenolol. *Journal of Consulting and Clinical Psychology, 62,* 350–358.

Üst, L. G., Salkovskis, P. M., & Hellström, K. (1991). One-session therapist directed exposure vs. self-exposure in the treatment of spider phobia. *Behavior Therapy, 22,* 407–422.

Wolpe, J. (1969). *The practice of behavior therapy.* New York: Pergamon Press.

Woody, S. R., & Sanderson, W. C. (1998). Manuals for empirically supported treatments: 1998 update. *The Clinical Psychologist, 51,* 17–21.

Evaluation of the RAINN National Sexual Assault Online Hotline

Jerry Finn
Penelope Hughes

This article discusses the evaluation and results of the first eleven months of the Rape, Abuse, and Incest National Network (RAINN) National Sexual Assault Online Hotline (NSAOH) (www.rainn.org), a new model for delivery of supportive and therapeutic services for those seeking help with issues of rape and sexual assault. Rape and sexual assault may have serious and long-lasting consequences for victims, especially when left untreated. In addition to the immediate physical and emotional injury caused by rape, symptoms suffered by victims of sexual assault include low self-esteem, depression, antisocial behavior, substance abuse, and self-mutilation. Rape survivors are also 13 times more likely to attempt suicide than noncrime victims and 6 times more likely than victims of other crimes (Miller, Cohen, & Wierama, 1996; Tjaden & Thoennes, 2006). Rape and sexual services must provide help for the immediate crisis situation as well as long-term support for victims and their significant others.

Rape crisis intervention services have evolved since their inception in the 1960 s (Byington, Martin, DiNitto, & Maxwell, 1991; Campbell & Ahrens, 1998). Interventions for rape and sexual abuse have thus far included emergency room assistance, rape crisis centers, and telephone hotlines (Byington et al., 1991). In 2005, there were 191,670 victims of rape, attempted rape, or sexual assaults according to the 2005 National Crime Victimization Survey (Catalano, 2006). The need for new rape crisis services continues to grow since reports are likely to substantially underestimate the actual number of sexual assaults occurring in the population due to victim's sense of shame, social stigma, and reluctance to use services. The National Violence Against Women Survey found that only one in five adult women (19 percent) reported their rapes to police (Tjaden & Thoennes 2006).

In order to reach out to those who may not have available services or who may be reluctant to seek face-to-face services, "hotline" telephone services have been developed to provide more anonymous services and to increase service access. For example, RAINN has provided a telephone hotline service to more than one million visitors since 1994 and currently receives more than 11,000 calls per month (Hughes, 2006). Telephone hotlines have also served the needs of those facing issues of suicide, mental illness, sexual orientation conflict, and being homeless (Gould, et al., 2004).

RAINN has recently expanded its services, and is the first to include the NSAOH (Finn, Hughes, & Berkowitz, in press). The hotline is funded by a combination of federal grants, in-kind technology-related gifts, and foundation support. Users (called "visitors" by RAINN) of the NSAOH may be sexual assault victims or their significant others in immediate crisis or may be dealing with unresolved issues related to longer-term effects of sexual assault. The goal of the hotline is primarily crisis intervention. Visitors are given crisis support and problem solving help as well as information and referral to local services. Visitors may access the NSOAH more than once, but calls are distributed to volunteers randomly, so an ongoing relationship with a specific volunteer is not possible. The NSAOH model includes (Finn, Hughes, & Berkowitz):

- A 24 hour, 7 days a week Internet-based one-to-one chat hotline. (Note: the NSAOH began with 2 hours of operation and is currently operating 12 hours a day. The NSAOH will become 24/7 as need dictates and as volunteers and supervisors can be trained and recruited.)
- Privacy protection through a secure server, automatic stripping by the AOL server of user's IP address to avoid collecting it and to assure user anonymity, and web-based information about maintaining online privacy and security
- Volunteers who are trained in crisis intervention, support skills, and information and referral at their affiliated local rape crisis center or at the RAINN office in Washington, DC. Volunteers have face-to-face supervisors at their local rape crisis center affiliate and online supervisors when in session. They also receive 10 hours of online training focused on online communication skills, including active listening online, culture of online communication (for instance, use of all caps, common abbreviations, and emoticons), protocols for starting and ending a session, guidelines on handling "difficult" visitors, mandatory reporting procedures, and practice with a simulated session.
- Professional supervisors (National Volunteer Supervisor—NVS) who are always available online when volunteers are online. NVSs volunteer their time to RAINN. They are professional rape crisis counselors. An NVS is reached by volunteers through a chat channel. The NVS can assist volunteers via chat during a session or take over a chat session when needed. They also randomly monitor chat sessions as part of quality control. Volunteers do not know when they are being monitored by an NVS, but they are told in training that the NVS may view their sessions on a random basis.
- Resource materials such as information and referral and educational materials regarding criminal justice, medical, and emotional issues are available to volunteers to supplement their own knowledge of rape crisis information. Information can be accessed by volunteers during a session and sent to visitors via cut-and-paste in a chat session.
- Support for mandatory reporting of suspected child abuse or neglect. Rape crisis volunteers are considered "mandatory

reporters" in most states; that is, they must report suspected child abuse or neglect, including sexual abuse. RAINN supports mandatory reporting through use of the strictest guidelines found among the states, mandatory reporting information on the RAINN website, training and protocols for volunteers in handling potential mandatory reporting cases, a designated RAINN legal staff who assesses mandatory reporting requirements in specific cases, and available legal consultation.

Operationally, the model works as follows:

- A visitor finds the RAINN online hotline through a number of ways, including a search engine, referral from another website, information on a social networking site such as Myspace, through a print media advertisement, by word of mouth, etc.
- Visitors access the NSAOH through a button on the RAINN website (www.rainn.org). They are also referred by text to 911 in an emergency or to the RAINN telephone hotline if the online hotline is not available.
- Visitors read a description of the service and its privacy policy and must check a box stating that they agree to participate before entering a chat session.
- Visitors then enter a chat session with a trained rape crisis volunteer. Volunteers begin with a brief explanation of confidentiality and an explanation of mandatory reporting requirements. They also ask whether a visitor is in immediate danger and refer to 911 if necessary. There follows a chat session based on the visitor's needs. This generally includes support, information and referral, and problem solving.
- As noted previously, if a volunteer is having difficulty in a session, the volunteer may summon an online supervisor through a chat channel for help. The supervisor can send messages to the volunteer or to the visitor directly.
- At the end of a session, a brief evaluation form pops up on the visitors screen.

The rationale for the NSAOH is based on (1) research that shows that the majority of victims of rape and sexual abuse are young people ages 14–24 (Catalano, 2006), (2) the reluctance of many victims to report victimization to traditional authorities (DOJ, 2002),

(3) the increasing use of the Internet, especially by young people, to obtain information and social support (Horrigan & Rainie, 2006; Lenhart, Madden, & Hitlin, 2005; Rideout, 2001), (4) the emerging evidence that therapeutic services can be effectively provided online (Barak, 2004; Barak & Bloch, 2006; Finn & Holden, 2000; Klein & Richards, 2001; Mallen, Vogel, Rochlen, & Day, 2005; Rochlen, Zack, & Speyer, 2004), and (5) many requests received by RAINN for Internet-based services from victims and their family through the RAINN website and telephone hotline.

In undertaking the NSAOH, RAINN simultaneously developed an evaluation of the program. Evaluation was considered essential since the emerging research on online therapy and other online helping services is relatively new and is currently limited in scope, sample size, and outcome measures (Barak & Buchanan, 2004). There is no research on online hotlines; however, elements of the hotline, such as provision of support and problem solving through chat have been shown to be effective in online practice and in online support groups (Griffiths, Lindenmeyer, Powell, Lowe, & Throgood, 2006; Golkaramnay, Bauer, Haug, Wolf, & Kordy, 2007). Furthermore, potential risks in providing online intervention that include greater chance for misunderstanding, disinhibited communication, and greater need for cultural competence have been described in the literature and warrant evaluation (Finn & Banach, 2000; Waldron, Lavitt, & Kelley, 2000). Thus, evaluation of the NSAOH is essential not only to promote program improvement, but also to establish the legitimacy of the service to consumers and to practitioners who may use or refer others to the hotline.

EVALUATION OF THE RAINN NATIONAL SEXUAL ASSAULT ONLINE HOTLINE

The NSAOH has three primary goals:

- The program will be delivered through a secure, anonymous, real-time online hotline on the RAINN website. Evaluation of this goal includes ease of use by visitors and volunteers, extent of program disruption due to technical difficulties, examination of user waiting time, and examination of volunteer self-scheduling process.

- The program will provide effective crisis intervention, information, and support to visitors. Evaluation of this goal includes user satisfaction and perceived helpfulness, user feedback, and volunteer perceptions of program usefulness.
- The program will be nationally known and widely used. Evaluation includes number of visitors and volunteers and extent of rape crisis center affiliations.

RAINN has conducted an evaluation of the first 11 months of its ongoing evaluation of NSAOH using a triangulation approach that includes feedback from visitors, volunteers, supervisors, and system data. Visitors provide feedback through a brief user satisfaction survey that pops up when they log off of their chat session. The survey focuses on the perceived helpfulness of the session, the user's reported intent to use information and resources provided by the NSAOH, perceived competence of the volunteer, and ease of use of the online hotline. The evaluation form is intentionally brief to promote user participation and to minimize the chance for identification of a user. Visitors are provided with a privacy policy that includes informed consent about the service and the evaluation that must be checked prior to receiving services. In addition, the feedback form states that submitting the form constitutes their consent to use the data for evaluation purposes.

Volunteers also fill out an online form at the end of their shift about their last session. This reduces volunteer time in answering surveys and provides a randomizing procedure for data collection. The survey focuses on perceived helpfulness of the session from the volunteer's viewpoint, type of issues discussed in the sessions (e.g. rape, family communication, health), extent of infrastructure difficulties, and types of service-related difficulties encountered in the session.

Supervisors can be called through chat by volunteers when the volunteer is experiencing difficulties. When this occurs, supervisors fill out a brief form indicating the type of difficulty encountered and the extent to which the problem was resolved successfully. Supervisors also randomly observe volunteer chat sessions to promote quality control. Supervisors fill out a quality control form that assesses the quality of the volunteer's activity during the observed period.

Finally, the NSOAH collects ongoing system data such as number of chat sessions, time of visits, and length of sessions. These data are useful in assessing program growth and planning future resource needs, but were not available for this evaluation.

RESULTS

Visitor Evaluation

Visitor evaluation is based on feedback from 623 RAINN online hotline (NSAOH) visitors for approximately 11 months of operation, from August 15, 2006, to July 23, 2007 (See Table 1). During that period, the RAINN online hotline (NSAOH) received 2,081 visitors, a 30 percent response rate. Feedback is focused on five research questions. Questions are scored on a five-point Likert-type scale: 1 = strongly disagree, 2 = disagree, 3 = neither agree nor disagree, 4 = agree, and 5 = strongly agree. Higher scores indicate stronger agreement and more successful outcomes. Questions include:

- I will use the services recommended by RAINN during my session.
- I am satisfied with the trained specialist's (counselor's) knowledge and skills.
- I would recommend the online hotline to someone else.
- The online hotline was easy to use.
- Overall, I am satisfied with this service.

Visitors found the NSAOH easy to use. The mean agreement that the NSAOH is easy to use (N = 621) is 4.4 (SD = 1.1), with 85.4 percent agreement (4 or 5) and only 9 percent who disagree (1 or 2). Ease of use is moderately associated with overall satisfaction (r = .64, p < .0001). Cross-tabulation found that of 621 sessions, 89.3 percent who did not find the NSAOH easy to use also reported low satisfaction.

The majority of visitors reported that they will use the services recommended by the NSAOH volunteers. On a five-point scale, the mean agreement that visitors will use services recommended by the NSAOH is 3.8 (N = 622) with standard deviation of 1.4. Approximately two-thirds of visitors, 64.9 percent, reported that they will use the services recommended by RAINN, and 19.2 percent believed they will not use the services. (These services include local rape crisis centers, health and mental health centers, police, departments of social services, family planning, and other social service agencies.)

The majority of visitors are satisfied with the volunteer's knowledge and skills. The mean satisfaction with the volunteers' knowledge and skills (N = 622) is 3.9 with standard deviation of 1.4. Approximately

TABLE 1. Visitor Evaluation Inter-Item Correlations

		Overall satisfaction	Will use recommended services	Volunteer's knowledge and skills	Would recommend hotline to someone else	Hotline easy to use
Overall satisfaction	Pearson correlation	1	.778*	.901*	.908*	.645*
	Sig. (2-tailed)		.000	.000	.000	.000
	N	623	620	622	622	621
Will use recommended services	Pearson Correlation	.778*	1	.741*	.762*	.587*
	Sig. (2-tailed)	.000		.000	.000	.000
	N	620	620	619	619	618
Volunteer's knowledge and skills	Pearson correlation	.901*	.741*	1	.872*	.630*
	Sig. (2-tailed)	.000	.000		.000	.000
	N	622	619	622	621	620
Would recommend hotline to someone else	Pearson Correlation	.908*	.762*	.872*	1	.664*
	Sig. (2-tailed)	.000	.000	.000		.000
	N	622	619	621	621	620
Hotline easy to use	Pearson Correlation	.645*	.587*	.630*	.664*	1
	Sig. (2-tailed)	.000	.000	.000	.000	
	N	621	618	620	620	621

*Correlation is significant at the 0.01 level (2-tailed).

two-thirds, 70.3 percent, reported high satisfaction (4 or 5) with the volunteer's knowledge and skills; however, almost 1 in 5 (19.5 percent) disagree. Volunteer's knowledge and skills is related to whether a visitor reports that they will use the referrals recommended by the volunteer. Cross-tabulation found that of 101 visitors who would not use the recommended referrals, 74.4 percent reported low satisfaction (1 or 2) with the volunteer's knowledge and skills. The volunteer's knowledge and skills and use of referrals show a moderately high correlation ($r = .74$, $p < .0001$).

The majority of visitors would recommend the NSAOH to others. The mean agreement that a user would recommend the NSAOH ($N = 622$) is 4.1 with standard deviation of 1.4. Approximately three-fourths, 74.4 percent, agree that they would recommend the NSAOH to others (4 or 5), and 16.2 percent disagree.

Overall, the majority of the visitors are satisfied with the NSAOH. The mean overall satisfaction ($N = 623$) is 4.0 ($SD = 1.4$), with 72 percent reporting high satisfaction with the NSAOH (4 or 5). Approximately 1 in 6 visitors, 17.6 percent, are not satisfied (1 or 2). Satisfaction is strongly associated with visitor perceptions of volunteer knowledge and skills ($r = .90$, $p < .0001$) and, as noted previously, to ease of use.

Volunteer Evaluation

Volunteers represent 105 affiliated rape crisis centers in 33 states. A total of 360 sessions were reported by 54 different volunteers. The number of sessions per volunteer ranged from 1 to 44, with a median of 13 sessions; 22.7 percent of volunteers had 5 or fewer sessions and 35 percent had 20 of more sessions. The length of sessions ranged from 0 minutes (a dropped call or hang up) to 240 minutes, with a median of 25 minutes. Approximately 20 percent of sessions were 10 minutes or shorter, and 14.4 percent was one hour or longer. Pearson correlation found no relationship between session length and perceived helpfulness of the session.

The vast majority (86.6 percent) of sessions ($n = 344$) involved communication with the victim of sexual abuse; 6.7 percent were family members of a victim, 5.2 percent were friends, and 1.5 percent were "other." In addition, 306 sessions reported the time frame of the assault. The majority, 60.1 percent, involved a past event (longer than 3 months ago), 25.5 percent involved the recent past (within the past three months), and 14.4 percent involved an immediate incident, within the past few days.

Volunteers reported the primary topic of the session. Approximately half of sessions (n = 344) discussed rape as the primary topic (52 percent). The primary topics also included child molestation (9 percent), other sexual assault (8 percent), incest (8 percent), and "other" topics (22 percent). The "other" category included a variety of issues: attempted rape, adult molestation, sexual exploitation, legal issues, flashbacks, suicide and self-harm, emotional outcomes of abuse such as panic attacks and nightmares, family caretaker abuse, relationship issues, assault, and other forms of abuse.

Table 2 show the percent of sessions (N = 327) in which a topic was discussed, whether or not it was the primary topic. Rape was most frequently discussed (52.2 percent). In addition, family issues (33.3 percent) and depression (33 percent) were discussed by 1 in 3 respondents. Approximately one-fourth of sessions discussed issues of sexual assault and dealing with anger. Note that more than 10 percent of sessions discussed issues related to children: child molestation (18.3 percent) and incest (13.1 percent). Cross-tabulation found that 1.4 percent of incest and 2.7 percent of child molestation sessions involved an immediate event, that is, within the past few days. One case was deemed to meet mandatory reporting requirements and was reported to the appropriate local protective services office by the RAINN supervisor. In addition, 13.8 percent of sessions discussed suicide, of which 2.1 percent involved an immediate event.

TABLE 2. Topics Discussed in the Sessions

Topic (N = 327)	Percent yes
Discussed rape	52.2
Discussed attempted rape	4.0
Discussed sexual assault	28.1
Discussed incest	13.1
Discussed child molestation	18.3
Discussed sexual exploitation	1.8
Discussed depression	33.0
Discussed anger	24.8
Discussed substance abuse	5.5
Discussed suicide	13.8
Discussed family issues	33.3
Discussed other issues	29.4

Table 3 reports the mean and standard deviation of the extent to which specific kinds of information or interventions were provided. Empathy and problem solving were provided to the greatest extent, followed by providing local referrals and general information. Empathy and problem solving were provided in 95 percent of sessions. General information about rape and information about rape and referral to local resources were provided in approximately 80 percent of sessions. Referrals to police and legal resources were provided in the 36 percent of sessions. Referrals to local 911 were given in 8 percent of sessions. "Other" areas of services included emotional support, safety planning, and discussion of the hotline operating procedures.

Difficulties. Approximately 1 in 5 (82 of 361, 22.7 percent) volunteers reported difficulties in their session. The most frequently reported difficulty was technical problems (22.9 percent) followed by "visitor stopped responding" (18.1 percent). There were a variety of other difficulties reported by fewer than 5 percent of volunteers, including: visitor became angry, not enough time to chat, not enough volunteers, "user closed chat when I disclosed I am male," possible "crank call," caller did not want to end session, abrupt session ending, suicidal threats from user, and not knowing how to handle a unique situation such as "visitor was the perpetrator, not a victim" or "visitor was from the Netherlands."

Perceived helpfulness. Volunteers were asked to rate their perception of the helpfulness of the session on a five-point scale from 1 (not at all) to 5 (a great deal). The mean helpfulness rating (N = 334) was

TABLE 3. Extent of Services Provided by Volunteers

	N	Mean	Std. Deviation	Percent Provided
Provide general information	342	2.70	1.3	79.8
Provide police and legal	342	1.70	1.1	35.7
Provide medical issues	343	1.38	.9	10.7
Provide local referral	341	3.15	1.4	79.4
Provide 911 referral	341	1.21	.8	7.9
Provide empathy	342	3.85	1.2	95.3
Provide problem solving	341	3.51	1.2	94.7
Provide other	43	2.72	1.1	94.7

3.5 (SD = 1.1). Approximately half of the volunteers (54 percent) rated the session as very helpful (4 or 5), 25 percent viewed the session as somewhat helpful (3), and 21 percent rated the session as not helpful (1 or 2). Cross-tabulation found that having difficulties was related to perceptions of helpfulness to visitors. High usefulness ratings (4 or 5) were reported by 64 percent of volunteers who reported no difficulties, compared with only 28 percent who reported difficulties ($\chi^2(2)$ 37.17, p < .0001). Perceived helpfulness was not related to the topic of discussion. While not a significant difference, note that in relation to suicide, 14 (32.6 percent) volunteers who discussed suicide rated their session as not helpful compared to 51 (18.5 percent) who did not discuss suicide.

Supervisor Evaluation

National volunteer supervisors (NVSs) are available to volunteers through a chat screen to assist when volunteers have difficulties. Supervisors may also intervene if they feel it is necessary when they are routinely monitoring volunteers' sessions as part of quality control. The data presented represents 14 NVSs who observed or intervened in 91 sessions by 33 volunteers. Supervisor interventions ranged in length from 1 to 300 minutes, with a mean of 27 minutes (SD = 37) and median of 15 minutes. 37 percent of interventions were 10 minutes or less, and 7.9 percent were one hour or longer. Of 89 sessions reported, the vast majority of supervisor assistance was at the volunteers' request (86.5 percent), and 13.5 percent was part of a supervisor regular "check in."

Supervisors were asked to check why they intervened. The reason for intervention was given in 72 sessions. The vast majority of intervention was because the volunteer needed assistance. Of these, supervisors reported that the volunteer needed "support" in 40 percent of sessions. Support included reminding volunteers to use protocols, providing advice on what to say to an angry visitor, giving suggestions about how to ask open-ended questions, providing positive feedback at the end of a session, and generally providing information, suggestions, and encouragement in a variety of situations. In addition, the volunteer needed help with a suicidal user in 18 percent, the volunteer was not following protocols in 14 percent, and the volunteer was inappropriate in 13 percent of sessions. Intervention due to technical difficulties accounted for

3 percent of sessions. In 13 percent of sessions, intervention occurred because the visitor was being "difficult."

Perceived helpfulness. Supervisors were asked to rate their perceptions of how helpful their intervention was for the volunteer on a five-point scale, from 1 (not at all) to 5 (a great deal). Overall, supervisors believed their intervention was very helpful for volunteers. For 87 rated sessions the mean was 4.2 (SD = 1.0), with 75 percent rating the intervention very helpful (4 or 5) and only 7 percent rating it not helpful (1 or 2). Supervisors also rated their perceptions that their intervention was helpful for the visitor. For 86 rated sessions the mean was 4.0 (SD = 1.3), with 70 percent rating the intervention as very helpful (4 or 5) and 13 percent rating the intervention as not helpful (1 or 2).

Difficulties. Supervisors were asked whether they experienced any difficulty during their session. Of 91 sessions, 10 (11 percent) reported some difficulties; 3 were related to technical problems such as dropped sessions or inability to transfer a session to someone else. The remaining 7 difficulties were related to volunteer interactions with visitors such as providing help with an "aggressive" visitor, helping a volunteer find online resources, correcting inappropriate discussion of religious issues, and helping a volunteer handle a visitor's self-injury behavior.

DISCUSSION

RAINN's NSAOH is a new model for the delivery of sexual assault intervention services, using the Internet to deliver sexual assault crisis services through instant messaging with trained volunteers and online volunteer supervision. After 11 months of operation, evaluation of the NSAOH suggests that the RAINN model is viable and useful for a majority of visitors and is meeting the needs of volunteer service providers as well. Overall, visitors find the online hotline easy to use and are satisfied with services and referrals they receive. Three-fourths would recommend the NSAOH to others. Volunteers and supervisors also believe that their interventions are helpful. The results are similar to consumer satisfaction outcomes found in face-to-face mental health services (Campbell, 1998), where consumer satisfaction is approximately 70 to 80 percent satisfied.

The initial evaluation shows that the infrastructure of the NSAOH, instant messaging, volunteer online scheduling, and online supervisory intervention is working well, although some technical difficulties related to dropped sessions and inability to transfer a visitor from one volunteer to another were reported. "Technical difficulties" was the most frequently reported difficulty of all of the difficulties listed by volunteers. In addition, users who reported that the NSAOH was not easy to use also reported low satisfaction with services. Ease of use may have been related to technical difficulties, although this is not directly addressed by the data. It is not surprising to have some technical difficulties at the beginning of a new online service. Focus groups of volunteers, supervisors, and technical support personnel are needed to further examine the nature and cause of technical difficulties. To improve services, every effort must be made to minimize disruptions due to technical difficulties. In addition, both volunteers and the website should warn users that the service is still in its initial phase and that technical difficulties may occur. Note that the phone number for the RAINN telephone rape crisis hotline is prominently available on the RAINN website as an alternative method of communication.

This study suggests that 86 percent of visitors are not in an immediate crisis. Examination of the timeframe of the assault show that only 14 percent discussed an incident that occurred during the past few days and only 1 percent required a referral to 911. More than half of visitors discussed an event that had taken place longer than three months previous. This suggests that the NSAOH is reaching many who have not previously sought services or did not resolve issues through other means. It also points to the importance of training volunteers in a wide variety of long-term issues related to rape. Rape and sexual assault were discussed most frequently by visitors; however, other topics such as family issues, feelings of anger and depression, suicide, and a wide range personal and health issues were also frequently topics of discussion. Volunteers were able to meet a variety of long-term health and mental health needs through provision of empathy, problem-solving, and information and referral.

User satisfaction with volunteer's knowledge and skills is generally high, and satisfaction with volunteers is strongly related to overall satisfaction with the NSAOH. The RAINN model, which includes local training by rape crisis centers as well as online training in online communication and the RAINN infrastructure, appears to be working very well. In the future, it will be important to identify the reasons that a small minority of visitors are not satisfied with the knowledge and skills of the volunteers. Since visitor satisfaction is very highly related to perception of volunteer knowledge and experience, the program should focus on refining and improving training for volunteers. Future evaluations might ask for open-ended comments from visitors about their experience in addition to the brief rating scales currently used. In addition, focus groups of volunteers and supervisors should identify training needs and deficits.

Online supervision appears to be working well. Supervisors are able to monitor sessions for quality control and to intervene in sessions when "called" by volunteers. The availability of online supervisors provides support to volunteers and visitors as well as continuous training and quality control of volunteers. It is an important part of the NSAOH and should be considered by other online services. Further evaluation of the online supervisory process through focus groups with volunteers and supervisors would be useful.

Although relatively infrequent, issues relating to children such as incest and molestation were discussed by visitors. The NSAOH has developed procedures for dealing with issues of mandatory reporting that include an introductory discussion with visitors about privacy and mandatory reporting, use of reporting standards that conform to the strictest state standards, and use of a specially trained RAINN staff member to assess and report cases deemed to involve mandatory reporting. Thus far, one case has received enough information for a report to be filed. The protocols, which include notification of the online supervisor and referral to a RAINN supervisor who is responsible for mandatory reporting issues, worked well in this case. Further evaluation of the mandatory reporting system is warranted.

Suicide was discussed by more than 1 in 10 visitors, and 6 (1.2 percent) visitors discussed an immediate event. RAINN volunteers and supervisors are trained in suicide prevention and intervention; however, almost one-third of volunteers rated their intervention when discussing suicide as not helpful for the visitor. Further evaluation, perhaps using focus groups of volunteers and supervisors, would be useful in better understanding volunteer's perceptions and needs related to working with suicidal visitors. In addition, online crisis services should put a link to the National Suicide Prevention Lifeline on their website for those in immediate crisis.

Limitations of the Evaluation

RAINN is able to obtain data about the process of service delivery and the perceived effectiveness and usefulness of the services through a triangulation approach. While visitor, volunteer, and supervisor perceptions are important, they are unable to provide information about the outcomes of services since user information is not collected for follow-up. The extent to which visitors actually are helped by RAINN volunteers and the extent to which they follow through on RAINN referrals is unknown. In addition, due to privacy concerns, no demographic information is collected so it is not possible to assess for whom (e.g. age, race, and gender) the services are most beneficial. It is also not possible to see if certain demographic groups are more likely to answer the feedback survey. Similarly, since visitors are not identified, visitor data cannot be analyzed in conjunction with volunteer or supervisor data. These limitations are inherent in an online hotline service that views user confidentiality as one of its highest values. Future research should consider a study in which visitors are asked to voluntarily agree to allow their data to specific volunteer information.

User participation in the evaluation is voluntary. Only 30 percent of users filled out evaluation forms. The reason that only some users fill out the evaluation form is unknown. It may be lack of interest, lack of time, focus on more pressing needs, or other reasons. In an effort to increase the response rate, RAINN has asked volunteers to request by chat that users fill out the evaluation form at the end of a session. Generally, voluntary satisfaction surveys are more likely to be filled out by those who are very happy or very unhappy with the services they receive (Royce, 2004), creating some bias in the sample. In addition, visitors who are in crisis when they use the NSAOH may be less likely to take time to fill out a satisfaction survey. The data may reflect those who are not in immediate crisis, thus missing a significant segment of the user population. The extent to which this happens is unknown.

One program goal is to be nationally utilized. No demographic information is available about visitors, so it is difficult to know the extent to which the service is used on a national level. Volunteers are associated with rape crisis centers in 33 states.

Volunteers fill out a session form at the end of each shift. Evaluations done only at the end of a shift may introduce some bias into the data if volunteers are tired or in a hurry at the end of the shift. In addition, some volunteers are more conscientious about filling out the end of session form than others. This may also create some bias in the data.

Finally, volunteers are asked to check the nature of the services that are provided. This includes items such as "support" and "problem solving." These are vague terms. More specific behavioral descriptions of types of support or problem solving as well as the issues to which they are addressed should be a focus of future evaluations.

CONCLUSION

The NSAOH is a new practice model for providing information, support, and therapeutic services to victims of rape and sexual assault. Initial evaluation suggests that the model is viable and useful, although further refinements in infrastructure development and volunteer training may enhance its effectiveness. The evaluation suggests that the NSAOH may be a useful model that can be applied to other crisis services, including domestic violence, teen runaway, mental health, teen pregnancy, and sexual exploitation through prostitution. Given the ubiquitous use of the Internet, online hotlines have the potential to supplement current services and reach a wider audience. The online hotline is not intended to replace current face-to-face services or telephone hotlines; rather, it is intended to promote greater access to services, serve as a convenient source of information and referral to more traditional services, and supplement traditional services in areas in which their availability is limited. The use of online hotlines may reduce health and mental health consequence of mental health crises and provide cost-effective support for those who need it.

A number of questions remain unanswered and will need further research and evaluation. From where do visitors originate? To what extent does the NSAOH meet service needs in areas in which they are not otherwise available? What is the motivation for visitors to use the NSAOH rather than other types of services? For whom and under what circumstances are online hotlines effective? What topics are best *not* handled by online hotlines? How do online hotline services compare to face-to-face services or telephone hotlines in terms of content discussed, user and volunteer satisfaction, and costs? What other than technical difficulties, ease of use, and volunteer knowledge and skill accounts for the perceptions that a small percent of visitors do not find their session useful? Will an online hotline be able to recruit enough trained volunteers and sustain volunteer's interest so that 24/7 services are available with a reasonable wait time for visitors? How much training and in what areas should volunteer training be focused? How effective is the mandatory reporting process? How effective is the online supervision process? How do volunteers integrate supervision from their local rape crisis center supervisor and their online supervisor? The answer to these questions will require multiple sources of data, including online evaluation forms, focus groups and in-depth interviews with volunteers and supervisors, and reports of user referral and satisfaction from local rape crisis centers and other local service providers who see RAINN-referred visitors. Given the online hotline's potential for use in a variety of online crisis services and its unique features, rigorous further evaluation of the program's process and outcomes is essential. The NSAOH services, training, and evaluation are a work in progress. This evaluation suggests that there is a solid foundation on which to build.

REFERENCES

Barak, A. (2004). Internet counseling. In C. E. Spielberger (Ed.), *Encyclopedia of applied psychology* (369–378). San Diego: Academic Press.

Barak, A., & Bloch, N. (2006). Factors related to perceived helpfulness in supporting highly distressed individuals through an online support chat. *Cyberpsychology and Behavior, 9*(1), 60–68.

Barak, A., & Buchanan, T. (2004). Internet-based psychological testing and assessment. In R. Kraus, G. Stricker, & J. Zack (Eds.), *Online counseling: A handbook for mental health professionals* (pp. 217–239). San Diego, CA: Elsevier Academic Press.

Byington D. B., et al. (2006). Teenagers' attitudes about seeking help from telephone crisis services (hotlines). *Suicide & Life-Threatening Behavior, 36*(6), 601–614.

Byington D. B., Martin P. Y., DiNitto D. M., Maxwell M. S. (1991). *Administration in Social Work, 15*(3), 83–103.

Campbell, J. (1998). Consumerism, outcomes, and satisfaction: A review of the literature. In R. W. Manderscheid, & M. J. Henderson (Eds.), *Mental health, United States, 1998.* DHHS Pub. No. (SMA) 99–3285.

Campbell, R., & Ahrens, C. (1998). Innovative community services for rape victims: An application of multiple case study methodology. *American Journal of Community Psychology, 26*(4), 537–527.

Catalano, S. M. (2006). Criminal victimization, 2005. National Crime Victims Survey. Washington, DC: U.S. Department of Justice, Bureau of Statistics.

Finn, J., & Banach, M. (2000). Victimization online: The downside of seeking services for women on the Internet. *Cyberpsychology and Behavior, 3*(2), 776–785.

Finn, J., & Holden, G. (Eds.) (2000). *Human services online: A new arena for service delivery.* Binghamton, NY: The Haworth Press.

Finn, J., Hughes, P., & Berkowitz, S. (in press). RAINN National Sexual Assault Online Hotline: An Internet-based model for delivery of rape crisis intervention services. Accepted, Violence Against Women, June, 2007.

Golkaramnay, V., Bauer, S., Haug, S., Wolf, M., & Kordy, H. (2007). The exploration of the effectiveness of group therapy through an Internet chat as aftercare: A controlled naturalistic study. *Psychotherapy & Psychosomatics, 76,* 219–225.

Gould, M. S., Velting, D., Kleinman, M., Lucas, C., Thomas, J. G., & Chung M. (2004). Teenagers' attitudes about coping strategies and help seeking behavior for suicidality. *Journal of the American Academy of Child and Adolescent Psychiatry, 43*(9), 1124–1133.

Griffiths, F., Lindenmeyer, A., Powell, J., Lowe, P., & Throgood, M. (2006). Why are health care interventions delivered over the internet? A systematic review of the published literature. *Journal of Medical Internet Research, 8,* www.jmir.org/2006/2/e10/.

Horrigan J., & Rainie, L. (2006). *The Internet's major role in life's major moments.* PEW Internet and American Life Project (2006). Retrieved October 23, 2006, from http://www.pewinternet.org/.

Hughes, P. (2006). Personal communication, December 20, 2006. Vice President, RAINN Online Services, Washington, DC.

Klein, B., & Richards, J. C. (2001). A brief Internet-based treatment for panic disorder. *Behavioural & Cognitive Psychotherapy, 29,* 113–117.

Lenhart, M., Madden, M., & Hitlin. (2005). Teens and technology. Washington, DC: The Pew Internet & American Life Project. Retrieved November 30, 2005, from http//www.pewinternet.org/pdfs/PIP_Teens_Tech_July2005web.pdf.

Mallen, M. J., Vogel, D.L, Rochlen, A. B., Day, S. X. (2005). Online counseling: Reviewing the literature from a counseling psychology framework. *Counseling Psychologist 33*(6), 819–871.

Miller, T. R., Cohen, M. A., & Wierama, B. (1996). *Victim costs and consequences: A new Look.* U. S. Department of Justice, Office of Justice Programs, National Institute of Justice. Rockville, MD: U.S. Department of Health and Human Services.

Rideout, V. (2001). *Generation Rx.com: How young people use the Internet for health information.* Menlo Park: Henry J. Kaiser Family Foundation.

Rochlen, A. B., Zack, J. S., & Speyer, C. (2004). Online therapy: Review of relevant definitions, debates, and current empirical support. *Journal of Clinical Psychology, 60,* 269–283.

Royce, D. (2004). *Research Methods in Social Work* (4th ed.). Pacific Grove, CA: Brooks/Cole.

Tjaden P., & Thoennes, N. (2006). Extent, nature, and consequences of rape victimization: Findings from the National Violence Against Women Survey. Washington, DC: National Institute of Justice; Report NCJ 210346. Retrieved June 21, 2007, from http//www.ncjrs.gov/pdffiles1/nij/210346.pdf.

Waldron, V., Lavitt, M., & Kelley, D. (2000). The nature and prevention of harm in technology-mediated self-help settings: Three exemplars. *Journal of Technology in Human Services, 17*(1,2,3), 267–294.

A Safe Place for Predators: Online Treatment of Recovering Sex Offenders

Poco D. Kernsmith
Roger M. Kernsmith

In recent years, the trend in treatment of perpetrators of sexual crimes has been toward stricter sentencing as well as increasing public knowledge of local sex offenders through mandated registration (Edwards & Hensley, 2001). In 2002, it is estimated through the National Crime Victims Survey (NCVS) that almost 250,000 people in the United States ages 12 and older were the victims of rape or sexual assault

(Rennison, 2003). Jones and Finkelhor (2001) report that in 1998 there were 103,600 substantiated cases of child sexual abuse in the United States. The current practice in all 50 states is to grant public access to the identity of convicted sexual offenders either through a publicly accessible registration system or through public notification (Tewksbury, 2002). These laws have been viewed as designed to punish and incapacitate sex offenders and to protect public safety (Farkas & Stichman, 2002). However, they do little to change the attitudes, thoughts, and behaviors of sex offenders.

Mandatory reporting laws require most helping professionals to report sex offenders to the child protection agencies, which may prevent many offenders from seeking help to change their behavior (Edwards & Hensley, 2001). However, the Internet has provided a new avenue for offenders to confidentially receive support and connect with others in a safe environment. The Internet provides an important opportunity for those who may feel shame or fear about seeking help in a setting that is not anonymous (Rochlen, Zack, & Speyer, 2004).

Traditional rehabilitation approaches often use a cognitive-behavioral model, focusing on building empathy for the victims and relapse prevention (Pithers & Gray, 1996), adapted from traditional substance abuse models. Pithers (1999) identified that building empathy for victims and potential victims can assist in relapse prevention by disrupting cognitive distortions (Mihailides, Devilly, & Ward, 2004) that neutralize social and emotional barriers to sexual offending. These distortions include the belief that they cannot control their sexuality, they are entitled to have the sexual relationships they desire, and that children are sexual beings. Offenders also identify behaviors that put them at risk for future perpetration and replace them with more appropriate thoughts and actions (Pithers & Gray, 1996). These interventions are found to be generally successful; however, motivation among mandated participants is noted as an important barrier (Mihailides et al., 2004; Pithers & Gray, 1996). This study examines an online self-help group that attempts to work with sex offenders using this same approach.

METHOD

The goal of the research was to explore an online self-help group as a means of promoting recovery of sex offenders. In addition, the study explores the process of change and barriers to rehabilitation for adult sex offenders, as demonstrated through their online behavior. The study consists of a qualitative content analysis of the written interaction of an online self-help group. All of the group members are voluntary participants. Most have no history of conviction for sex-related crimes based on self-report. This process analysis focuses on the nature of support and confrontation as they relate to the rehabilitation of offenders, similar to research conducted in prison-based treatment groups (Frost & Connolly, 2004).

Retrospective data were collected, totaling 3,401 messages, between June 1, 2004, and April 1, 2005. Approximately 86 individuals participated in the group during that time. The majority (81 percent) were males who had offended against one or more children. Prior to the onset of the study, the group facilitators gave permission for the researchers to observe the interaction. From the inception of the group, the moderators determined and participants were made aware, that professionals, including social workers and researchers would be allowed to participate in or observe the group.

Data were copied from the online group into the database program Claris FileMaker Pro 7.0. Messages contained no identifying information, except perhaps a first name, so the anonymity of participants was ensured. Those names posted were stripped from the data at the time of data collection in order to further protect participants. All procedures were approved by the university committee for the protection of human participants in research.

Ethical issues were an important consideration in the design of the study. As the researcher, as well as any other professionals who may choose to observe the group, are mandated reporters of child abuse, concern was expressed that a report of perpetration could result in severe legal and emotional consequences for that member. For this reason, the group takes its own precautions to protect the identity of all members. No identifying information is available in the group, including names, e-mail addresses, or locations. Moderators take care to screen messages prior to allowing them to be posted to the group. For this reasons, there were few risks that a breach of confidentiality in the research would be possible.

Messages posted to the board were coded by a team of six trained MSW students and two supervising faculty researchers. Each message was coded by two to three different people to ensure the reliability of results. Differences were resolved to the satisfaction of all coders. Reliability of coding was analyzed by calculating the percentage of agreement for each category and found to be quite high (ranging from 84 percent to 100 percent), with most discrepancies due to entry error and not disagreement on content or meaning.

Some coding categories were developed prior to the onset of the analysis of these data due to the purposes of this study; for example, the presence of group confrontation of unhealthy or dangerous thoughts and feelings. However, the flexibility of coding category creation allowed the analyst to generate the coding frame based on the content of the discussion, including such things as cognitive distortions, social supports, and barriers to change. In addition, threads were coded to determine what types of posts are more likely to elicit support, confrontation, or informative responses, allowing for an exploration of the process of the interaction.

Coding categories for this study included an examination of the dynamics of the group. These included such things as empathy, attacks, and positive confrontation. In addition, indicators of level recovery included such variables as acceptance of cognitive distortions (Mihailides et al., 2004), accountability, recognizing harm to victims, and obsessive thoughts. Appendix A offers a list of coding definitions.

Description of the Group

The online self-help group is moderated by two members, who are themselves recovering offenders. The moderators were the two individuals who developed the group. Neither is a trained psychologist or social worker, but instead they are individuals who had progressed through their recovery through the help of therapy and support groups many years prior. For this reason, the term self-help is used to describe this group instead of support group. Self-help groups are designed to help people in similar circumstances using holistic and empowerment approaches (Katz, 1992). The group facilitates a supportive environment but does not provide therapy. On many occasions, group participants were encouraged by other members to seek face-to-face support through Sex Addicts Anonymous or individual therapy in their own community.

The group was created by the moderators in 2003 and uses an asynchronous format, meaning members post messages to the discussion board for others' responses at a later time. The advantage of this format is the ability for many members to participate without needing to be online at the same time. The disadvantage is the lack of immediate support should a member be in a state of crisis.

RESULTS

The members posted an average of 46 times during the six month study period. However, there is a wide range with many members rarely participating. The number of posts per author ranged from 1 to 385 with a median of 10 posts. Only approximately 15 of the members could be considered active based on their level of participation, likely due to the voluntary nature of the group. These members posted to the group nearly every day and often several times a day. Analysis of activity revealed that members either posted to the discussion board fewer than 50 times (N = 54) or more than 100 times (N = 32) during the data collection period.

Preliminary analysis indicated that the group did function to help those members who chose to actively participate, based on changes in the number of fantasies or cognitive distortions present in the posts over time. No members in the group reported actual perpetration during the time of the study. However, this may reflect a dynamic of the group, such as fear of legal consequences if a breach of confidentiality occurred, and not actual behavior. The majority of the authors (52 percent) reflected accountability for their behavior. Relatively few described feelings of empathy for the victims (18 percent), although they did recognize that their behavior was harmful to the children (49 percent). In addition, the participants discussed the impact on their own families. Table 1 provides the number of posts in which indicators of recovery were present. In interpreting the table, it is important to recognize that the percentages reflect the percent of all posts. Because conversation was often off-topic or responses to others, the percentage is expected to be low in comparison to the data on the characteristics of authors.

The discussion largely focused around attempts to change their thoughts and desires, therefore cognitive distortions represented a higher proportion of posts (21 percent). Barriers to change, such as

TABLE 1. Frequency of Indicators of Offender Recovery*

Indicators of Recovery	Frequency (N = 3401)	Percent of Messages (%)
Accountability	288	9
Shame	82	3
Remorse	54	2
Recognize harm	219	6
Any cognitive distortions	716	21
Compulsion	93	3
Obsessive thoughts	102	3

*Categories are not mutually exclusive, therefore percent will not equal 100%.

fear of seeking counseling and lack of social supports, were also common themes. Those who had experience with the legal system were more likely to report being in traditional, face-to-face counseling or support groups, often reporting a negative experience in those groups. The following participant expresses this sense of stigma as a pedophile even with respect to his Sex Addicts Anonymous sponsor:

> I feel like I need a lot of time before I am ready to talk to my sponsor about my pedophilia.... I think that I would be a lot more comfortable working with these issues here in this support group [referring to the online group] with people that understand the issues. As we all know, people despise pedophiles. The term recovering offender does little to curb the hatred.

These individuals also reported being ostracized by friends and family, as well as negative reactions and even violence as a result of being identified from sex offender registries.

The group was generally a supportive environment, characterized by empathy and positive confrontation. Attacks or criticism were rare in this group. In those cases where participants presented cognitive distortions or rationalizations for their behavior, they were equally likely to be responded to with advice or empathy. An illustration of this supportive, yet challenging, environment is provided by a response posted to the previous message:

> I think you are absolutely right to be cautious, but I notice you are operating on your expectations of what your new sponsor's

TABLE 2. Frequency of Forms of Group Interaction*

Group Interaction	Frequency (N = 3401)	Percent of Messages (%)
Positive confrontation	448	13
Attack	98	3
Empathy	839	25
Inspirational material	68	2
Provide information/referral	342	10
Advice	613	18
Collusion	207	6

*Categories are not mutually exclusive, therefore percent will not equal 100%.

reaction would be to revelations about your paedophilia [sic], rather than objective evidence. Isn't there some way you could sound out your sponsor on what his reaction might actually be without getting too hurt?

Positive confrontation was also common, particularly from the moderators and more active members (78 percent of active members exhibited this characteristic). When potentially dangerous thoughts or behaviors were responded to with collusion, these responses were typically challenged by other members. Table 2 provides descriptive data on the types of responses given to group members. The following message, posted in response to a group member who expressed a desire to strike up a "safe" relationship with a young boy whom he encounters at work, provides a clear example of such a confrontation:

> ... Safe is a matter of perception. The thoughts that drive your attraction are not safe. Therefore, your interactions with this child, in ways, are not safe as they could lead to abuse if given the right circumstances. .... You need to step back and examine the thoughts behind why you let this child respond the way you have. The way to enjoy the innocents of this child is place your self back in the roll of store clerk and allow this child to experience life in a safe environment. As a store clerk, what is your roll in this child's life? What interactions are expected of a store clerk, in the eyes of a primary caretaker? If you compare your actions with the actions expected of you, you might find them to be quite different. Basically, what I am trying to say is, you

TABLE 3. Change in Indicators of Offender Recovery over Time

Category	Correlation with Time
Individual Indicators	
Accountability	.125*
Shame	.005
Remorse	.002
Recognize harm	.024
Any cognitive distortions	−.154*
Compulsion	−.059*
Obsessive thoughts	−.048*
Group Dynamics	
Attack	−.038*
Empathy	.096*
Positive confrontation	.006
Collusion	−.232*

*p < .05.

have over steeped [sic] a boundary. From here, there are but a few obstacles standing between you and a victim that you can act out with. Now is time to take control of your thoughts and actions.

Based on the data in Table 3 the attitudes and thoughts of the active members appeared to progress in a positive direction during the time period analyzed. Using a correlation of time with reports of several indicators of recovery, members showed positive change over time in many areas over the 10 month duration of the study. To analyze this, the number of days from the onset of the study was correlated with the frequency that an author exhibited such characteristics as "accountability." In analyses of threaded conversation such as this, the number of messages exhibiting any specific characteristic is typically quite low due to the conversational nature of the data. More simply, authors tend not to repeat similar content in multiple successive messages. In addition, when responding to others or discussing content unrelated to their own offenses, these characteristics typically do not occur. Thus, there is a high degree of variability in message characteristics and therefore a relatively low rate of occurrence of any one particular characteristic. This can result in unrepresentatively low correlation coefficients, which would not normally be considered clinically significant, when all messages are included as data points.

In addition, several other factors would be expected to be important predictors of change, such as personal motivation and social support outside the group. As participation in this group is only one factor influencing these changes, participation in the group itself cannot necessarily be viewed as responsible for these changes. However, examination of other influential factors is beyond the scope of this study.

Over time, it was found that factors that may be associated with recidivism, including cognitive distortions, obsessive thoughts, and compulsive behavior (Mihailides et al., 2004), were found to decrease. Accountability for ones behavior and actions was found to increase. See Table 3 for significant correlations.

Active and inactive members showed distinct differences in these indicators. To analyze these differences each member was coded as high activity or low activity based on the number of posts. Then the posts of each member were analyzed to determine if the member ever exhibited the behavior coded. This dichotomy was created because high activity members would by definition exhibit each characteristic more frequently in their postings. The dichotomy allows for an examination of differences in proportion. A t-test was conducted to analyze group differences in number of posts related to the message categories. Active members were found to exhibit nearly all of the characteristics of interest. The percentage of messages reflecting the characteristics indicates that high activity members not only posted more frequently, but their messages reflected more substantive content than low activity members. This indicates more engagement with one another as well as more self-disclosure (See Table 4).

Although it is impossible to draw a direct causal link to the impact of the group, members reported feeling the group was helpful to them in providing support and changing beliefs. All of the high activity members and 55 percent of low activity members reported in the group discussion that they felt the group was helpful.

DISCUSSION

The data indicates that this group is working to actively tackle difficult issues and support members through the change process. This is

TABLE 4. Differences in Indicators of Offender Recovery by Activity Level (N = 86)

Category	Percent of High Activity Members (%)	Percent of Low Activity Members (%)	T	df	Sig.
Individual Indicators					
Accountability	69	36	3.45	85	.003
Shame	56	18	3.79	85	.001
Remorse	28	24	0.93	85	.645
Recognize harm	59	44	2.88	85	.016
Any cognitive distortions	78	69	2.62	85	.010
Compulsion	47	25	3.13	85	.041
Obsessive thoughts	47	25	2.60	85	.041
Group Dynamics					
Attack	41	20	2.42	85	.038
Empathy	81	47	5.21	85	.002
Positive confrontation	78	34	4.27	85	.000
Collusion	47	29	2.35	85	.021

indicated by the frequency with which the group tackles issues of cognitive distortions (Mihailides et al., 2004). These cognitive distortions are commonly responded to with positive confrontation, providing support to the finding that the group holds the members accountable and supports each through the process of change.

In general, the group dynamics appear positive, with empathy being the most common response, followed by positive confrontation and advice. As expected, high activity group members are more likely to exhibit all forms of responding. This indicates that high activity members are more engaged and therefore more likely to respond to others. Conversely, low activity members are less engaged with the community and primarily post their own thoughts and experiences, with fewer responses to the posts of others.

Over time, positive change in the group is indicated by improved group dynamics. The group evolves to become more empathetic over time. Attacks, criticism, and collusion become less common. This may indicate that the group is not only becoming more close knit, but also is improving in the ways members encourage recovery through appropriate responding.

Individual indicators of recovery show statistically significant improvement. This included increased accountability of group members, as well as decreases in cognitive distortions, compulsive behaviors, and obsessive thoughts. Each of these is an important indicator in relapse prevention (Mihailides et al., 2004; Pithers & Gray, 1996). Although there are limitations to the data, they seem to be encouraging and suggest further research is needed. Specifically, a more extensive evaluation of the intervention, perhaps in comparison to traditional approaches, would expand understanding of the impact. In addition, interviews with the participants would provide greater insight into the process and barriers to change.

High activity and low activity group members show significant differences in terms of indicators of recovery. High activity members were more likely to demonstrate accountability for their behavior, recognize the harm to victims, and report feelings of shame. However, they were also more likely to report compulsive behavior and obsessive thoughts. It is possible that this may be due to greater feelings of comfort and trust in the group. It may also be important to note that both of these indicators were found to significantly decrease over time, possibly indicating positive change for these group members.

Limitations of the Study

The data source has several inherent limitations. Most notably, participants may not always be truthful in their posts, possibly omitting thoughts or behaviors that are not socially acceptable. However, the unobtrusive observation may have minimized any researcher effects. As a self-selected, voluntary group of offenders, it is also likely that this intervention may not be effective with another group of offenders who do not share similar characteristics, such as motivation to change. For several reasons, the group may appear more effective than it actually is. For example, it is possible that those offenders who are not successful in their recovery may stop participating in the group. In addition, members may learn what is not acceptable to say in the group and change what they post without actually changing how they think.

Implications

It is unclear if the participation of a professional facilitator would help or hinder the group. It is likely that the facilitator could be helpful in such things as challenging cognitive distortions and providing alternative cognitions. However, data indicates that group members are holding one another accountable and responding appropriately in most cases. The facilitator could also be helpful in processing childhood trauma, which most report. However, it is also possible that the presence of a professional, who is a mandated reporter of child abuse, may discourage some from choosing to participate. Further research could explore the differences and similarities in these types of online interventions.

The existence of the group without a professional facilitator poses some important ethical questions. Most notably, without a mandated reporter known to be participating in the group, there may be the risk that someone would disclose the intent to harm a child and no one would take responsibility for reporting the act to authorities. Following is an example of one such quote that may raise concerns about mandated reporting.

> Today after seeing the doctor I really felt the urge to go find a little girl and in fact I walked past the school just so I could look. One of them recognised me cos [sic] she waved and I waved back. I went back home and masturbated and then I slept. I don't think that was ideal but it kept me off the streets.... I didn't try and find out who the kid was who waved and start making friends with her family–although as I write that I am feeling the temptation–so I'm doing much better than I used to ... ps I think she goes to my church.

Because the research and other observers do not have access to any identifying information, reporting this to the appropriate authorities would not be possible. However, in a group facilitated by a mental health professional, that facilitator may be mandated to report this or other comments.

Since 1974, legislation has required mental health professionals to report suspected child abuse or the threat of it to a child protection agency (U.S. Department of Health and Human Services, 2005). Laws vary between states in the types of individuals required to report, including teachers and photo processing personnel. In some states, all people, regardless of occupation, are mandated to report. However, even if a mandated reporter were to participate in the group, the anonymous nature would prohibit the individual from making a report unless the group member had disclosed his or her actual name and other identifying information. In actuality, the group welcomes professionals, including those who may be mandated reporters, to participate in the group, as evidenced by the welcome letter on the home page, "We accept all comers here. Offenders & Victims & Social workers, etc. are welcome."

It is also possible that the group could become an avenue for offenders to network to share child pornography or otherwise support the abusive behavior of others. However, in the group studied here, the group members and the moderators work to ensure that the group functions only for the intended purpose of recovery. Group policies indicate that members can be removed from the group for inappropriate behavior. These are important risks of this type of intervention that should not be understated. However, given the reluctance of members to fully disclose in a setting that is not anonymous, the benefits of this available support may outweigh the potential risks.

Further research in this area may include interviews or surveys of members of online and face-to-face counseling groups in order to investigate the relative effectiveness of the intervention. This line of research could also examine the impact of the presence of a professional facilitator. In addition, this research could be replicated as it relates to intervention with similarly stigmatized groups, such as sexual minorities, people dealing with addiction, or other criminal populations.

CONCLUSION

The preliminary analysis indicates that this group is helpful for those who choose to actively participate. Given the reluctance of members to divulge their behaviors to others, this anonymous group offers one of a limited number of opportunities for predators to get support. Lack of social support has been identified as a risk factor for recidivism of sexual offenders (Cesaroni, 2001), highlighting the need for such online services. Because this group provides an opportunity to discuss feelings and struggles in a safe environment, as well as to form bonds with others, it may be a promising intervention.

REFERENCES

Cesaroni, C. (2001). Releasing sex offenders into the community through "Circles of Support"—A means of reintegrating the "worst of the worst." *Journal of Offender Rehabilitation, 34*(2), 85–98.

Edwards, W., & Hensley, C. (2001) Contextualizing sex offender management legislation and policy: Evaluating the problem of latent consequences in community notification laws. *International Journal of Offender Therapy & Comparative Criminology, 45*(1), 83–101.

Farkas, M. J., & Stichman, A. (2002). Sex offender laws: Can treatment, punishment, incapacitation, and public safety be reconciled? *Criminal Justice Review, 27*(2), 256–283.

Frost, A., & Connolly, M. (2004). Reflexivity, reflection, and the change process in offender work. *Sexual Abuse: Journal of Research & Treatment, 16*(4), 365–380.

Jones, L., & Finkelhor, D. (2001). *The decline in child sexual abuse cases.* Washington, DC: U.S. Department of Justice. NCJ #184741.

Katz, A. H. (1992). *Self help: Concepts and applications.* Philadelphia: Charles Press.

Mihailides, S., Devilly, G. J., & Ward, T. (2004) Implicit cognitive distortions and sexual offending. *Sexual Abuse: Journal of Research & Treatment, 16*(4), 333–350.

Pithers, W. D. (1999). Empathy: Definition, enhancement, and relevance to the treatment of sexual abusers. *Journal of Interpersonal Violence, 14*(3), 257–284.

Pithers, W. D., & Gray, A. S. (1996). Utility of relapse prevention in treatment of sexual abusers. *Sexual Abuse: Journal of Research & Treatment, 8*(3), 223–230.

Rennison, C. M. (2003). *Criminal victimization, 2002.* Washington, DC: U.S. Department of Justice. NCJ # 199994.

Rochlen, A. B., Zack, J. S., & Speyer, C. (2004) Online therapy: Review of relevant definitions, debates, and current empirical support. *Journal of Clinical Psychology, 60*(3), 269–283.

Tewksbury, R. (2002). Validity and utility of the Kentucky sex offender registry. *Federal Probation, 66*(1), 21–26.

U.S. Department of Health and Human Services (2005). Mandatory reporters of child abuse and neglect. Retrieved April 28, 2007, from www.childwelfare.gov/systemwide/laws_policies/statutes/manda.cfm.

APPENDIX A. Coding Definitions

Indicators of Change

Accountability	Author takes responsibility for his or her own behavior.
Shame	A strong sense of dishonor, disgrace, or unworthiness. May be related to perpetration or own victimization.
Remorse	Author expresses remorse (a feeling of deep regret) for previous behaviors.
Recognize harm	Author identifies the real or potential negative consequences of his or her behavior to self or others.
Cognitive distortions	*Children as sexual beings*: Children are sexual and may initiate, want, or enjoy sexual experiences with adults. Children may be attracted to the group members.
	Uncontrollability of sexuality: Author is unable to control his or her sexual behavior because of sexual addiction, victimization experiences, etc.
	Sexual entitlement: Author feels that he or she should be able to have sex with whomever and whenever he or she pleases because he or she is more important than others.
	Children unharmed: Victims are not hurt by the sexual experiences and may even enjoy them.
	Dangerous world: Author believes that the world is a dangerous place in which he or she must fight to regain control because others are abusive and/or controlling.
	Deny sexual intent: The author did not mean for the relationship to be sexual and instead it just happened that way.
	Misinterpreting own abuse: Author describes feeling loved, valued, etc. by those who committed childhood abuse against them.
	Other distortions: Authors thoughts are irrational or interpretations seem strange or incorrect.
Compulsion	Author expresses a drive or need to perform a behavior (offending, masturbation, etc.) that is strong and he or she feels is difficult to control or ignore.
Obsessive thoughts	Author has excessive repeated thoughts (preoccupation) about children, sexuality, or other topics related to offending.

Group Interaction

Positive confrontation	Author confronts the thoughts, feelings, or behavior of another member in a way that is constructive or therapeutically appropriate.
Attack	Author confronts a member in a way that is hostile, aggressive, or otherwise not constructive.
Empathy	Author responds in a manner that is supportive, caring, compassionate, etc.
Inspirational material	Author posts something intended to inspire other members of the group, such as quotes, poetry, religious references, etc.

(Continued)

APPENDIX A. Coding Definitions (*Continued*)

Information or referral	Author provides information about or from other sources, such as television, websites, books, movies, etc. The post may either direct them to the source or provide information from it.
Advice	Author provides suggestions or advice on how to deal with something. This advice may or may not have been solicited.
Collusion	Author responds in a way that reinforces the cognitive distortions, rationalization, or justifications of another member.

The Need for Web-Based Cognitive Behavior Therapy Among University Students

Ove K. Lintvedt
Kristian Sørensen
Andreas R. Østvik
Bas Verplanken
Catharina E. Wang

Depression is a leading cause of disability in today's Europe and the United States (World Health Organization [WHO], 2001b), and the age of onset of depression seems to be decreasing (Lewinsohn, Hops, Roberts, Seeley, & Andrews, 1993; Ministry of Health, 1997). This adds strains to the younger individuals in our society. Internet-based self-help tools may particularly benefit the high-risk young adult population because they are more likely to be aware of and use new technologies. An important question is whether those who would otherwise not seek mental health support would make use of such services.

Depression is common in our society and currently affecting about 340 million people worldwide (WHO, 2001a), with incidence of depressive symptoms increasing in all age groups and in all Western cultures (Moussavi et al., 2007; Wang et al., 2007). The rate of treatment is increasing at the same time as most patients with a mental disorder problem do not receive treatment (Kessler et al., 2005). Furthermore, the possible benefits of early intervention are evident when keeping in mind that most people suffering from depression do not make contact with health services or have unmet needs for treatment (Wells, Burnam, Rogers, Hays, & Camp, 1992; Wang et al., 2007). Accordingly, these findings clearly show the importance of a prevention focus in the treatment of depression. According to Beck's (Bech, 1967, 1976) cognitive theory of depression, negative thoughts play a central role in depression. The aim of cognitive-behavior therapy (CBT) is to change negative patterns of thinking and dysfunctional attitudes in vulnerable individuals to prevent depressive symptoms from developing. This will in turn facilitate positive coping skills when faced with stressful situations (Bech, Rush, Shaw, & Emery, 1979). Individuals with depression are reluctant to seek professional help. Estimates indicate that more than half of subjects with major depression in the community do not consult a health professional (Mental Health Norway, 2004).

Becoming a student implies major life changes. The entry into higher education adds challenges to students' lives at a time when they try to cope with the transition from adolescence into adulthood. In addition, students may encounter various major life events. In Norway only 1 of 10 students lives with their parents while they attend higher education (Løwe & Sæthe, 2007). More than 6 percent of first-year students report homesickness, and they are at the greatest risk of developing mental health problems of all university students (Adlaf, Glicksman, Demers, & Newton, 2001). These can be compounded by the lack of a confiding relationship and a subjective feeling of loneliness, which has shown to be associated with symptoms of anxiety, depression, alcohol and drug misuse, and suicidal ideation (Stecker, 2004). Some students mention stigma as a reason not to access counseling services (Royal College of Psychiatrists, 2001). All these are factors that increase the risk of developing mental disorders including depression (Walden, 2003). Helping these individuals is a difficult and challenging task for providers of mental health services. Self-help web sites developed for these particular age groups may be a way to provide services or information that may not otherwise be sought.

A recent study (Skarsvåg, 2004) concerning mental health problems among students found that among a sample of 741 students from a Norwegian university, one-third had felt a need for psychological help. As many as two-thirds of these subjects refrained from seeking help. When asked about alternative help resources more than 57 percent with a felt need for psychological help were positive toward using an Internet-based counseling service. Thus, there may be a significant segment of students who are in the need of mental health support who do not seek help from traditional services but may make use of Internet-based self-help programs.

Internet-based intervention programs often make use of CBT to increase self-help ability. A large number of applications are available on the Internet or as computerized cognitive-behavioral therapy (CCBT). For people with mild to moderate depression, Beating the Blues (Ultrasis, 2007), MoodGYM (Australian National University, 2007), and Good Days Ahead (MindStreet, 2007) are well-known programs. FearFighter (CCBT, 2007) is a program developed for people with panic and phobia, while Mastering My Life (Interactive Health Systems, 2007) is developed for helping people with stress-related aspects of their life. It is not the use of the computers or

Internet per se which proves effective but rather the therapeutic techniques on which the programs are built (Proudfoot et al., 2004). The aim of CBT is to change negative patterns of thinking and dysfunctional attitudes in vulnerable individuals, thereby reducing or preventing depressive symptoms. This in turn should facilitate positive coping skills in face of stressful situations (Butler, Chapman, Forman, & Beck, 2006; Chambless & Ollendick, 2001). CBT has been shown to be especially effective in treating people with mild to moderate depression, also with regard to preventing relapse (Frazer, Christensen, & Griffiths, 2005; Churchill et al., 2001; Department of Health, 2001). In addition, it can be adapted to different self-help procedures. Therefore, CBT seems to be a well-suited tool for self-help interventions.

One of the unique qualities of Internet-based counseling is that therapeutic changes can take place in an anonymous or pseudo-anonymous context (Grohol, 2001), which may minimize psychological distress. People who feel themselves stigmatized by their problems, diagnosis or the counseling process are more likely to seek help online where they feel less ashamed than in a personal encounter with a therapist (Rochlen, Zack, & Speyer, 2004).

Before establishing an Internet-based counseling service based on CBT at a university in Norway, we decided to assess the need for Internet-based mental health services among a sample of students, mapping the mental health status of prospective users and investigating willingness and intentions to use such a program. We choose to use MoodGYM (Christensen, Griffiths, & Jorm, 2004) as an example of an Internet-based intervention program because it is a free self-help program developed with the age group 15–25 as primary target group, it is well structured, and based on CBT. MoodGYM has been found to be effective in randomized controlled trials to reduce depressive symptoms and negative thinking (Christensen et al, 2004).

To assess students' intentions we applied the theory of planned behavior (TPB; Ajzen, 1991), widely used within consumer and health psychology (Francis, Johnston, Eccles, Grimshaw, & Kaner, 2004). In a meta-analysis of 10 meta-analyses comparing 422 correlational studies describing intention-behavior relationships documented in the extant social-psychological literature, Sheeran (2002) found that intention explained on average 28 percent of the variance in future behavior. He found an R^2 of .28 and an $r+$ of .53, indicating a large effect size, corresponding with a large effect based on Cohen's (1992) conventions for quantifying effect size. As a result there has been a great enthusiasm for social cognitive theories of health behavior and for the predictive primacy of behavioral intention. The TPB assumes that performing behaviors are strongly associated with beliefs about the outcome of the behavior ("what I expect to occur"), normative beliefs (social pressure) about the expectations of others, and control beliefs ("things I can do") about facilitating or inhibiting factors of the behavior in question. The beliefs about the possible outcome of the behavior form an attitude toward the behavior. Perceived social pressure or subjective norm is the result of normative beliefs about the behavior. The control beliefs result in a perceived behavioral control in the individual. The concepts of attitude, subjective norm, and perceived behavioral control together result in a behavioral intention. Behavioral intention is thought to be the immediate antecedent of behavior. The stronger a person's intention, the more likely he or she is to enact a behavior (Armitage & Conner, 2001). Consumers are more likely to adopt a new technology if they have used similar technologies in the past (Korgaonkar & Moschis, 1987; Jarvenpaa, Tractinsky, & Vitale, 2000) and have developed favorable attitudes toward using similar technologies (Dabholkar, 1992, 1996). Therefore, it is proposed that positive attitudes toward using the Internet in general will have a direct, positive effect on attitudes toward the use of mental health care services on the Internet. It was hypothesized that symptoms of depression and negative thinking, TPB measures, attitude toward the Internet, and previous help seeking behavior would account for a significant portion of variance in intention to make use of an Internet-based mental health service that is not yet implemented.

The research questions in this paper are divided in two parts: (1) What is the need for using MoodGYM in a university population? and (2) What are the predictive factors for the intention to use MoodGYM?

METHOD

Participants

Questionnaires were randomly handed out at various lectures to 630 students at the University of Tromsø and the University College of Tromsø, Norway. The sample represented 6.3 percent of the total student population. The number of students who returned the questionnaire was 367, representing a response rate of 58.3 percent with a clear female majority of 263 (71.9 percent) and 103 (28.1 percent) males. For comparison, the distribution of gender at the university is about 61 percent females and 39 percent males (reported from student registry in September 2006). The mean age in the sample was 23.10 years ($SD = 5.7$) and median age was 21.00 years ($SD = 5.7$). Almost all students in the sample studied full time (99.7 percent). The mean semester for the students was 3.1 and median number of semesters was 1.0. Students were bachelor students (51.6 percent), master students (20.5 percent), professional students in psychology and law (15.8 percent), and students with other fields of study (17.1 percent). There were no measures for racial or cultural differences. The study was approved by the Regional Committee for Research Ethics.

Measures

The demographic variables selected in this study were age and gender. Depressive symptoms were assessed by the Centre for Epidemiological Studies–Depression Scale (CES-D; Radloff, 1977). This 20-item self-report scale records symptoms according to 4-point Likert-type response scales (0–3), allowing a range from 0 to 60, with scores 16 or higher reflecting symptoms of depression. A full description of the inventory, including psychometric properties, can be found in Radloff (1977, 1991). The sum of all of the items were computed and used in all of the analyses (Cronbach's alpha = .87).

Habitual negative self-thinking was assessed by the Habit Index of Negative Thinking (HINT; Verplanken, Friborg, Wang, Trafimow, & Woolf, 2007). This 12-item self-report scale asks for the degree of negative thinking on a 7-point Likert-type response scales (1–7), allowing a range from 12 to 84, with higher scores indicating a stronger negative thinking habit. A full description of the inventory, including psychometric properties can be found in Verplanken and colleagues (2007). The sum of all of the items were computed and used in all the analyses (Cronbach's alpha = .95).

The intention to use an Internet-based counseling service based on CBT (i.e., MoodGYM) was assessed by using the theory of planned behavior (TPB; Ajzen, 1991, 2002). The TPB questions developed for this study comprise different scales measuring perceived behavioral control (4 items), subjective norms (5 items), attitudes toward using MoodGYM (7 items), and intentions to use MoodGYM (5 items), all to be scored along a 7-point Likert-type response scale, items ranging from 1 (totally agree) to 7 (totally disagree). Attitudes toward using MoodGYM were scored along a 7-point semantic differential scale. The scale contains 7 semantic differential pairs of adjectives, each pair scored from 1 (negative adjective) to 7 (positive adjective). The scale includes pairs of adjectives such as whether MoodGYM is negative or positive, harmful or beneficial, bad or good, etc. The sum of all of the items were computed and used in all of the analyses (Cronbach's alpha: subjective norm = .80; perceived behavioral control = .76; intention to use MoodGYM = .95; attitudes toward MoodGYM = .86).

Other measures used in this study. Previous help-seeking and mental health was assessed by asking whether the participants had felt need for help with psychological problems during the previous 12 months but refrained from seeking help. Answers were categorized as 0 (no need for help), 1 (sought help), and 2 (unmet need for help). This linear scale is based on a previous study (Skarsvåg, 2004) that found increased symptoms of depression with increased need for help. Previous use of Internet for health-related purposes during the previuos year was assessed by 3 questions (whether the participants have used the Internet to search for health-related information; search for information regarding mental health; discussed their own mental health on the Internet), with scores ranging from 1 (never) to 5 (more than 20 times). These three questions are thought to reflect the participant's prior behavior and experiences using the Internet seeking both somatic and mental-health-related information. Self-reported need for help by an Internet-based service such as MoodGYM was assessed by asking the participants if they feel the need for MoodGYM for themselves, for others they know, have other reasons for using MoodGYM, or if they are not interested in using MoodGYM. The items were scored "yes" or "no." This is thought to reflect mainly the participant's motivation for using a service such as MoodGYM. The participants were provided with a written general description about an Internet-based self-help program based on the characteristics of MoodGYM. The description focused specifically on features such as anonymity, low threshold services (from home), availability, and easy access. Finally, the purpose of MoodGYM as a program for preventing depression was elaborated.

Statistics

Statistical analyses were performed with Statistical Package for the Social Sciences (SPSS for Windows, version 13; SPSS, Inc.). For comparison between groups, ANOVA with post hoc Bonferroni was employed for continuous and chi-square test for nominal variables. To study interrelationship between continuous variables linear regression was carried out. Pearson correlations were conducted to investigate covariation between variables. A significance level of .05 was chosen. Listwise deletion was applied to missing data. The total N therefore varied in the analyses.

RESULTS

Feeling Need for Help, Depression, Negative Thinking, and Web Experience

The results show that 45.8 percent of the participants have felt a need for help with psychological problems. Both participants who have sought help for their problems and participants who have not are represented in this group. The total sample can therefore be divided into three groups according to their help-seeking behavior. More than half ($n = 195$, 54.2 percent) of the participants in the sample reported no need for help (no-need group). About one-third ($n = 115$, 31.9 percent) of the respondents have felt a need for help but refrained from seeking help and therefore have an unmet need for help (unmet-need group). The rest of the respondents ($n = 50$, 13.9 percent) have sought help for their problems (sought-help group).

One-way ANOVA was used to compare symptoms of depression (CES-D) in the three groups (Table 1). The unmet-need group and the sought-help group reported significantly more symptoms of depression than the no-need group ($F(2,333) = 19.90$, $p = .000$). There was no significant difference in symptoms of depression between the unmet-need group and the sought-help group. The ANOVA results also show that 40.4 percent of the unmet-need group reported a CES-D score above the cutoff (value = 16) for depressive

TABLE 1. Center for Epidemiologic Studies-Depression Scale (CES-D) and Habit Index Negative Thinking (HINT): Means, Standard Deviations, and One-Way Analyses of Variance (ANOVAs) for Effects of Three Help-Seeking Groups

	Unmet-need group		Sought-help group		No-need group		ANOVA			
	n	*M (SD)*	*n*	*M (SD)*	*n*	*M (SD)*	*n*	*df*	*F*	*p*
CES-D	104	14.80^a (9.40)	43	12.40^b (7.90)	186	9.00 (6.40)	333	2	19.90*	.000
HINT	111	43.50^c (20.30)	47	40.30^d (21.20)	191	31.10 (17.50)	349	2	16.20*	.000

Note: Post hoc Bonferroni was carried out to show what classes differed between one another. Significant differences are marked with separate specific notes.
[a]Unmet-need group differed from no-need group. $M_{diff} = 5.80$ $p = .000$.
[b]Sought-help group differed from no-need group. $M_{diff} = 3.40$ $p = .026$.
[c]Unmet-need group differed from no-need group. $M_{diff} = 12.40$ $p = .000$.
[d]Sought-help group differed from no-need group. $M_{diff} = 9.10$ $p = .010$.
*$p < .001$.

symptoms. In the sought-help group, 30.2 percent ($n = 15$) had a CES-D score above cutoff for depressive symptoms. In the no-need group, 13.4 percent ($n = 26$) of the participants score above the cutoff for depressive symptoms. There is a significantly greater percentage of participants in the unmet-need group and sought-help groups than in the no-need group, who have a CES-D score above the cutoff for depressive symptoms ($\chi^2(2, N = 333) = 27.6, p < .001$).

One-way ANOVA was conducted to compare the intergroup differences of negative thinking (Table 1), according to help seeking behavior ($F(2,349) = 16.20$, $p < .001$). The unmet-need group reported significantly more negative thinking than the no-need group ($M_{diff} = 12.40$, $p = .000$). The sought-help group also reported significantly more negative thinking than the no-need group ($M_{diff} = 9.1$, $p = .01$). There was no significant difference between the unmet-need group and the sought-help group.

A total of 92.4 percent of the participants had used the Internet to search for health information during the previous year. No significant difference between the groups occurred. As regards searching for mental health information, the sought-help group (54.1 percent) and the unmet-need group (45.1 percent) have used the Internet to a larger degree to search for mental health information than the no-need group (27.0 percent) ($\chi^2(2, N = 257) = 12.84, p < .002$).

Participants in the unmet-need group also reported discussing their own mental health on the Internet more often than the no-need group ($\chi^2(2, N = 257) = 7.20, p < .027$).

Participants in the unmet-need group ($n = 115$, 50.0 percent) and the sought-help group ($n = 50$, 38.8 percent) reported significantly more need for MoodGYM for themselves than the no-need group ($n = 195$, 13.9 percent) ($\chi^2(2, N = 357) = 48.27$, $p < .001$). Regarding the need for others, 38.9 percent ($n = 139$) of the participants reported that someone they know would be in need of MoodGYM. There were no significant intergroup differences on this measure. Most of the participants ($n = 300$, 84.1 percent) have a positive evaluation of this web-based CBT program.

Intention to Use MoodGYM

Correlations between intention to use MoodGYM and other variables assumed to be associated with use are presented in Table 2. The correlations show that the intention to use MoodGYM is

TABLE 2. Means, Standard Deviations, and Intercorrelations of Variables in the Study Affecting Intention to Use MoodGYM ($N = 217$)

Variable	1	2	3	4	5	6	7	8	9
1. Intention to use MoodGYM	–	.24**	.33**	.43**	.24**	.15*	−.01	.28**	.64**
2. HINT			.54**	.24**	−.05	.03	−.10	.19**	.22**
3. CES-D				.36**	−.14*	−.05	−.24**	.23**	.29**
4. Previous help-seeking					.07	.11**	−.04	.21**	
5. Attitude						.38**	.41**	.01	.23**
6. Perceived behavioral control							.37**	.09	.08
7. Subjective norm								.01	−.04
8. Sought mental health info on web									.14*
9. Need for help: MoodGYM									–
M	3.50	3.04	11.16	.74	5.55	6.11	6.16	1.57	2.74
SD	1.68	1.71	8.42	.89	.95	.95	.98	.93	1.10

Note: $^*p < .05$; $^{**}p < .01$.

significantly associated with all selected variables, except for subjective norms. The strongest correlation emerged between intention to use MoodGYM and need for an Internet-based self-help service like MoodGYM.

A hierarchical, multiple-regression analysis was conducted to investigate the effects of the psychological, previous help-seeking, attitude toward the Internet, and TPB variables on intention. In step 1, intention was regressed on negative thinking (HINT), which obtained a significant beta ($\beta = .24$, $p < .001$). The R^2 was significantly raised in step 2 when intention was regressed on depressive symptoms (CES-D), with a significant beta ($\beta = .29$, $p < .001$). The beta weight of HINT was no longer significant in step 2 ($\beta = .09$). In step 3, intention was regressed on need for help with psychological problems in the past (previous help-seeking). R^2 increased significantly in step 3 with a significant beta ($\beta = .36$, $p < .001$). The CES-D retained a significant beta ($\beta = .17$, $p < .05$) in this step. In step 4, intention was regressed on attitude ($\beta = .26$, $p < .001$), perceived behavioral control ($\beta = .05$, $p > .40$) and subjective norm ($\beta = .05$, $p > .40$). R^2 increased significantly, where only attitude had a significant beta. CES-D and previous help-seeking retained significant beta (CES-D: $\beta = .22$, $p < .01$; previous help seeking: $\beta = .327$, $p < .001$). The R^2 increased significantly in step 5 when intention was regressed on seeking information about mental health on the Internet, with a significant beta ($\beta = .16$, $p < .01$). The beta of CES-D ($\beta = .19$, $p < .01$), previous help-seeking ($\beta = .30$, $p < .001$), and attitude ($\beta = .26$, $p < .001$) retained significance. In step 6, intention was regressed on need for help by Internet-based intervention (MoodGYM), with a significant beta ($\beta = .50$, $p < .001$. R^2 increased significantly. Previous help-seeking ($\beta = .20$, $p < .001$), attitude ($\beta = .11$, $p < .05$), and seeking information about mental health on the Internet ($\beta = .14$, $p < .01$) retained significant betas. Interestingly, the beta of CES-D is no longer significant in step 6 ($\beta = .10$). R^2 in the final step was .51. The results are presented in Table 3.

The variables that remained substantial and statistically significant were then used in a final regression analysis. The overall regression model accounted for 49.0 percent of the variance of the intention to use an Internet-based self-help service such as MoodGYM. The psychological background variable (previous help-seeking) explains 16.6 percent of the variance, the

TABLE 3. Hierarchical Multiple Regression Analysis Predicting the Intention to Use MoodGYM (N = 217)

Predictor	B	SE B	β	Final β	R^2	ΔR^2
Step 1:						
HINT	.24	.06	.24***	.01	.06	.06***
Step 2:						
CES-D	1.15	.30	.29***	.10	.12	.06***
Step 3:						
Previous help-seeking	.67	.12	.35***	.20***	.23	.11***
Step 4:						
Perceived behavioral control	.08	.12	.05			
Attitude	.45	.12	.25***	.11*		
Subjective norm	.06	.12	.06	.02	.29	.06***
Step 5:						
Sought mental health info on Internet	.29	.11	.16**	.14**	.31	.02**
Step 6:						
Need for help: MoodGYM	.75	.08	.49***	.49***	.51	.20***

Note: *p < .05; **p < .01; ***p < .001. The dependent measure is the mean score of intention to use MoodGYM. $\Delta R^2 = R^2$ change.

TPB variable (attitude) explains 6.4 percent of the variance, use of Internet for health-related purposes explains 4.7 percent. Finally, the need for MoodGYM was the most important predictor of the intention to use MoodGYM, explaining 21.6 percent of the variance. In step 1, intention was regressed on previous help-seeking, which obtained a significant beta ($\beta = .41$, $p < .001$). In step 2, intention was regressed on the TPB measure of attitude, which obtained a significant beta ($\beta = .25$, $p < .001$). The R^2 was significantly raised in step 2. Intention was regressed on use of Internet for health-related searching in step 3, which obtained a significant beta ($\beta = .22$, $p < .001$), and R^2 increased significantly. In step 4, intention was regressed on need for Internet-based intervention (MoodGYM), which obtained a significant beta ($\beta = .51$, $p < .001$). R^2 increased significantly. All variables remained substantial and statistically significant, suggesting that the effect of these variables was largely independent (see Table 2). R^2 in the final step was .49. The variance inflation factors varied from 1.00 to 1.21, indicating that there was no reason to suspect multi-collinearity problems. The Durbin-Watson observer is 1.96, indicating no dependency among residuals.

DISCUSSION

The results of this study show that a substantial number of students with an unmet need for help have positive attitudes about using MoodGYM. This means that web-based CBT has the potential of reaching a group of students with psychological problems who traditional mental health services have not been able to reach in the past. Considering the proportion of students in this study with an unmet need for help (31.9 percent) and the proportion of these with positive feeling about using MoodGYM (91.2 percent), it might be possible to reach many of the students with an unmet need for help, using Web-based CBT.

The findings from our study reveal that almost half (45.8 percent) of the students have felt a need for help with psychological problems, and that only 43 percent of those in need have actually sought help. The relatively high number of participants with a felt need for help with psychological problems is not limited to clinical conditions but is reflecting a subjective need for help. In a relatively recent epidemiological study from Norway (Kringlen, Torgersen, & Cramer, 2001) it was found that about 3 percent of the population met the diagnostic criteria for a mental health condition during one year. Furthermore, both students with a met and an unmet need for help report symptoms of depression and negative thinking more frequently than participants with no need for help. Accordingly, offering MoodGYM, which focuses primarily on depressive symptoms and negative thinking, to the student population, which focuses primarily on depressive symptoms and negative thinking, may be an optimal intervention to reduce such kinds of symptoms and thinking in this group of young adults. Furthermore, our findings indicate that seeking health information on the Internet is a relatively common behavior among students, especially among those with a need for help with psychological problems. These are important findings because we know that consumers are much more likely to adopt a new technology if they have used similar technologies in the past (Korgaonkar & Moschis, 1987; Jarvenpaa et al., 2000). Accordingly, almost one-third (28.9 percent) of the students reported a need for MoodGYM for themselves, while even more (38.9 percent) regarded MoodGYM as a possible helping tool for others. While students seem to have an overall positive attitude toward an Internet-based self-help service like MoodGYM, we also wanted to measure students' intention to use MoodGYM, and to find out the predictors of their intention.

Negative thinking and depressive symptoms differed significantly between the groups based on need for help. However, in the final regression model the beta weights of these predictors were not significant. The intercorrelation between depression (CES-D) and negative thinking (HINT) is also relatively high, indicating that these measures might explain some similar factors related to intention, which is an established finding in the literature on depression and negative thinking (Beck, 1967, 1976). The need for help with psychological problems appeared to be a stronger predictor of intention than negative thinking (HINT) and depression (CES-D). Actual felt need for help, in this respect an unmet need for help with psychological problems, indicates stronger intention to use MoodGYM. Consequently, some students with a high degree of depressive symptoms or negative thinking but with no felt need for help might not use MoodGYM.

The results reveal attitude in the TPB model is a predictor that remains significant through all steps of the regression analysis. Perceived behavioral control and subjective norm represent no main factors for the intention to use MoodGYM. For perceived behavioral control, it might be a problem that the behavior in question (i.e., the use of a Norwegian version of MoodGYM), did not exist as a service when the study was carried out. Accordingly, the participants had to consider statements about control over behaviors that they had never performed themselves. The fear of stigma and consequences of seeking help are important factors in avoiding help-seeking (Halter, 2003). However, by using Internet as a medium the possibility of personal anonymity is high. Accordingly, in the aspect that subjective norm include social pressure, confusing MoodGYM is interesting because it can be applied in one's own home. Consequently, social pressure and the beliefs of others might be of less importance to users.

Seeking mental health information on the Internet is also a contributor to the final model. Implicit is the notion that individuals who are accustomed to using the Internet as a tool for finding information are also slightly more inclined to use the Internet as a tool to diminish psychological distress. This is in line with previous research showing that consumers more readily adopt new technologies if they have used similar technologies before (Korgaonkar & Moschis, 1987; Jarvenpaa et al., 2000).

The empirical model of the intention to use MoodGYM explained almost 5 percent of the variance in intention to use MoodGYM, with

FIGURE 1. Empirical Model of the Intention to Use Web-Based CBT

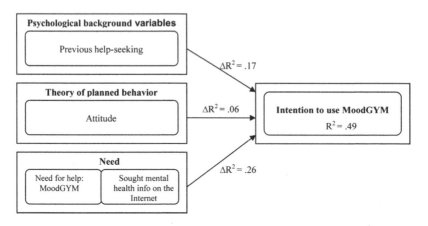

the need for an Internet-based self-help service like MoodGYM as the strongest single predictor of intention. MoodGYM is an alternative mental health service designed for helping people who for a variety of reasons do not seek help from other mental health services. There are a number of students with an unmet need for help who feel positively toward using MoodGYM. This is encouraging as it supports that MoodGYM will fulfill its intended purpose. The empirical model is illustrated in Figure 1.

CONCLUSIONS, SHORTCOMINGS, AND FURTHER RESEARCH

There are currently some problems associated with Internet-based interventions concerning the nature and ethics of the services. Many websites offer counseling, but the degree of professionalism differs widely (Griffiths & Christensen, 2000). A general review of this critique has not been included in the current study, as the main focus was assessing the need and use of a specific unattended Internet-based counseling service. Another possible shortcoming is the fact that aspects such as personality and demographic variables are not taken into consideration in predicting the intention to use MoodGYM. The importance of these variables represents issues for further research. Some shortcomings also concern the use of TPB in this study. The theory is based on the assumption that human beings are usually rational and makes systematic use of information available to them (Ajzen & Fishbein, 1980). Unconscious motives are therefore not considered directly. In online interventions the aspect of subjective norm needs further exploration since norms, social pressure, and the beliefs of others might be of less importance to users. Usually, in TPB research, a follow-up measurement of the participants' actual behavior is included. This might constitute a problem in the current study since the actual behavior (using MoodGYM) cannot possibly be executed before MoodGYM is implemented. TPB has still been selected as an appropriate method of predicting use of MoodGYM since the model has proven robust and stable during years of research. The relatively high number of participants with a felt need for help with psychological problems could be a result of sampling. Although the lectures were selected by random, most of the participants were in their first year at the university. Based on knowledge that more than 60 percent of first-year students report homesickness and have other adjustment issues, this result could to some degree be a result of a biased sample. The very high correlation ($r = .64$) between need for help by Internet self-help (e.g., MoodGYM) and intent to use MoodGYM suggesting that one variable is an indicator of the other or that the two variables may be capturing a similar construct. There might have been a response bias, in particular a bias to respond in a consistent fashion. Replication of this concept could be necessary to unravel the effect of the measures on the outcome.

It is evident that many students with a need for help do not intend to use Internet-based services or other mental health services. Several factors will have to be taken into account to explain this. Severity of depression, lack of motivation, lack of knowledge about effective treatment, and lack of insight into one's own problems are possible areas for exploration. Increasing the availability of information about alternative help resources such as MoodGYM might be a possible approach to reaching out to individuals who do not seek help.

An important distinction between different Internet-based interventions is whether they are unattended or offer/require additional support from mental health personnel. Both kinds of interventions are proven effective in reducing symptoms of mild to moderate depression (Andersson et al., 2005; Christensen et al., 2004; Clarke et al., 2005). All of these Internet-based interventions are based on CBT, but little is known about the effect of support or feedback versus no feedback. Operating costs would obviously be higher for interventions with support. A goal for further research could be to investigate the effect for unattended systems with automatic tailored e-mail feedback, focusing on cost-benefit, personal variables, and demographics.

In conclusion, the results of this study lend support to the implementation of an Internet-based counseling service to students of higher education.

REFERENCES

Adlaf, E. M, Glicksman, L., Demers, A., & Newton, T. B. (2001). The prevalence of elevated psychological distress among Canadian undergraduates: Findings from the 1998 Canadian campus survey (editorial). *Journal of American College Health*, *50*, 67–72.

Ajzen, I. (1991). The theory of planned behavior. *Organizational Behavior and Human Decision Processes*, *50*, 179–211.

Ajzen, I. (2002). *Constructing a TPB questionnaire: Conceptual and methodological considerations*. Retrieved March 1, 2007, from http://www.people.umass.edu/aizen/pdf/tpb.measurement.pdf.

Ajzen, I., & Fishbein, M. (1980). *Understanding attitudes and predicting social behavior*. Englewood Cliffs, NJ: Prentice-Hall.

Andersson, G., Berström, J., Holländare, F., Carlbring, P., Kaldo, V., & Ekselius, L. (2005). Internet-based self-help for depression: Randomised controlled trial. *British Journal of Psychiatry*, *187*, 456–461.

Armitage, C. J., & Conner, M. (2001). Efficacy of the theory of planned behaviour: A meta-analytic review. *British Journal of Social Psychology*, *40*, 471–499.

Australian National University. (2007). The MoodGYM training program. Retrieved September 4, 2007, from http://www.ehub.anu.edu.au/research/moodgym.php.

Beck, A. T. (1967). *Depression: Clinical, experimental, and theoretical aspects*. New York: Harper and Row.

Beck, A. T. (1976). *Cognitive therapy and the emotional disorders*. Madison, CT: International University Press.

Beck, A. T., Rush, A. J., Shaw, B. F., & Emery, G. (1979). *Cognitive therapy of depression*. New York: Guilford Press.

Butler, A. C., Chapman, J. E., Forman, E. M., & Beck, A. T. (2006). The empirical status of cognitive-behavioral therapy: A review of meta-analyses. *Clinical Psychological Review*, *26*, 17–31.

CCBT (2007). FearFighter. Retrieved September 4, 2007, from http://www.fearfighter.com/index.htm.

Chambless, D. L., & Ollendick, T. H. (2001). Empirically supported psychological interventions. *Annual Review of Psychology, 52,* 685–716.

Christensen, H., Griffiths, K. M., & Jorm A. F. (2004). Delivering depression interventions using the Internet: Positive results from a large randomised controlled trial. *British Medical Journal, 328*(7434), 265–269.

Churchill, R., Hunot, V., Corney, R., Knapp, M., McGuire, H., Tylee, A., et al. (2001). A systematic review of controlled trials of the effectiveness and cost-effectiveness of brief psychological treatments for depression. *Health Technol Assess, 5*(35), 1–173.

Clarke, G., Eubanks, D., Reid, E., Kelleher, C., O'Connor, E., DeBar, L. L., et al. (2005). Overcoming depression on the Internet (ODIN) (2): A randomized trial of a self-help depression skills program with reminders. [Electronic version]. *Journal of Medical Internet Research, 7*(2), e16.

Cohen, J. (1992). A power primer. *Psychological Bulletin, 112,* 155–159.

Dabholkar, P. A. (1992). The role of prior behavior and category-based affect in on-site service encounters. In Sherry, J. F., & Sternthal, B. (Eds.), *Diversity in consumer behavior* (pp. 19, 563–569). Provo, UT: Association for Consumer Research.

Dabholkar, P. A. (1996). Consumer evaluations of new technology-based self-service options: An investigation of alternative models of service quality. *International Journal of Research in Marketing, 13*(1), 29–51.

Department of Health. (2001). *Treatment choice in psychological therapies and counselling. Evidence-based clinical practice guidelines.* London: Department of Health Publications.

Francis, J. J., Johnston M., Eccles, M. P., Grimshaw, J., & Kaner, E. F. S. (2004). *Constructing questionnaires based on the theory of planned behaviour: A manual for health services researchers.* Retrieved March 1, 2007, from http://www.rebeqi.org/ViewFile.aspx?itemID=212.

Frazer, C. J., Christensen, H. & Griffiths, K. M. (2005). Effectiveness of treatments for depression in older people. *The Medical Journal of Australia, 182*(12), 627–632.

Griffiths, K., & Christensen, H. (2000). Quality of web based information on treatment of depression: Cross sectional survey. *British Medical Journal, 321*(7275), 1511–1515.

Grohol, J. M. (2001). *Best practices of etherapy: Clarifying the definition of etherapy.* Retrieved March 1, 2007, from http://psychcentral.com/best/best5.htm.

Halter, M. J. (2003). The influence of stigma on help seeking attitudes for depression. *Dissertation Abstracts International: Section B: The Sciences & Engineering, 64*(3), B0: 1178.

Interactive Health Systems. (2007). Mastering my life. Retrieved September 4, 2007, from http://www.masteringmylife.com/mml.asp?p?0.

Jarvenpaa, S. L., Tractinsky, N., & Vitale, M. (2000). Consumer trust in an Internet store. *Information Technology Management, 1,* 45–71.

Kessler, R. C., Demler, O., Frank, R. G., Olfson, M., Pincus, H. A., Walters, E. E., et al. (2005). Prevalence and treatment of mental disorders, 1990 to 2003. *The New England Journal of Medicine, 352*(24), 2515–23.

Korgaonkar, P., & Moschis, G. P. (1987). Consumer adoption of videotex services. *Journal of Direct Marketing, 1*(4), 63–71.

Kringlen, E., Torgersen, S., & Cramer V. A. (2001). Norwegian psychiatric epidemiological study. *Archives of General Psychiatry, 158,* 1091–1098.

Lewinsohn, P. M., Hops, H., Roberts, R. E., Seeley, J. R., & Andrews, J. A. (1993). Adolescents psychopathology: 1. Prevalence and incidence of depression and other DSM-III disorders in high school students. *Journal of Abnormal Psychology, 110*(2), 203–215.

Løwe, T., & Sæthe, J. P. (2007). *Studenters inntekt, økonomi og boforhold. Studenters levekår 2005. [Students income, economics, and housing situation. Students circumstances 2005].* Statistics Norway, 2. Retrieved September 20, 2007, from http://www.ssb.no/emner/00/02/rapp_200702/rapp_200702.pdf.

Mental Health Norway. (2004). *Den nye folkesykdommen. [The new public disease].* Retrieved May 19, 2006, from http://www.mentalhelse.no/?module=Articles; action=Article.publicOpen;ID=4046.

Mindstreet (2007). Good days ahead. Retrieved September 4, 2007, from http://www.mindstreet.com/.

Ministry of Health (1997). *Åpenhet og helhet. Om psykiske lidelser og tjenestetilbudene.* Stortingsmelding nr. 25 (1996–1997) *[Openness and Comprehensiveness. Mental Disorders and Mental Services.* White Paper No. 25 (1996–1997)]. Oslo, Norway: Ministry of Health and Social Affairs.

Moussavi, S., Chatterji, S., Verdes, E., Tandon, A., Patel, V., & Ustun, B. (2007). Depression, chronic diseases, and decrements in health: Results from the World Health Surveys. *Lancet, 370,* 851–858.

Proudfoot, J., Ryden, C., Everitt, B., Shapiro, D., Goldberg, D., Mann, A., et al. (2004). Clinical efficacy of computerised cognitive- behavioural therapy for anxiety and depression in primary care: Randomised controlled trial. *British Journal of Psychiatry, 185,* 46–54.

Radloff, L. S. (1977). The CES-D: A self-report depression scale for research in the general population. *Applied Psychological Measurement, 1*(3), 385–401.

Radloff, L. S. (1991). The use of the center for epidemiologic studies depression scale in adolescents and young adults. *Journal of Youth and Adolescence, 20*(2), 149–166.

Rochlen, A. B., Zack, J. S., & Speyer, C. (2004). Online therapy: Review of relevant definitions, debates, and current empirical support. *Journal of Clinical Psychology, 60,* 269–283.

Royal College of Psychiatrists, Royal College of Physicians of London, & British Medical Association. (2001). *Mental illness: Stigmatisation and discrimination within the medical profession* (Council Report CR91). London: Royal College of Psychiatrists.

Sheeran, P. (2002). Intention-behavior relations: A conceptual and empirical review. *European Review of Social Psychology, 12,* 1–36.

Skarsvåg, H. A. (2004). Seeking treatment or not? A study on mental helpseeking and its relation to needs, symptoms, person characteristica, experiences and attitudes in a student population. Master's thesis, University of Tromsø. Retrieved September 4, 2007, from http://www.ub.uit.no/munin/handle/10037/1164.

Stecker, T. (2004). Well-being in an academic environment. *Medical Education*, *38*(5), 465–478.

Ultrasis (2007). Beating the blues. Retrieved September 4, 2007, from http://www.ultrasis.com/products/product.jsp?product_id=1.

Verplanken, B., Friborg, O., Wang, C. E., Trafimow, D., & Woolf, K. (2007). Mental habits: Metacognitive reflection on negative self-thinking. *Journal of Personality and Social Psychology*, *92*(3), 526–541.

Walden, C. (2003). *The mental health of students in higher education* (Council Report CR112). London: Royal College of Psychiatrists. Retrieved March 1, 2007, from http://www.rcpsyc.ac.uk/files/pdfversion/cr112.pdf.

Wang, P. S., Aguilar-Gaxiola, S., Alonso, J., Angermeyer, M. C., Borges, G., Bromet, E. J., et al. (2007). Use of mental health services for anxiety, mood, and substance disorders in 17 countries in the WHO world mental health surveys. *Lancet, 370*, 841–850.

Wells, K. B., Burnam, M. A., Rogers, W., Hays, R., & Camp, P. (1992). The course of depression in adult outpatients: Results from the medical outcomes study. *Archives of General Psychiatry*, *49*, 788–794.

World Health Organization. (2001a). Mental and neurological disorders, 2001. Retrieved May 20, 2006, from http://www.who.int/mental_health/evidence/en/prevention_of_mental_disorders_sr.pdf.

World Health Organization (2001b). *The World Health Report 2001—Mental health: New understanding, new hope*. Retrieved March 1, 2007, from http://www.who.int/whr/2001/en/index.html

Issues in the Evaluation of an Online Prevention Exercise

Bhavana Pahwa
Dick Schoech

PREVENTION RESEARCH

Much research has been conducted in the past 20 years on how best to prevent substance abuse in youth (Bosworth, 1998; Schinke, Brounstein, Gardner, 2002; Substance Abuse and Mental Health Services Administration [SAHMSA], 2000; National Institute on

Drug Abuse [NIDA], 2004). Prevention programs make a difference. Research-based prevention programs are effective not only in stopping youth from initiating substance use, but also in reducing the number of individuals who become dependent. Current model prevention programs show an average reduction in substance use by program participants of 25 percent (NIDA, 2003). The literature also suggests that prevention strategies based on information alone or "one shot" methods that utilize scare tactics are not effective (Tobler, 1992; Bosworth, 1998). Programs that strictly adhere to an intervention model based on developing social skills and skills for managing negative feelings are best (Gonet, 1994; Skiba, Monroe, & Wodarski, 2004). Booster sessions are important in establishing initial progress and in maintaining effects over time (NIDA, 2004).

According to the Monitoring the Future survey of 8th, 10th, and 12th graders, illicit drug use between 2001 and 2006 among students declined 23 percent (from 19.4 percent to 14.9 percent) (NIDA, 2006). Increased intolerance of drug use by the teen's friends has been cited as an important factor linked to the decrease in substance abuse among youth. Parental drug and alcohol use, failure of the adolescent to bond to school, problems in ability to regulate emotion, and poor interpersonal skills and peer relations are cited as factors increasing the risk of drug problem development (Brook, Whiteman, Nomura, Gordon, & Cohen, 1988; Hilarski, 2004). Family influences found to be related to the risk of alcohol and other drug abuse include modeling of drug using behavior and parental attitudes toward children's drug use. In addition, poor parenting practices, high levels of conflict in the family, and a low degree of bonding between children and parents appear to increase teens' risk for the abuse of alcohol and other drugs (Dyer, 2005; Minuchin & Fishman, 1981; Hilarski, 2004).

In early adolescence, when teens begin spending less time at home and more time with friends, peers become a significant source of support and intimacy (Berndt & Perry, 1990). Research has consistently shown that young adolescents with positive lifestyles are apt to select pro-social peers, whereas young adolescents oriented toward antisocial or problem behavior are likely to select similarly deviant peers (Bush, Weinfurt, & Ianotti, 1994). The literature also suggests that demographic factors, such as age and gender, are directly linked with substance abuse or with delinquent behavior. According to Svensson (2003), environmental factors, such as parental monitoring and peer delinquency, were directly linked with age and gender. Younger children and girls were more closely supervised and controlled by parents, and therefore tended to have less involvement with delinquent peers. This in turn reduced the likelihood that younger children and girls would get involved in substance abuse and other delinquent behavior.

ADVANTAGES OF ONLINE PREVENTION

Various features of the Internet make it suitable for prevention programming for teens. Supporting the constructivist approach to learning, the Internet can be used to create prevention programs that are interactive, under user control, and individually tailored to the user's demographic and risk profile (Tsai, 2008; Herie, 2005). Online prevention programs can also take advantage of multimedia and game features of the Internet that attract teens. The Internet also lends itself to maintaining intervention fidelity (Christensen & Griffiths, 2002). Follow-up sessions, which may be required to maintain intervention effects, can also be designed and delivered at predetermined times. Use of online interventions can be easily tracked and data collected more efficiently compared to traditional methods. In addition, modifying and distributing paper-based prevention curriculum is slower and more resource intensive than changing online curriculum. Finally, online prevention interventions may generate more honest and candid responses because of the user's perception of anonymity. This perception of anonymity is especially important in areas such as teen substance abuse, where recipients may be reluctant to share personal information due to embarrassment or fear of negative reprisals (Christensen & Griffiths, 2002).

PREVENTION WEBSITES

Currently, the Internet offers many prevention programs for problems, including AIDS (TeenAIDS-PeerCorps, n.d.), teen pregnancy (Advocates for Youth, n.d.), and bullying (PACER National Center for Bullying Prevention, n.d.). Providing a summary of these online prevention programs is beyond the scope of this article given their diverse foci and the variety of curricula formats.

To help design the evaluation of the anger management exercise presented in this article, teen and young adult online substance abuse prevention sites were reviewed with specific attention given to evaluative information (Table 1). Table 1 does not include online interventions that were not focused on youth substance abuse prevention, even those with strong evaluations. For example, not included is re-Mission, an online 3D adventure game with research showing effectiveness in helping teens fight cancer (HopeLab, 2007).

Most sites did not report the theoretical model used to develop content. The majority of the sites relied on text rather than on multimedia and other interactive tools that are thought to enhance user involvement (United Nations Office on Drugs and Crime, 2002). Column three in Table 1 indicates the type of content each site contained, for example, news, frequently asked questions (FAQs), links to resources, discussion forums, screening, games, and arty efforts such as pictures, storytelling, animations, and music.

EVALUATIONS OF ONLINE PREVENTION

Column 4 of Table 1 presents evaluative information that was found on the websites or from a Google search. Typically, sites in Table 1 that were free-form, multimedia oriented, interactive, designed to be fun, and that took advantage of advanced Internet features lacked evaluative information. Evaluations were primarily available for sites that presented traditional prevention curricula, for example, a series of lessons that could be downloaded and used in a classroom or accessed from the website.

The majority of evaluations used a randomized pre-post design based on the theory of planned behavior (Glanz, & Rimer, 2005; Ajzen, 2006). The theory of planned behavior (TPB) suggests that behavioral intention determines actual behavior. Behavioral intention is influenced by

TABLE 1. Online Prevention Programs Reviewed for this Evaluation

Name and URL	Focus	Content Present	Evaluation
AlcoholEdu for College, www.alcoholedu.com/	Alcohol use by college students	3-hour text-based course including assessments and tests	Pre-posttest self-report from students on knowledge, attitudes, social norms, and behavior regarding alcohol use
Champion of Hope http://championofhope.homestead.com/Hope1.html	Educating, preventing, and supporting teens affected by addictions	Moderated support group via chat	No evaluations found
Consider This www.considerthisusa.net/	Change social influence about smoking in youth, grades 6–9	Modules on media, relationships, body-mind, decision making, and resistance strategies	Randomized pre-posttest controlled trials with 3,311 students in the United States and Australia
The Cool Spot www.thecoolspot.gov/	Give teens 11–13 a clearer picture about peer alcohol use and resisting peer pressure.	Quizzes, information, and animation	No evaluations found
e-CHUG—High School www.e-chug.com/hs/	Motivate and support youth to abstain or reduce the risks of alcohol consumption	Detailed self-assessment followed by personalized feedback on how to reduce use and risks.	6 controlled studies on 5 campuses. No evaluative information found on the high school version.
Freevibe http://freevibe.com/	Provides knowledge and personal empowerment to help teens reject drugs and risky behavior	Multimedia-based media campaign approach including art, stories, news, ads, interviews, and user feedback	Part of overall evaluation of the National Youth Anti-drug Media Campaign. TPB type model used
Girl Power www.girlpower.gov/	Promoting positive body image, healthy choices for girls ages 10–15 years	Mostly text-based information and links	Limited evaluative information found. Most lacked controls

Website	Purpose/Audience	Content	Evaluation
Joe Chemo www.joechemo.org/	Tobacco use by 4th and 5th grade students	Mostly text-based information, screening, e-cards, and resources.	No evaluations found
My Student Body www.mystudentbody.com	Beliefs, behaviors, and consequences regarding alcohol, STDs, tobacco, eating disorders, and stress prevention for college students	Interactive information including flash animation peer stories	Randomized, controlled clinical trial with students' self-reports on behavior change, knowledge, attitudes, behavioral control, and intention
NIDA for Teens www.teens.drugabuse.gov/	Educate teens 11–15 on the science behind drug abuse and making healthy decisions.	Information, FAQs, animations, quizzes, stories, and games	No evaluations found
One Teen at a Time www.socialworkers.org/practice/oneteen/	Information on teen problems to help achieve healthy and positive outcomes	Informational pages and downloads for teens, professionals, and parents	No evaluations found
The Reconstructor http://reconstructors.rice.edu/recon1/	Making healthier choices by avoiding drugs that are abused	Interactive learning adventure game that uses music and sound effects	35 item pre-posttest distributed to 289 students resulted in a significant increase in knowledge. No theory specified but website design based on constructivist theory of knowledge gained
Science, Tobacco, & You http://scienceu.fsu.edu/	Tobacco use by 4th to 6th grade students	Hands-on, inquiry-based, science curriculum for teachers	Differences between pre-posttest of intervention and comparison group on beliefs, knowledge, attitudes, and other measures, but not on behaviors and intentions

(Continued)

TABLE 1. Online Prevention Programs Reviewed for this Evaluation *(continued)*

Name and URL	Focus	Content Present	Evaluation
StepOnline (**St**udents **T**eachers **E**mployers **P**arents) www.steponline.com/	Drug use by youth, peer pressure, media literacy, goal setting, and decision making	Information, videos, art, discussion boards, stories, and advice	No evaluations found
Teen Central www.teencentral.net/	Allow teens to discuss feelings and problems, find resources, and consult with professionals	Information, resources, stories, and celebrities' stories	No evaluations found
TeenNet CyberIsle www.cyberisle.org/	Teen choices concerning positive lifestyle behaviors	Information, discussion forums, assessments, simulations, links, and games	Surveys, focus groups, participatory action research. The online smoking booklet was evaluated in a randomized clinical trail assessing intentions and behaviors at pre, post, and 3/6 month follow-up.
There4me www.There4me.com	Help for teens 12–16 with issues such as bullying, exams, drugs, and self-harm	Information, message board, e-mail advice, and games	No evaluations found. Site contains satisfaction survey
Virtual Party www.virtual-party.org	Provides youth information about alcohol, other drugs, and mental health issues, emphasizing healthy choices and harm reduction.	Resource list of links and game where users attend a virtual party as one of several possible characters	No evaluations found. An on-site feedback form is available
Vstreet www.vstreet.com	To give youth the skills and support needed to live on their own.	E-mail, bulletin boards, chat, journaling, and interactive animated curriculum/stories	Randomized pre-post with control self reports of knowledge, change, and satisfaction.

a person's attitudes toward the behavior, feelings about one's ability to control a behavior (behavioral control), and perceptions of whether significant others approve or disapprove of the behavior (behavioral norms). Thus, most evaluative studies relied on self-report of behavioral intention and its predictors rather than measuring actual behavior change. Sites that allowed teens to come and go as they desired tended to not have evaluative information; for example, Freevibe.com.

Most websites in Table 1 with evaluations found the intervention effective in preventing substance abuse. However, the detailed measures for success varied substantially. While the TPB model typically does not view knowledge as a predictor of behavioral intent and subsequent behavior change, knowledge was seen as a success measure in most evaluations. TPB theorizes that knowledge does not prevent substance abuse; it just makes for more informed users (Glanz & Rimer, 2005). In addition, sites often were successful on some measures and not successful on others; for example, significant changes on intention to change and actual behavior change seem to be the most difficult to achieve. Many issues surfaced during the evaluations. Some issues concerned the sensitivity of scales or the fact that teens scored high on their pretests, making posttest significance difficult to obtain. Fidelity was often an issue; for example, sites such as Science, Tobacco, & You found the need for teacher training, because teachers were part of the implementation process. Three and six month follow-ups were not frequently part of the evaluation. Few tried to link evaluation success with actual future substance abuse, perhaps due to the long-term funding needed for such evaluations. Sites with school contracts had a captive audience that allowed for evaluations that are more formal. Sites that serve college students seem to have the best evaluative information, probably due to their long-term contracts with colleges to serve specific student populations; for example, entering freshmen or those in fraternities. Thus, current evaluation of online prevention sites are occurring, but due to limited funding and the time required for rigorous evaluations, most are inconclusive and imprecise.

EVALUATION OF AN ONLINE ANGER MANAGEMENT EXERCISE

This section describes the online intervention being evaluated, the theoretical model used, the hypothesized results, and the evaluation design.

Based on a review of the literature and the sites in Table 1, an evaluation was designed to determine the effectiveness of the anger management exercise of SubstanceAbusePrevention.org. For simplicity, the term SAPVC (substance abuse prevention virtual community) will be used for the site at www.substanceabuseprevention.org. SAPVC was for teens ages 13 to 18 at risk for substance abuse. SAPVC was based on the resiliency model of prevention where content focused on reducing risk factors and fostering protective factors (Vance & Sanchez, 1998). SAPVC provides a variety of content including links to resources, screening, psychoeducational games, telling of stories, rap music, and skill-building exercises in areas such as anger management, refusal skills, and handling difficult situations. The anger management exercise of SAPVC (Figure 1) was selected for evaluation because several studies have found a definite link between inability to regulate emotions and express anger appropriately to the increased risk of substance abuse. For example, Cautin, Overholser, and Goetz (2001) found that externalized anger is linked with increased risk of alcohol abuse.

In the anger management exercises, the teens are presented with an introductory video that sets up a situation in which anger management skills are needed. Teens then can listen to two or more teen stories and two or more adult experts, watch two video scenarios of

FIGURE 1. Screenshot of the Anger Management Exercise of SAPVC

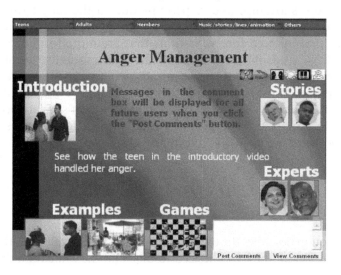

teens handling their anger preceded and followed by discussion from an expert, read or add comments in a discussion forum, and play a game on anger management. Teachers can have class discussion anytime during the exercise. If the exercise is completed alone outside of the classroom, teens type in their thoughts and reactions in the discussion forum, which are saved for peers and significant adults. No feedback is provided on postings in the discussion forum. Throughout the exercise, text-based help, guidance, and supportive messages appear in the center of the screen. Icons provide links to text containing additional help, discussion questions, future activities, and resources/references.

Theoretical Model and Hypotheses

The evaluation of the SAPVC anger management exercise used the Ajzen (2006) TPB model, which was modified to include the effect of various demographics and two environmental factors on the development of knowledge, attitudes, norms, and behavioral control (Figure 2). The two environmental factors were based on a review of the literature, which suggested that families and peers are major influences affecting teen drug use behavior. Knowledge was added to the model since it was the most frequently used measure in evaluating the online prevention sites in Table 1, and since some evidence exists that knowledge is important for online interventions (Schneider, Mataix-Cols, Marks, & Bachofen, 2005). Some factors considered but excluded in order to keep the model and measurement

FIGURE 2. Theoretical Model for the Evaluation

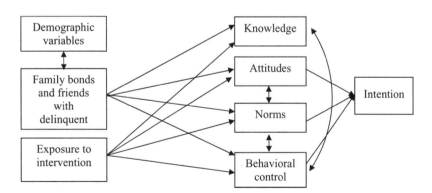

instruments from being overly complex were consistency in discipline, parental supervision, and parental and family history of drug use.

Based on the literature, it was hypothesized that one intervention of approximately 30 minutes was not sufficient to change attitudes, norms, behavioral control, or intention, but it could change knowledge. A significant change in knowledge along with the positive changes in attitudes, norms, behavioral control, and intention would indicate that the online exercise had the potential to change subsequent behavior. Thus, the evaluation was seen as not only a pilot study to obtain preliminary results of one exercise, but it was also seen as a way to test the potential of an evaluation design for future research on SAPVC.

Evaluation Design

The evaluation used nonrandomized treatment groups and a comparison group with a pre-posttest design. Although the randomized control trial is the "ideal" design, the nonrandomized comparison group with a pre-posttest design is cited as providing reliable results if the subjects in the groups are similar in demographic and other relevant characteristics (Isaac & Michael, 1977). For this evaluation, the issue was availability of teens. Teachers were on a tight schedule and were unwilling to participate in a study that had a complex research protocol. Subjects were selected from preassembled similar groups obtained from suburban middle schools and high schools and from after-school programs located in Texas and New York. Teens were assigned as availability permitted to the three separate experimental conditions and a comparison group as follows.

1. *Homework-only (HW) group* in which the teacher provided 21 middle school and 22 high school students in an after-school program with a brief introduction to the anger management exercise and its purpose and then allowed them to complete the exercise at their own pace independently in the school computer lab.
2. *Teacher-guided (TG) group* in which the teacher guided 23 middle school and 21 high school students through the online anger management exercises in a classroom setting. The middle school students were participants in a structured after-school program and the high school students were enrolled in a Peer Leadership class.
3. *Teacher-guided supplemented by homework (TG + HW) group* in which the teacher guided 12 middle school and 17 high school

students in an after-school program through the exercises class and then assigned the exercise as homework for the students to complete independently in the computer lab.

4. *Comparison group* in which 22 middle school students in an after-school program and 17 high school students in a peer leadership class were administered a survey at the beginning and end of a 1.5 hour class.

Students in each experimental group were administered a 60-item, paper/pencil survey before any verbal or online introduction/instruction was given about the exercise. A survey with the same questions was administered after students in each group completed the full exercise. Therefore, the TG + HW group was administered the survey on four separate occasions.

The survey was developed from the literature and administered by teachers. The survey could have been administered from SAPVC, but this would have required teachers and students to have access to computers and for SAPVC content to bypass school firewall, both of which would have added complexity to the research administration. Items for each variable in the survey were averaged to get an individual score for every respondent. The survey was pilot tested with 20 teens and items with low reliability and validity were removed. The resulting 60-item survey and Cronbach's Alpha reliability scores are reported in Table 2. In addition, reliability tests were run for the high school and the middle school teens. The high school survey had a pretest reliability of 0.88 and the middle school survey had a pretest reliability score of 0.75. It is possible that the junior high school reliability score was lower because junior high students have shorter attention spans and were enrolled in an after-school program rather than a school class. Thus, they may not have taken the evaluation less seriously and answered questions in a random manner. The combined sample reliability for the survey was .84 at pretest and .71 at posttest, which is considered good, although the drop between pre and post could indicate that test fatigue or other factors decreased reliability at posttest.

RESULTS

Results of the evaluation are presented in Tables 3, 4, and 5. Table 3 presents the pre and post means for each group. Table 4 presents the

TABLE 2. Measurement Instrument Reliability

Variable	Qs	Basis of Instrument Construction	Alpha
Knowledge	7	Developed from the contents of the anger management exercise	0.69
Behavioral control	5	Self-Efficacy Teen Conflict Survey[1]	0.85
Attitudes	9	Attitude Toward Conflict Scale[1]	0.67
Norms	7	Anger management for substance abuse and mental health clients http://kap.samhsa.gov/products/manuals/pdfs/anger2.pdf Controlling anger—a self help guide: http://www.welwynhatfield-pct.nhs.uk/comms/counselling/ Controlling%20 Anger.pdf.	0.76
Intentions	8	Violent Intentions—Teen Conflict Survey[1]	0.84
Friends' delinquent behavior	7	Delinquent Behavior-Adolescent Attitude Survey[1]	0.55
Family bonding	5	Family Bonding—Individual Protective Factor Index[1]	0.84

[1]*Source*: Dahlberg, Toal, Swahn, and Behrens (2005).

regression results. Table 5 presents the results from the Scheffe's post hoc test in the analysis of variance procedure in SPSS (Statistical Package for the Social Sciences), which shows which pairs of means were significant.

The data revealed that there was no significant gain in scores on any of the variables for the homework group. In fact, the regression scores in Table 4 show that the comparison group had a greater change in scores across all variables compared to the homework group. Table 4 also showed that the teacher-guided and the teacher-guided supplemented by homework group had significant changes in knowledge of anger management compared to the comparison group. However, in this study there was no significant gain in knowledge after the supplemented homework session compared to the teacher-guided session alone (Tables 3, 4, and 5). Although the change in attitude was significant for the TG + HW group, the negative regression score indicates that the comparison group had greater change than the experimental group. Furthermore, the results of the post hoc Scheffe's test in Table 5 reveal a significant difference between the HW group compared to the TG + HW group for both

TABLE 3. Pre- and Posttest means for Junior High and High School Students, Both Locations

Dependent Variables	Groups									Teacher guided plus homework (group 3)						
	Comparison group			Homework only (group 1)			Teacher guided (group 2)			Teacher guided			Homework			Tot Dif
	Pre	Post	Dif	Pre	Post	Dif	Pre	Post	Dif	Pre	Post	Dif	Pre	Post	Dif	
Knowledge	1.73	1.76	.03	1.71	1.68	-.03	1.63	1.84	.21	1.54	1.66	.12	1.67	1.75	.08	.21
Behavior control	3.77	3.79	.02	3.84	3.12	-.62	3.86	4.17	.31	3.46	3.35	-.09	3.28	3.52	.24	.06
Attitudes	3.56	3.68	.12	3.42	3.08	-.34	3.81	3.79	-.02	3.43	3.23	-.20	3.28	3.25	-.03	-.18
Norms	2.87	3.03	.16	2.80	2.88	.08	3.00	2.97	-.03	2.97	3.25	.28	3.11	3.40	.29	.43
Intentions	2.36	2.40	.04	2.56	2.49	-.07	2.43	2.63	.20	2.13	2.10	-.03	2.76	2.37	-.39	.24
Sample N	37,38	36,38		43	41,43		41,44	42,44		28	29		29	27,29		

TABLE 4. Regression of Treatment on Comparison Group

	HW vs. Comparison	TG vs. Comparison	TG + HW vs. Comparison
Knowledge	−.117 p = .304	.399* p = .00	.399* p = .001
Beh. control	−.370* p = .001	.205 p = .068	.040 p = .753
Attitude	−.305* p = .006	−.122 p = .285	−.244* p = .048
Norms	−.067 p = .557	−.157 p = .175	.213 p = .089
Intention	−.036 p = .760	.143 p = .218	.168 p = .184

*Significant at p = < .05

change in knowledge and change in behavioral control (Tables 3 and 5). These results, in addition to the difference in pre- and posttest scores (Table 3) indicate that the TG and the TG + HW groups had a greater impact in changing knowledge compared to the HW only and the comparison groups.

TABLE 5. Significance of Group Differences, Post Hoc Scheffe's Test

Groups	Groups and dependent variables		
	TG	TG + HW	Comparison
Change in knowledge			
HW	.000*	.004*	.816
TG		.993	.011*
TG + HW			.057
Change in behavior control			
HW	.000*	.032*	.004*
TG		.538	.634
TG + HW			.993
Change in attitudes			
HW	.123	.727	.24*
TG		.782	.897
TG + HW			.404
Change in norms			
HW	.941	.303	.952
TG		.118	.709
TG + HW			.619
Change in intention			
HW	.453	.390	.989
TG		.995	.691
TG + HW			.603

*=Significant at p < .05.

DISCUSSION

Program evaluations are different from pure research conducted to develop theories. The latter needs to adhere to strict research protocol. Program evaluations, on the other hand, are difficult to replicate with such stringent fidelity. As such, the results of this evaluation may be difficult to interpret and generalize. While study limitations will be discussed in the next section, it is important to remember that this pilot study was primarily conducted to not only explore the effects of the intervention but also to determine if the evaluation design was relevant for future evaluations of the prevention content of SAPVC. Second, it was also important to see if the online prevention content could be used independent of class work and if it could be effectively used to supplement the more traditional face-to-face classroom delivery.

Consistent with the hypothesis, knowledge was the only variable that showed significant increases following the 30-minute exercise. Changes in behavior control, attitudes, norms, and intentions were not significant and sometimes not in the predicted direction. One clear finding was that the delivery of the online program by assigning it as homework did not bring about change in any of the variables measured (Group 1 in Table 3). However, both the TG and the TG + HW groups showed significant gains in knowledge compared to the comparison groups. The results also demonstrate that online programs assigned as homework may effectively supplement the knowledge gained through traditional classroom prevention programs. That is, the data in Table 3 showed the gain in knowledge due to the classroom exercise was .12 while the knowledge gains from a repeating the exercise as homework was .08. This suggests that online prevention content may be useful in providing the booster sessions suggested by the literature. However, the booster session in this study immediately followed the intervention rather than occurring weeks or months after. More research is needed to explore the use of online prevention as a booster to classroom delivery.

LIMITATIONS

This study encountered many limitations that require the results to be interpreted with caution and that may help design future evaluative research for online prevention programs. The first limitation was the 60-item survey, which seemed to reliably measure the dependent variables but may have been was too long for teens, especially for younger teens in after-school programs and for the TG + HW group, which had to complete the instrument four times. In some cases, the length of the survey probably resulted in test fatigue and the haphazard answering of items. Visually inspecting and removing surveys answered haphazardly seemed not to eliminate this problem. Another limitation of the survey, especially for the statistical analyses, was that the comparison group experienced large increases in attitudes and norms, suggesting that problems may exist with the design or with those measures, even though they had high reliability.

One unexpected limitation was that the only in-school teens were those in the high school TG group and the high school comparison group. All others teens were in after-school programs. Typically, classroom teachers are better trained and work from a tighter structure than after-school programs. Even structured after-school programs are much less controlled than a classroom setting. Having teens either from only an after-school program or only from an in-school program might have eliminated some of the unexplained variance in the data. A final limitation is that the TPB was used to design the evaluation while the anger management exercise was based on resilience theory. Initial thinking was that exposure to prevention messages delivered by peers and through interactive methods might be sufficient to change attitudes, beliefs, and perceived behavior control. The evaluation suggests that change in attitudes, beliefs, and behavior control may require longer exposure than a 30-minute exercise or more targeted messages.

ISSUES AND IMPLICATIONS FOR THE EVALUATION OF ONLINE PREVENTION INTERVENTIONS

The experience of developing and conducting this evaluation has identified several issues. One of the first issues involves obtaining a sample. Teens in school and after-school programs are often selected because they are available. The majority of the teens who participated in this evaluation were participants in an after-school program. The researcher who collected the data observed that teens in an after-school program behave very differently than those in a school environment. Teens are more receptive to instructional messages in a school situation but want more interactive and entertaining activities in their after-school time. Thus, prevention programs for after-school programs may need to use different strategies to engage youth. This implies that online prevention programs that are proven effective in a school environment may have very different outcomes when implemented in an after-school program. Similarly, prevention programs that are effective with high school teens may not be effective with middle school teens. Online prevention program developers may need to explore the relative efficacy of programs in both school and after-school environments for various age groups.

Another issue concerns moving face-to-face, booklet-based classroom curriculum to the Internet, which is typically the first phase of moving prevention online. The second phase involves redesigning current curriculum to take advantage of the interactive multimedia nature of the Internet. Current evaluation models based on TPB work best for websites at the first online phase. The content of SAPVC was developed in close cooperation with teens in an inpatient substance abuse treatment program who pushed the developers into interactive multimedia content. Feedback from these teens, as well as presentations to many groups of at-risk teens, suggests that SAPVC exercises and games are useful in guiding discussions on prevention issues and in developing prevention skills. However, while useful, the evaluation of this 30-minute exercise did not increase teens' intention to change their behavior; TPB suggests intention is the best measure of effectiveness of prevention programs.

A similar issue concerns the difficulty of linking theory, program design, and evaluation. The online exercise was based on resiliency theory because it is frequently suggested for designing prevention programs. However, resiliency theory does not lend itself to a strong evaluation design. To elaborate further, resiliency theory identifies various risk and protective factors that need to be addressed or changed by prevention programs. While resiliency theory focuses actions on healthy and problem behaviors, it does not explain how or why behavior *change* takes place. The logic is that the more protective factors youth possess and the fewer risk factors they possess the more resilient they will be to drugs. In contrast, TPB posits the direct link of norms, attitudes, perception of behavior control, and intention to change future behavior with the probability of actual behavior change. It also provides a clear path to measurement of change

(Francis et al., 2004). Rather than measure all of the risk/protective factors a youth possesses, TPB just measures norms, attitudes, behavioral control, and intention. The implications of this research are that evaluative models and measures need to be considered at the very beginning of the design of any prevention intervention. Evaluations developed after programs are operational may focus on a few key factors and ignore a robust, rich, and coherent program design. The modification of the original TPB model in the present study to include and investigate the link between risk and protective factors (family and friends) and the attitudes, norms, etc. was an attempt to link these two important theories. This link may be worthy of further investigation by future researchers. This issue has surfaced in a national debate with the No Child Left Behind legislation, which imposes a national evaluation on local teaching curricula throughout the United States. Critics of No Child Left Behind suggest that teachers have abandoned well-balanced curricula containing things such as critical thinking skills and only "teach to the test" (National Center for Fair & Open Testing, n.d.). Some suggest the results may be teens with high test scores but who are poorly prepared for life.

Another issue is that as evaluative models become more robust by considering more variables, the measurement instruments become overly long for teens who have short attention spans. The 60-item survey developed to test the model used in this evaluation may have been too long, especially for teens in after-school programs and those in the TG + HW group who had to complete it four times. Some responses on the posttest of the TG + HW group suggest a pattern of random answering rather than reading each item. Future researchers might consider developing a much shorter measure for each construct or using several different evaluations with each evaluation addressing a different factor, such as norms (University of Washington, n.d.).

A similar issue is that teens typically do not participate in research or explore prevention websites of their own volition. Teens may cooperate more fully with research if (1) they are required to participate in a structured environment that is monitored by an adult; (2) they are provided with appropriate incentives to take the research seriously—for example, monitory incentives; (3) they are involved using small groups and the importance and significance of the research is emphasized; and (4) the intervention is interactive, entertaining, and challenging. Malone and Lepper (1987) identified seven key factors for creating an intrinsically motivating instructional environment: challenge, curiosity, control, fantasy, cooperation, competition, and recognition. While the anger management exercise evaluated in this study contained multimedia videos and teen stories, it did not hold teens' attention when they were instructed to explore the exercise in a school study hall environment. One method often suggested to make online prevention curriculum more attractive to teens is to use interactive games that incorporate prevention lessons and skill building. The researcher observed that teens were eager to play the "snakes and ladders" type game in the exercise to see how they scored. Some asked if they could just play the game and not do all of the video lessons in the exercise. While some prevention websites in Table 1 are game based, the evaluation of prevention games poses additional difficulties. For example, since most game content varies with each click or answer, two teens playing the same game might get very different interventions. Consequently, fidelity, a key issue in prevention research, is often compromised when prevention content is tailored to teens. We also found it difficult to develop prevention games based in the TPB. Funding agencies may have to allow researchers to develop evaluation models more suited to free-form, interactive, multimedia interventions that teens prefer on the Internet. One possible evaluation model, which is derived from the evaluation of television advertisements, uses body and brain sensors to measure propensity to act (Olsen, 2007).

One implication of the issues identified in this study is that costs for the evaluation of online prevention interventions may be much higher than most anticipate. Online prevention programming may be seen as a 5 to 10 year process of continuous development, evaluation, modification, and follow-up. Few funding sources are willing to make this kind of long-term commitment. In addition, web technology is changing so rapidly that it is difficult to develop a long-term strategy for designing and evaluating an online prevention intervention.

CONCLUSION

In an environment where schools are increasingly under pressure to deliver on academic outcomes, prevention providers find it more and more difficult to compete for adequate class time to deliver programs. Online programs are attractive options to deliver prevention curriculum consistently throughout the developmental years and with adequate frequency that would counter the effects of negative environmental messages and pressures. In addition, online prevention interventions can be attractive to teens if they take advantage of the free-form, interactive, multimedia, and gamelike features of the web that are so attractive to teens. While many web-based prevention programs exist, evaluations are more prevalent for those based on traditional prevention curricula in which lesson plans are delivered sequentially and both the intervention and the evaluations are based on a consistent theoretical model. The current study documents a struggle to evaluate a 30-minute, interactive, multimedia, online anger management exercise for teens using the TPB evaluation model. While the evaluation provided some support that web-guided prevention programs can be effective in increasing teens' prevention knowledge, and that completing the online exercise as supplemental homework reinforces the classroom experience, positive changes in other measures of behavior change were not supported. The study pointed to many issues that occur when developing online interventions and evaluating them in real-world environments. These include the consistency between the development and evaluative model, the problems with combining in-school and after-school program teens of various ages in the sample, the need for short measure of the many variables relevant to behavior change, and the high cost of evaluations. This study suggests that interactive, multimedia-based online intervention may require new evaluative models and measure in order for researchers to understand how and when they can effectively prevent substance abuse in teens.

REFERENCES

Advocates for Youth. (n.d.). *Welcome to the youth lounge!* Retrieved November 5, 2007, from http://www.advocatesforyouth.org/youth/index.htm.

Ajzen, I. (2006). *Interactive TpB diagram.* Retrieved August 10, 2007, from http://www.people.umass.edu/aizen/tpb.diag.html.

Berndt, T. J., & Perry, T. B. (1990). Distinctive features and effects of early adolescent friendships. In R. Montemayor, G. R. Adams, & T. P. Gullotta (Eds.), *From childhood to adolescence: A transitional period?* (Vol. 2; pp. 269–287). Newbury Park, CA: Sage.

Bosworth, K. (Ed.). (1998). *New directions in drug education programs: Hot topics series.* Bloomington, IN: Phi Delta Kappa International.

Brook, J. S., Whiteman, M., Nomura, A. S., Gordon, A. S., & Cohen, P. (1988). Personality, family and ecological influences on adolescent drug use: A developmental analysis. In R. H. Coombs (Ed.), *The family context of adolescent drug use* (pp. 123–162). Binghamton, NY: The Haworth Press.

Bush, P., Weinfurt, K., & Ianotti, R. (1994). Families versus peers: Developmental influences on drug use from grade 4–5 to grade 7–8. *Journal of Applied Developmental Psychology, 15*, 437–456. Cited in Szapocznik, J., Hervis, O., Schwartz, S. (2003). *Brief Strategic Family Therapy for Adolescent Drug Abuse.* Retrieved July 22, 2004, from http://www.nida.nih.gov/pdf/Manual5.pdf.

Cautin, R. L., Overholser, J. C., & Goetz, P. (2001). Assessment of mode of anger expression in adolescent psychiatric inpatients. *Adolescence, 36*(141), 163–170.

Christensen, H., & Griffiths, K. (2002). *The prevention of depression using the Internet.* Retrieved May 19, 2004, from http://www.mja.com.au/public/issues/177_07_071002/chr10370_fm.html.

Dahlberg, L. L., Toal, S. B., Swahn, M., Behrens, C. B. (2005). Measuring violence-related artitudes, behaviors, and influences among youths: A compendium of assessment tools. Atlanta, GA: Centers for Disease Control and Prevention, National Center for Injury Prevention and Control.

Dyer, F. J. (2005). *Developing resilience in children and adolescents.* Retrieved September 2, 2005, from http://www.counselormagazine.com/display_article. asp?aid=Resiliency.asp.

Francis, J. J., Eccles, M. P., Johnston, M., Wlaker, A., Grimshaw, J., Foy, R., et al. (2004). *Constructing questionnaires based on the theory of planned behaviour: A manual for health services researchers.* Retrieved December 10, 2007, from http://www.rebeqi.org/ViewFile.aspx?itemID=212.

Glanz, K., & Rimer, B. K. (2005). *Theory at a glance: A guide for health promotion practice* (2nd ed.). Washington, DC: U.S. Department of Health and Human Services, Public Health Service, National Institutes of Health, National Cancer Institute.

Gonet, M. M. (1994). *Counseling the adolescent substance abuser: School based intervention and prevention.* Pacific Grove, CA: Sage.

Herie, M. (2005). Theoretical perspectives in online pedagogy. *Journal of Technology in Human Services, 23*(1/2), 29–52.

Hilarski, C. (2004). Child and adolescent alcohol use and abuse: Risk factors, assessment, and treatment. *Journal of Evidence-Based Social Work, 1*(1), 81–99.

HopeLab. (2007). *About Hopelab: Our history.* Retrieved July 20, 2007, from http://www.remission.net/site/about/history.php.

Isaac, S., & Michael, W. (1977). *Handbook in research and evaluation for education and behavioral sciences.* Retrieved May 19, 2004, from http://nces.ed.gov/pubs2004/2004011.pdf.

Malone, T. W., & Lepper, M. R. (1987). Making learning fun: A taxonomy of intrinsic motivations for learning. *Aptitude, Learning, and Instruction, 3*, 223–253.

Minuchin, S., & Fishman, H. C. (1981). *Family therapy techniques.* Cambridge, MA: Harvard University Press. Cited in in Liddle, H. (2003). *Multidimensional Family Therapy for Early Adolescent Substance Abuse Treatment Manual.* Cannabis Youth Treatment Series (Vol. 5). Rockville, MD: U.S. Department of Health and Human Services. Retrieved June 7, 2004, from http://kap.samhsa.gov/products/manuals/cyt/pdfs/cyt5.pdf.

National Center for Fair & Open Testing. (n.d). *FairTest*. Retrieved November 27, 2007, from http://www.fairtest.org/nclb%20flaw%20fact%20sheet%201-7-04.html.

National Institute on Drug Abuse. (2003). *25 years of discovery to advance the health of the public*. Retrieved May 14, 2004, from http://www.drugabuse.gov/STRC/STRCindex.html.

National Institute on Drug Abuse. (2004). *Monitoring the future survey*. Retrieved June 20, 2004, from http://www.drugabuse.gov/DrugPages/MTF.html.

National Institute on Drug Abuse. (2006). *Monitoring the future survey, Overview of findings 2006*. Retrieved December 3, 2007, from http://www.drugabuse.gov/newsroom/06/MTF06Overview.html.

Olsen, S. (2007, August 21). *This is your brain on video games, ads*. Retrieved August 21, 2007, from http://news.com.com/2102-11395_3-6203560.html?tag=st.util.print.

PACER National Center for Bullying Prevention. (n.d.). *Overview*. Retrieved November 4, 2007, from http://www.pacer.org/bullying/index.asp.

Schinke, S., Brounstein, P., & Gardner, S. (2002). *Science-based prevention programs and principles, 2002*. DHHS Pub. No. (SMA) 03-3764. Rockville, MD: Center for Substance Abuse Prevention.

Schneider, A. J., Mataix-Cols, D., Marks, I. M., & Bachofen, M. (2005). Internet-guided self-help with or without exposure therapy for phobic and panic disorders. *Psychotherapy and Psychosomatics*, *74*, 154–164.

Skiba, D., Monroe, J., & Wodarski, J. (2004). Adolescent substance use: Reviewing the effectiveness of prevention strategies. *Social Work*, *49*(3), 343–353.

Substance Abuse & Mental Health Services Administration. (2000). *Effective prevention principles and programs*. Retrieved May 20, 2004, from http://model programs.samhsa.gov/.

Svensson, R. (2003). Gender differences in adolescent drug use: The impact of parental monitoring and peer deviance. *Youth and Society*, *34*(3), 300–329.

TeenAIDS-PeerCorps. (n.d.). *Teens*. Retrieved November 5, 2007, from http://www.teenaids.org/Teens/tabid/52/Default.aspx.

Tobler, N. (1992). Drug prevention programs can work: Research findings. *Journal of Addictive Diseases*, *11*(3), 1–28.

Tsai, C. (2008). The preferences toward constructivist Internet-based learning environments among university students in Taiwan. *Computers in Human Behavior*, *24*, 16–31.

United Nations Office on Drugs and Crime. (2002). *Using the Internet for drug abuse prevention*. New York: United Nations.

University of Washington. (n.d.) *Social Norms and Alcohol prevention (SNAP)*. Retrieved December 17, 2007, from http://depts.washington.edu/abrc/snap.htm.

Vance, E., & Sanchez, H. (1998). *Creating a service system that builds resiliency*. Retrieved August 31, 2007, from http://www.dhhs.state.nc.us/mhddsas/childandfamily/technicalassistance/risk_and_resiliency.htm.

The LivePerson Model for Delivery of Etherapy Services: A Case Study

Jerry Finn
Sharon Bruce

Research suggests that etherapy is becoming widely available on the Internet and that it can be an effective treatment option for a variety of mental health and relationship issues. The studies of etherapy are primarily anecdotal reports by individual practitioners or research-based studies from hospital or university-based programs. Many etherapy services, however, are offered over the Internet in a variety of models that seek to advertise and deliver the services of private practitioners. There is very little research about the structure, processes, use, consumer satisfaction, or outcomes of etherapy offered through private practice. Even less is known about the therapists who choose to make their services available online. No study has investigated their qualifications, motivation, satisfaction, effectiveness, and concerns. The purpose of this paper is to present a case study of one model for the delivery of online services, describing the infrastructure that supports etherapy and the experiences of an online therapist with several years of etherapy experience.

The use of etherapy, providing supportive and therapeutic mental health services by professionals over the Internet, continues to grow, and new models of service delivery are emerging. Professionals such as psychiatrists, psychologists, social workers, marital and family therapists, and counselors are providing therapeutic services by e-mail, chat, video conferencing, and unassisted web-based behavioral programs (Benderly, 2005; Finn, 2006; Newman, 2004; Tate & Zabinski, 2004). The number of online practitioners in unknown, but appears to be increasing rapidly. In an early report, Ainsworth reported that fee-based etherapy has been provided by individuals in private practice as early as 1995, and found that by 1999 there were more than 250 private practice etherapy websites (Ainsworth, 2001). By 2006, Lavallee noted that *one* online therapy company MyTherapyNet (http://www.mytherapynet.com/) had more than 1,000 registered therapists who provided services to more than 5,000 users per month. Similarly, Freeny (2001) reported that between 5,000 and 25,000 messages per day were sent in online counseling sessions. More recently, the *Wall Street Journal* reported that *one* therapist estimated that he had documented more than one million words, the equivalent of 17 doctoral dissertations, between himself and his online clients between January 2004 and December 2006 (Mulhauser, 2006). Researchers attribute the rapid growth of etherapy in the United States to the geometric expansion of Internet use by the general population, as well as to convenience, desire for anonymity, stigma associated with traditional services, ease of communication, accessibility for isolated or stigmatized groups, lack of service availability in a local area, desire for continuity in a mobile society, and lower costs (Finn & Holden, 2000; Grohol, 2004; Hsiung, 2002; Suler, 2004; Zelvin & Speyer, 2003).

The rapid growth of etherapy may also be related, in part, to increasing acceptance of etherapy by practitioners and consumers as a result of accumulating research evidence generally showing positive outcomes for etherapy intervention. Many anecdotal reports and some controlled studies have found etherapy to be as effective as face-to-face therapy and more effective than wait-list control groups for treating a variety of issues including depression, anxiety, panic disorder, weight loss, smoking cessation, eating disorders, and problem drinking (Barak, 2004; Hirai & Clum, 2006; Spek et al., 2007; Wantland, Portillo, Holzemer, Slaughter, & McGhee, 2004).

The growth of etherapy is also taking place despite ethical, legal, and practical concerns related to etherapy being unresolved (Kraus, Stricker, & Zack, 2003). Recommendations for ethical online practice have been published by the American Counseling Association (2005), the Clinical Social Work Federation (2001), the American Psychological Association (1997), American Mental Health Counselors Association (2000), and the International Society for Mental Health Online (2000). While technological stability of communications and the security and confidentiality of online client information can now be reasonably assured through encryption and secure servers, issues related to establishing client identity, ability to intervene in a crisis, lack of visual cues for assessment, mandatory reporting, and jurisdiction remain problematic (Barnett & Scheetz, 2003; Finn & Banach, 2002; Manhaul-Baugus, 2001; Mitchell & Murphy, 2004; Ragusea & Vandecreek, 2003).

ETHERAPY INFRASTRUCTURE

Etherapy is being offered through a variety of models on the Internet. These include:

- **Private practitioner website.** A private individual practitioner or group posts a website that provides information such as fees, methods, services, and forms of service delivery (e.g. e-mail, chat, video conferencing). The individual entity is responsible for maintaining the website, fees and billing, and meeting the requirements of ethical practice (See, for example, Marriage Matters at http://www.marriagematters.com/).

- **Information and referral website.** A website posts the name, address, phone number, and e-mail address of practitioners offering their services. Services may be face to face, telephone, and/or online. The website posts information about the provider such as credentials, experience, and methods. The site is searchable by criteria such as name, location, and service offered. In many cases, the website will check the credentials of a practitioner before posting a listing. The website, however, does not provide a platform for service delivery. See, for example, Therapist Locator (http://www.therapistlocator.net/), Network Therapy (http://www.networktherapy.com/), or Psychology Today (http://therapists.psychologytoday.com/rms/prof_search.php).
- **University or hospital-based clinics.** A university or hospital may offer online services to the public or to its members. Services may be a structured, web-based program without interaction with a clinician or may also include direct interaction though chat, e-mail, or phone with clinical staff. Services may be completely online or may be part of supplemental or follow-up services. (See, for example, Andersson, Strömgren, Ström, & Lyttkens, 2002; Carlbring, Furmark, Steczkó, Ekselius, & Andersson, 2006). These offer consumers a specific treatment program and confidence that comes from working with a known professional organization.
- **Nonprofit crisis line.** A nonprofit organization offers a chat-based help line for information and referral as well as for supportive counseling. The help line is staffed by trained volunteers who are supervised online by professionals. Transactions are completely anonymous since the service strips in internet protocol (IP) address so the user cannot be identified and no transcripts are kept of consumer/volunteer interactions. See, Rape, Abuse and Incest National Network (http://www.rainn.org).
- **Private hosting service.** A private hosting service is a for-profit company that provides the infrastructure for professional therapists to offer their services to the public. The company develops and maintains the website; provides data security, storage, and backup; and handles fees, billing, and collections. The website posts information about the therapist such as credentials, experience, methods, and

fees, and often provides a picture of the therapist as well. In many cases, the website will check the credentials of a practitioner before posting a listing. The site is searchable by criteria such as therapist name and services offered. The hosting service provides the infrastructure for the delivery of services, which may include e-mail, chat, and video conference. Fees are set by the individual practitioner. Fees may be based on the cost of an individual or set of e-mail transactions, a time period for e-mail (e.g., one month's e-mail transactions), or a specific session length (e.g., half hour of chat time). The hosting service may receive a percentage of the fees earned by the practitioner and in some cases charges the therapist an initial fee and/or monthly fee. Consumers are assured that their information is private and confidential through a service agreement contract that must be "checked" before receiving services. The hosting service, however, has access to consumer's identifying information as well as to stored transcripts of e-mail and chat sessions with therapists. A variety of disclaimers about privacy and security of records, guarantees of availability, and effectiveness of services offered are generally included in the service agreement as well. (See, for example, HelpHorizons (http://www.helphorizons.com/) and MyTherapyNet (http://www.mytherapynet.com/).

No research has investigated the relative effectiveness of these models of online service delivery. Little is known about the number of consumers that seek each model of service delivery, their motivation for doing so, their consumer satisfaction, or the relationship between service models and treatment outcomes.

A CASE STUDY OF THE LIVEPERSON MODEL

Information in this section is based on analysis of publicly accessible information posted on the LivePerson website. (Note: Until April, 2008 the website was called Kasamba with the URL www.kasamba.com. This is a change in name only and the policies remain as described.) In addition, the author corresponded by e-mail with Arthur Fuhrer, MD, co-founder of Kasamba, to gain additional information and clarification of policies. LivePerson (www.liveperson.com) is a relatively new model for providing etherapy services. Etherapy is offered through a private hosting service similar to that described previously; however, there are additional features that make it unique. Professional Counseling is a subsection of LivePerson (http://www.liveperson.com/experts/professional-counseling). In addition to counseling, experts can be found in the categories of Shopping and Style, Coaching and Personal Development, Spirituality and Religion, Computers and Programming, Education and Tutoring, Health and Medicine, Business and Finance, Arts and Creative Services, Legal Service, Home and Leisure, and Other Expertise. The website states that there are more than 30,000 experts working with LivePerson. As of February 2008, 118 were listed in the Professional Counseling area. Subareas within Counseling include: Addictions, Coping with Crisis and Physical Conditions, Eating Disorders, Parenting, Personal Development, Personality and Emotional Disorders, Relationship Issues, Supervision for Professional Counselors, and Website partners. In addition, these subareas have further delineations. For example, clicking on the Parenting area shows: ADD/ADHD, Adoption, Child Development, Children with Special Needs, Coping with Adolescents, Education Specialists, Family Therapy, and Single Parenting. Users can find an expert by performing a keyword search or by browsing through the categories of experts on the homepage.

In the LivePerson model, experts provide services either through an online chat program, via e-mail, or by phone. The website states that in some countries, such as the United States, clients must be at least 18 years old to obtain services from a mental health professional on LivePerson. A parent or legal guardian seeking online therapy for a child can fax LivePerson a signed consent form so that services can be legally provided to the child.

In order to select a counselor, a user can review information about the service provider. The website shows whether a counselor is currently online and allows a user to sort experts by those who are currently available as well as by price and rating. The website posts a brief description of an expert's services and credentials, the expert's suggested per minute and e-mail fees, consumer ratings from one to five stars (discussed later), and brief descriptions of consumer satisfaction statements.

Number of Sessions

The LivePerson website lists the number of rated sessions for each expert. At the time of this review, the number of sessions ranged from 0 (new) to 779 with a median of 12 sessions. Approximately one-fifth

(21.2 percent) were experts with no ratings, 22 percent had more than 100 ratings, and 12.7 percent had more than 200 ratings. The number of ratings, however, underestimates the volume of services, because ratings are optional and not all consumers choose to rate their session. The percent of consumers who rate services is approximately 50 percent (Furher, 2008).

Demographics

Of the 118 counselors, 79 (66.9 percent) were female and 39 (33.1 percent) were male. Based on the name and picture on the LivePerson site, it is estimated that the vast majority, 90.6 percent are white. In addition, 5 (4.3 percent) are Southeast Asian, 4 (3.4 percent) are African American, and 2 (1.7 percent) are Latino.

Credentials

The website posts the expert's credentials. LivePerson states that all counselors fill out a release form enabling LivePerson to verify both their degree and professional licensure before being approved as an active LivePerson expert. A graphic in the expert's description indicates that their credentials have been checked. The degrees accepted by LivePerson are listed in the Help section of the website (http://www.LivePerson.com/help/help-popup.aspx?ID=456&Type=1). In the Counseling section, the academic degree of counselors includes PhDs in clinical psychology and in counseling; EdD in counseling; master's degrees in social work, psychology, marriage and family therapy, counseling psychology, and counseling; and bachelor's degree in Psychology. One psychiatrist is listed on the website. Professional licensure includes Licensed Marriage and Family Therapist (LMFT), Licensed Clinical Social Worker (LCSW), Licensed Mental Health Counselor (LMHC), Certified Addiction Professional (CAP), and others. Of the experts listed, 5 (4.2 percent) do not list their degree, 3 (2.4 percent) have a bachelor's degree, 83 (70.3 percent) have a master's degree, 21 (17.8 percent) have a doctorate, and 6 (5.1 percent) have a degree from a foreign country, including degrees from England, Scotland, Ireland, and India.

Fees

Fees for chat per minute range from $.25 to $3.00 per minute ($15 to $180 per hour), with a mean of $1.36 (SD .44) and median and mode of $1.25 per minute. E-mail-based fees are negotiated separately and vary widely. For example, one expert charges "$50 per business week," another charges $15 per e-mail, and still another lists a range of $10 to $80 per e-mail depending on the complexity of the issue. E-mail fees ranged from $5 to $100 per e-mail with a median fee of $15 per e-mail. Of 118 experts, 68 (58 percent) provided a specific e-mail price. The remainder provided a range for e-mail services or stated that the price varies depending on the complexity of the issue.

Fees are paid by consumers via credit card or PayPal on a secure server. Live sessions start in free mode. Consumers are not charged until they agree to hire an expert by pressing the Hire button on the website. For the client's first session on LivePerson, the first three minutes are free, and "hired" mode starts automatically after that time. After the first session, the session is free as long as the consumer has not clicked a Hire button while in session. This means that the time is free for as long as the client and counselor wish it to be. In most cases, the client clicks Hire after a few minutes into the session.

There is no fee for experts to list their services. LivePerson charges experts 30 percent of their e-mail fees and 30 percent plus 17 cents per minute of live session fees.

Consumer Ratings

LivePerson uses a rating system similar to the eBay auction (www.e-bay.com) model in which consumers can rate their satisfaction with sellers. Experts are rated by consumers with from 1 (unacceptable) to 5 (outstanding) stars. The average star rating and total number of ratings are shown next to the expert's name. Consumers must rate an expert within 30 days of a session in order for the rating to be posted. Viewers can read the rating comments given by previous users. For example, an expert may show 213 ratings with an average 4.5 stars. Rating comments tend to be brief and lack specificity. For example, a reviewer might write, "Very compassionate and helpful," or, "patient and caring, listens to you carefully," or "not really helpful." In addition, not all comments are posted for public viewing. The LivePerson website states that their quality assurance team reviews all of the comments on a daily bases and removes any statements that are not directly related to the expert's service. The LivePerson website states the policies regarding comments in the help section for experts and for consumers. All publicly displayed ratings are for paid sessions only; ratings for free sessions are seen by the client and expert, and are not made public.

The website states that the quality assurance team will not remove a rating given legitimately by a consumer. If an expert feels that a low rating was received as a result of a technical problem or for any other reason not directly related to their practice, the expert may dispute the rating. LivePerson states they will investigate the matter. Dr. Fuhrer stated that ratings are very seldom removed, and only in cases where it is believed that the rating is undeserved (e.g., if there has been a documented technical problem with the session, or if the rating comment suggests that the consumer was dissatisfied with something other than the service received by the expert). The quality assurance team's reasons for not posting a comment and the extent to which this occurs warrants further research.

Of 92 (78 percent) experts that were rated with stars, all except one were given high ratings, between 4 and 5 stars. The remainder of experts was "new" and had not yet been rated. Of the rated experts, 57 (62 percent) were rated with 5 stars, 31 (33.7 percent) were given 4.5 stars, 3 (3.3 percent) were rated 4 stars, and 1 (1.1 percent) was rated with 1 star. The mean rating for all experts was 4.76 (SD .48).

Language

The website also lists the languages in which the expert offers services. For example, a search using the site search engine found 10 counselors that provide Spanish language counseling, 3 in French, 2 in Hebrew, 1 in Greek, and 1 in Farsi. A search for German, Italian, Russian, Arabic, Mandarin, Cantonese, Korean, or Japanese yielded no experts.

Privacy, Security, and Confidentiality

Steps are taken to promote privacy, security, and confidentiality of records. LivePerson uses the industry standard secure socket layer (SSL) encryption and firewalls to protect against loss, misuse, and alteration of any personal data. Both chat-based and e-mail transactions are carried out through the secure website. To further promote privacy, users go to the LivePerson website to read their e-mail from the LivePerson server rather than having e-mail sent to a user's e-mail address. Session transcripts of chat-based sessions and e-mails are stored and available to the consumer who initiated the session and to the expert who provided the service. In addition, in their Help section, LivePerson warns consumers, "NEVER pass on any personal contact information, such as a personal e-mail address or telephone number to our experts. Such actions compromise your privacy and are beyond our control and responsibility. At LivePerson, you can communicate with our experts and safely pay session fees while maintaining complete confidentiality."

LivePerson states that communication between experts and consumers is confidential; however, there are exceptions. The Expert Service Agreement section of the website states:

> LivePerson does not screen or edit the content of communications between Clients and Experts. Such communications are personal and private unless both parties agree to additional distribution, for example by posting questions or services on the Public Board.... All communications between Experts and Clients are NOT encrypted and thus may be subject to unauthorized interception and monitoring. LivePerson may screen, copy, transmit and review all communications conducted by or through LivePerson.com for technical support and/or in order to enforce these Terms of Service.

With regard to enforcing terms of service, LivePerson screens transactions between experts and consumers in order to be sure that experts do not refer consumers to their own practice outside of Live-Person. LivePerson seeks to ensure the confidentiality of communications between experts and consumers in this process. In an e-mail statement to the authors Dr. Fuhrer stated,

> We have a very strict policy that absolutely prohibits anyone from LivePerson from accessing session transcripts. Since we do not permit experts to exchange contact information with clients, we do run routine automated searches on session transcripts to find expressions such as email addresses and phone numbers. The output of these searches is handled without reading session transcripts.

With regard to mandatory reporting, LivePerson notifies clients through a posted confidentiality statement that in specific safety- related circumstances, therapists are required by law to report to local authorities in situations that include the perpetration of emotional, physical, or sexual abuse; homicidal or suicidal intentions; or any other case in which an individual's life is in imminent danger. In addition, in an emergency or in case of reported abuse, LivePerson enables the expert to get the consumer's physical address and IP address from the system at the click of a button. LivePerson then sees it as the expert's professional obligation to report the incident to the appropriate authorities since LivePerson is only a venue for service delivery. The extent to which mandatory reporting takes place and the process for doing so warrants further study.

The exact nature of the privacy and storage of communication between experts and consumers is not clear to the authors after reading the privacy statement. The website states, "Certain communications may be recorded and maintained by LivePerson. LivePerson does not screen or edit the content of communications between Clients and Experts. Such communications are personal and private unless both parties agree to additional distribution." What is not clear on the website is what communications may be recorded, who has access to them, and for how long they will remain on the server. In an e-mail, Dr. Fuhrer (2008) explained that every communication via e-mail and chat is recorded automatically on secure servers. It is company policy that no one is allowed to access these records. This is not reflected in the legal agreement and privacy statement because it does not apply to categories other than Professional Counseling. The records are kept indefinitely, although from time to time they may be archived to save server space.

LivePerson maintains a record of the user's IP addresses to analyze trends, administer the site, track user's movement, and gather demographic information for aggregate use. The site also notes that IP addresses are linked to personally identifiable information such as credit cards "in order to better the user's experience." LivePerson also states in its agreement with experts that it has the right to use any material that is transmitted on the site. The agreement states,

> Expert agrees that any information or content that he [or she] posts or transmits through LivePerson.com will not be considered confidential. Expert grants LivePerson.com an unlimited,

irrevocable, royalty-free license to use, reproduce, display, edit, copy, transmit, publicly perform, create derivative works, communicate to the public any such information and content on a world-wide basis

Finally, LivePerson, through a "Disclaimers of Warranties" statement notes that there is no guarantee that the service will be secure:

> DISCLAIMER OF WARRANTIES... LIVEPERSON ENTITIES MAKE NO WARRANTY THAT (I) THE SERVICE WILL MEET YOUR REQUIREMENTS; (II) THE SERVICE WILL BE UNINTERRUPTED, TIMELY, SECURE OR ERROR-FREE; (III) THE RESULTS THAT MAY BE OBTAINED FROM THE USE OF THE SERVICE WILL BE ACCURATE OR RELIABLE; OR (IV) THE QUALITY OF ANY PRODUCTS, SERVICES INFORMATION OR OTHER MATERIAL PURCHASED OR OBTAINED BY YOU THROUGH THE SERVICE WILL MEET YOUR EXPECTATIONS.

With regard to these statements, Dr. Fuhrer commented that,

> This is a very general legal statement that is supposed to protect the company's interests. As far as session data is concerned, we do not permit anyone to access session transcripts (in the professional counseling categories), and surely we do not intend to make any other use of such information which we deem private, confidential and highly sensitive.

LivePerson provides information related to emergencies. The site states that online counseling is not appropriate for all problems and is not a replacement for face-to-face therapy. Specifically, material states that online counseling is not suitable for psychiatric disorders and severe psychopathologies. Those with suicidal thoughts are encouraged to seek professional help immediately through other channels of communication. They are also directed to a telephone crisis line and to 911 for help. Users outside the United States are directed to Befrienders Worldwide (http://www.befrienders.org/) to find support in their specific country.

CASE STUDY OF A LIVEPERSON EXPERT

Case study is used in research to provide in-depth, detailed qualitative information and examples about a phenomenon, especially when little is known about the area (Krysik & Finn, 2007). In order to better understand motivation, practice, and experiences of an online counselor using the LivePerson model, a case study was conducted using open-ended questions via e-mail. Information presented is based on the experiences of one online counselor and cannot be generalized. It is presented in order to highlight issues associated with online etherapy practice and to highlight issues for further research.

The counselor, "MJ" (identity for this paper) was selected from the LivePerson website because she had a master's degree and had considerable experience on LivePerson. The website noted that she had conducted more than 400 sessions and was rated 5 stars. The authors e-mailed MJ at the LivePerson website. She was the first counselor approached for the study and she agreed to participate. The authors then e-mailed MJ 47 closed and open-ended questions about her experience at LivePerson, including questions about background, motivation, consumers, treatment methods, perceptions of online therapy, ethical issues, and evaluation. After reading MJ's responses, the authors asked additional questions by e-mail to provide more detail or to cover issues not previously addressed. The following is a summary of MJ's responses. MJ has reviewed this summary and states that it accurately reflects her comments.

Background

MJ is a white female with more than 20 years experience in professional counseling. Her practice settings have included inpatient and outpatient hospital psychiatric social work, public and private agencies, public schools, and private practice in individual, group, and family therapy. She has both bachelor's and master's degrees in social work and is licensed as a clinical social worker, LCSW. She does not do face-to-face counseling at this time due to a need to be home for caregiving responsibilities. She had not received formal training as an online counselor when she began providing services on LivePerson. Since that time, she has received informal training in online counseling through reading the literature and discussions with more experienced online colleagues. She uses an eclectic approach, relying most heavily on cognitive-behavioral approaches.

Beginnings

MJ's association with LivePerson began in early 2006 after a review of online therapy resources. She was in need of work that she could do from home due to family circumstances. The idea to join an online counseling organization was based on her belief that counseling must be happening online, and she explored her options. She did not find LivePerson through referral from colleagues or previous knowledge of its services. She initially decided to join LivePerson on a trial basis, to determine if online counseling was a good fit. The reasons for choosing LivePerson had to do with the ease of joining, the simplicity of the contractual arrangement, and it's relatively high presence on searches of the Internet for online counselors.

Consumers

MJ estimates that she has worked with approximately 1,000 consumers online. Approximately 50 percent of her consumers chose to rate their session. She states that approximately 60 percent of consumers are female and they range between ages 18 and 60, with the majority between 25 and 40 years old.

Building an online practice may be a developmental process. It is similar to face-to-face private practice in that a therapist must build a reputation and a consumer base. It is different in that many consumers engage for only one session and services are offered in the context of an open marketplace. MJ stated that the number of people requesting help varied greatly when she initially started with LivePerson. It depended on the number of hours she made herself available, the time of day or night she was available, the number of other counselors available at the same time, and her place in the ranking of counselors. At first, when she was ranked low in number of sessions, she knew that she needed to be available for a great number of hours and to receive positive feedback from clients in the ranking system in order to receive clients. As she moved up in the ranking system and received regular clients, she was able to stay open for fewer hours and have a more regular schedule. Over the first few months MJ provided services to approximately 25 to 35 people per month. The number of consumers varied greatly. On some days, when available for 4 or more hours she has received requests from 5 consumers. Other days, 8 hours may go by with only one request. She states that the variation in consumers initially makes it difficult to rely on etherapy alone for regular financial benefit. Most consumers receive services one time, requesting specific help dealing with situations that are immediate. Others may ask for help for 10 or 12 sessions. She has one client who has been in regular sessions online for more than two years. In addition, she has also seen one particular client once or more a day for a period of one month during a very stressful period of time in his life where frequent support was very helpful to him. She currently sees primarily ongoing consumers on a specific schedule.

MJ states that the number of minutes spent with a client really depends on the issue, whether or not the client is benefiting from the time, and on finances. She estimates an average session is 45 minutes, but the range is great. The longest session she had on LivePerson was 150 minutes. She tries to assess the situation before the client hires her in order to be sure she can be of help. Sometimes, however, the client hires before explaining, or at other times the client or MJ decide that MJ is not able to be helpful and the session ends after only 5 or 10 minutes.

Treatment Issues

Overall, MJ believes that online counseling can hold a very important place in the field of the helping professions. She describes accessibility for two clients:

> I have one very successful client with a traumatic history of abuse and of failure in face-to-face counseling. For many years she did not receive treatment, due to her fear of people which was based in her past trauma and in her poor treatment in face-to-face counseling as an adolescent. She reached out to me in an e-mail, very hesitantly I might add. She agreed to one week of daily e-mails. That week allowed her to build some trust. Yes, it was trust in someone that she couldn't see and didn't have to feel responsible to because I did not know her real name or where she lived. But that was why any trust at all was able to be built. And from that small beginning she has built a strong therapeutic relationship in e-mail therapy and has made tremendous strides overcoming her fear of people, her

depression related to old thinking patterns developed during her abuse, and in her sense of self-worth. It is extremely gratifying to work with someone like this client. The next step for her was a live chat session and we are working toward a phone session in the future. At some point she will be ready for face-to-face therapy, with another therapist in her area.

Another client comes to mind who was tortured in her mind by a rape that occurred 20 years ago. She struggled with this daily, and had never had the courage to talk about it with anyone. She reached out to me in a live chat session from a hotel room, far from her home. It was only by being far from her family, from the place of the rape, and in the anonymity of the online contact that she was able to talk about it at last and start to get some relief from carrying the burden of the shame of this trauma by herself for 20 years. I believe that she might never have shared it if her only option was to do so in person.

MJ states that the vast majority of sessions with clients are for a single session. She believes that a single session can be very useful. She provides the following example:

For instance, a mother might contact me upset because she found her son smoking pot in his room and can't figure out what to do about it. I might offer her some compassion first, a listening ear, in order to help her calm down. I also might try to normalize this experience for her so that her anxiety doesn't escalate. And then, I can offer her specific suggestions on how to confront her son in a way that will do less harm to the relationship and that will both let him know that his behavior is outside of the limits of the household but that he is still loved and that his well-being is her concern. Often, that's all it takes to really help someone in this situation.

MJ is not without concerns about online treatment and states that she has encountered many of the same problems in treatment of consumers online as those that occur in person. Treatment issues are also similar. For instance, she has worked with consumers with issues of borderline personality who, at times, will try to monopolize time, frequently present with crises requesting immediate help, or will attempt to cross professional boundaries inquiring into her personal life. Other issues such as false identity, seeking inappropriate services, dishonesty, or financial troubles may impede treatment.

MJ believes that careful assessment is important but not always possible in etherapy. Sometimes she sends an assessment tool to a client to be completed and e-mailed back to her before the first session. This is typically true if she is approached by e-mail in the first contact. The assessment tool is a standard psychosocial assessment that she has utilized in many face-to-face settings. If a consumer's first contact is through chat, she states that they are typically feeling in need of immediate support and so she does a more general assessment prior to and during the session, determining if the issue is appropriate for online treatment. In addition, she always discusses the limitations of online counseling.

MJ states that she takes her work with clients very seriously, as the vast majority of clients come to her seeking real help for real problems. Once engaged, she provides the services she feels are needed. If she believes a consumer would be better served by referral elsewhere, she helps them move on to other services. She notes that this is not as easy as it is in person, as her clients are worldwide and it is not possible for her to know all of what is available to them for services in their area. She has a list of referral sources that she gives out in those circumstances. She has referred clients elsewhere when she felt that someone else, with more experience or training in a certain area, would be better able to help them, or if the issue they present with is not one which she believes can be treated well in online therapy.

Evaluation

MJ believes that she is fairly successful in treating clients online. This was also true in her face-to-face work, but she believes that because she responds well to formulating and presenting help with the written word, she may actually be more helpful to specific clients online than she may have been in person. MJ states that supervision is also very useful in helping her be clear about her success in treating clients. MJ states that she uses client feedback as a means of determining her success with clients. This is tempered with her own assessment of the true need and the true benefit. Finally, MJ gets regular feedback from the reviews of her sessions. As noted, she has a mean of 5 (stars) on a 5-point scale for more than 400 sessions.

Fees

MJ initially scanned the fee range of other therapists and set her fees near the low end when she was first starting online therapy. As she developed more ratings and a more consistent consumer base, she raised her fees to be in conjunction with therapists of similar experience and credentials. She notes that the fees she posts on site are determined for the most part, by the "competition" or going rate among other therapists working at that time. She states that some therapists with higher fees did not continue with LivePerson and the newer therapists have held their rates at a lower level. While she has reduced her rate somewhat in response to the other counselor's lower rates, she believes that a lower rate can draw less than serious clients, sometimes clients who are not in true need of help or are actually looking for sexual services. She estimates that 90 percent of her consumers are serious about getting counseling services and 5 percent are seeking sexual services. Because LivePerson's Experts also include a great number of psychics in the Spirituality and Religion section, she is sometimes mistaken as a psychic and asked for a psychic reading. This happens approximately 25 percent of the time, and she refers them to the Spirituality and Religion section. She feels that as a professional that her services are somewhat devalued by the association with psychics on another part of the site.

MJ notes some difficulties with collecting fees online. She states that LivePerson allows clients to input their credit card information but is not able to assess the amount of credit available. A session can run for over an hour, but the consumer may not have the funds available on the card to pay for the entire session. This has happened several times to MJ, and she was not paid for the sessions initially and later was not paid beyond the credit limit on the card. She notes that LivePerson does continue to try to bill the card, and in all except one case they have been successful in receiving payment. This sometimes takes a month or more.

The other funding issue that can affect session length happens when a client puts a specific amount of funds into their LivePerson account. MJ states that in a dozen or more sessions, a session has ended abruptly with no notice when the consumer's funds ran out.

If a consumer lets her know ahead of time that there is a limited amount of dollars in their account, MJ may then decide to adjust her rate in order to give the consumer a certain number of minutes for a session. For instance, if a client tells her that they are feeling very much in need of help dealing with anxiety over a pressing situation but that they have only $20 in their account, she may choose to adjust her rate in order to give them a half hour or 45 minute session for that price. In addition, MJ states that she offers a reduced fee to regular consumers and to consumers who are in need financially.

Perceptions of What is Useful About LivePerson

Overall, MJ is very satisfied with her relationship with LivePerson and with etherapy as a practice modality. MJ believes LivePerson's strengths are its ease of use for consumers, anonymity, and convenience. She notes that signing up is a simple process and once done, accessing a therapist is quite easy. It takes merely a click of the mouse on the "Contact Live" icon. In addition, the therapist is not privy to identifying information, even the client's name, unless the client chooses to make that known or there is need for emergency contact or mandatory reporting. While MJ is available on a limited basis, typically there is a counselor available at almost all hours of the day. She believes that this is useful in providing help at the time it is needed.

Concerns

MJ has a number of concerns about online therapy and about the LivePerson model itself. She states:

> I think that training regarding the limitations of practice would be the most important factor in a training program for online counselors. There is a quote about philosophy that I like very much but cannot recall entirely accurately. Basically, it states in life that we must learn to trust our feelings least, our reason more, and our limitations most—very good advice in the work of online therapy.

She notes that some of the things mentioned earlier that are benefits of online counseling can also be detriments. The relative anonymity that allows people to feel freer in reaching out for help also opens up the potential for trouble. She states:

> I've encountered this with a client who, by my professional esti-
> mation, was assuming an identity not his or her own. No real help
> can be offered in this situation as the issue lies within the deception
> itself and that deception is not easily identified or dealt with within
> the confines of an online therapeutic relationship.

She also believes that another drawback arises in situations where
the client might be in danger to themselves or others, something
encountered by all seasoned professionals at one point, in all forms
of counseling. She knows that LivePerson does have a system wherein
the counselor can contact administration and report a concern, pre-
sumably to allow them to contact authorities with personal information in the system regarding this client. But, she asks, What if
that client has used another person's information in signing up for
services? Or, if there is a delay in response by LivePerson, clients
could potentially not receive help in time to prevent harm to themselves or others. For this reason, she makes it very clear to each client
through a standard form that she cannot ethically treat someone with
issues of suicide, and also makes clear the limitations of treatment
online.

Similarly, MJ has concerns about mandatory reporting:

> My concern here is that I cannot report an offense as I am man-
> dated to do because I do not have contact information. I would
> never leave a person asking for help hanging. I would try to get
> them to see the benefit of contacting someone in person for help.
> LivePerson should be responsible for reporting abuse; however,
> when I have contacted them with concerns over a client, I did
> not receive a response for many days. This is unacceptable, as
> was their response, which did not confirm that they would
> report my concerns.

MJ also notes that online therapy does not provide the important
feedback of body language, voice inflection, or the many other indicators that a therapist can utilize in assessing and treating a client in
face-to-face therapy. For this reason, she believes careful screening
must be done before offering help. She sends e-mail clients a standardized intake form. She also attempts to assess the type of problem to
be discussed and the client's ability to communicate online when
working with chat-based consumers.

She is very concerned about issues of confidentiality on LivePerson. She states that supposedly confidential communication between counselor and consumer is regularly screened by LivePerson staff. She explained that she knows of counselors who were contacted and reprimanded by LivePerson for providing contact information to the consumer other than the LivePerson contact information. LivePerson does not allow this, since it has potential for taking clients away from their site. She states that she was informed by LivePerson that they use a "screening tool" and do not actually read the sessions. (This was confirmed by Dr. Furher, as noted previously.) She is unclear about how this works. MJ believes that professional counselors need to provide private e-mail addresses or other contact means to consumers in case the consumer is unable to reach them through LivePerson due to technical troubles or other issues that do occur. MJ also notes that LivePerson does not utilize encryption to add further security to communication in sessions. Her understanding of privacy on the website is only partially correct. According to Dr. Furher, all live chat sessions are encrypted using industry standard SSL. E-mail sessions, while not encrypted, are located in a password protected area that is accessible only to the client and expert. LivePerson's servers are hosted in a secure and guarded facility, behind a firewall.

MJ states that she is also concerned about verification of the credentials of professionals, which she believes is *slack* at times. She stated that when she first began at LivePerson she repeatedly asked where and when to send her license information. LivePerson did not respond and did not request verification of her licensure for several months after she began practicing on the site. (Note: Dr. Fuhrer stated that LivePerson began checking credentials only in mid-2006. It is now standard policy to check all credentials.) In addition, MJ's license was up for renewal last May, and although LivePerson would know this by the date listed on the copy of her license, they have not asked her if she has renewed her license. MJ notes that this creates questions because a counselor could potentially be unable to renew their license due to malpractice or other reasons. She states, "LivePerson should want to know that all counselors are still practicing legally." In addition, she states that the quality and ethics of the professional counselors on the site may be unknown since LivePerson does not interview or ask for references from potential counselors; at least they did not when she applied in the first quarter of 2006.

MJ commented on the challenge of meeting the needs of consumers across state lines and the international clients. Regarding U.S. consumers, she is aware that state regulations differ and that some states require licensing in the state in which the consumer resides. She states:

> I try to contact the boards involved and find out what is required legally for me to practice with the specific clients. This is of course impossible to do with a live, drop-in session, which is one reason why I rarely do that any more. Frankly, it is a concern to me though, and one which I need to further explore. Of particular concern are the cases of false identity or the situations in which the client does not wish to let me know the state in which they are living.

With regard to international consumers, MJ has worked with consumers from South Africa, the Punjab, Great Britain, and South America. She states:

> It is critical to be aware of ethnic and cultural differences in order to fully meet the needs of the individual client, in all settings. This is never more so anywhere than it is in online counseling.... Interestingly, I have not, to my knowledge, treated anyone within my home state of [Deleted] where I hold my license! Dealing with language and cultural barriers is intriguing and challenging, and must be approached in the greatest humility if any help at all is to be had by the client. That being said, these clients are out there, right now, asking for help through this medium. We must decide as a profession, how we can best meet their needs.

Resolving Ethical Conflicts

MJ was asked how she decides to practice online given the ethical concerns she has raised about working on LivePerson. Her response indicates her weighing the benefits and risks of online practice, and belief that the profession should continue to pursue this approach.

> I see this as an emerging field of practice, one in which all the bugs have not been worked out. I'm hoping that solutions to

these problems will be found, over time. I'm also aware that there are risks in all forms of social work practice and that if I'm diligent about assessing the risk to the best of my ability and careful about determining the appropriateness of online intervention in each particular instance, I can feel okay with offering help in this way. As I mentioned already, people are asking for help online. And for some of these people, this may be the only opportunity they have for receiving help, for a variety of reasons. I'd like to think we can meet that need as a profession, working out the ethics and pragmatics.

DISCUSSION

This case study of the LivePerson model for service delivery high-lights many of the benefits and concerns previously discussed in the literature related to etherapy. There appears to be a strong demand for etherapy services and a growing number of practitioners providing their services online. The LivePerson model offers ease of use, convenience, and anonymity to those seeking services, and a convenient and reliable infrastructure for practitioners. The case study supports the proposition that some people who would otherwise not seek services will engage in etherapy. In addition, the model promotes the globalization and access of etherapy services with both service providers and consumers coming from countries outside the United States.

The model also promotes consumer choice in selecting practitioners since credentials, areas of expertise, experience, and consumer satisfaction ratings are readily available and searchable. In addition, the model makes it easy to "shop" for a therapist since consumers may easily terminate a session and quickly engage a new e-therapist at any time. While consumers have always had the ability to select professionals based on credentials and costs, the LivePerson model greatly increases information and choice. In order to promote consumer education, research is needed to understand how and why consumers chose their therapist in this new kind of entrepreneurial model. Research is also needed to examine the impact of the ease with which a professional relationship can be ended.

Public rating of services is common on retail sites on the Internet but is a new procedure for etherapy services. The mean rating of 4.76 for all therapists is very high. It may be that consumers will not engage a therapist who has received a low rating given so many choices with high ratings. Thus, initial ratings may carry great power to influence a therapist's ability to work on the site. The influence of ratings on a therapist's work is unknown. For example, would fear of low ratings reduce the amount of confrontation in therapy sessions? Would fear of low ratings result in denial of service for certain types of problems or consumers? The reasons that ratings are given and their impact on services warrants further research.

In this case study, the vast majority of consumers engaged the professional for only one session. This raises many questions. To what extent can issues be resolved in one session? What is the long-term outcome of such brief treatment? Or, do consumers engage in "just-in-time" counseling? Do they seek services when they perceive the need, engaging for several sessions spread over time, perhaps with many different counselors? Further research is needed to understand the process and impact of this new model of service delivery.

Fees for face-to-face counseling vary by profession, location, and marketplace conditions. Fees for e-mail also vary based on length, number of e-mails, and variation among service providers. All of these fees involve a set price for a specific amount of service. LivePerson presents a new model for fees based on per-minute fees for chat-based therapy services. This means that a consumer will not know how long a session will last at the outset and consequently will not know the exact fee that will be charged. This may work in a consumer's favor if an issue is resolved quickly, or it may lead to unexpected charges if sessions run longer than expected. This presents interesting challenges for both therapists and consumers. To what extent does worry about the length of session (and mounting charges) influence the content and process of a session? Will consumers feel "rushed"? Will therapists be influenced to shorten or lengthen sessions given the fee structure? Further research is needed to examine the impact of the per-minute fee model on the therapeutic process.

The case study underscores some of the legal and ethical dilemmas previously reported in the literature related to confidentiality, ability to intervene in a crisis, mandatory reporting, establishing the identity of a consumer, ability to do appropriate assessment, and jurisdiction issues. They are compounded by a model in which the operating company may have a conflict of interest with professional values.

While the company will want to assure confidentiality because it is good for business, it is not bound by the ethics of a helping professional. For example, the company wants all transactions to take place within the company infrastructure while a professional might want the consumer to have multiple ways of contact in case of an emergency. Similarly, a professional is obligated to report child abuse or neglect; however, the professional must rely on the company to provide identifying information so that the professional can report the suspected abuse. The extent to which this process functions smoothly warrants further investigation. In addition, a professional is obligated to keep information confidential, but the company's interests are to monitor transactions to be sure that professionals are not engaging in business outside of the host site. In the case of LivePerson, monitoring is automated based on algorithms looking for expressions such as phone numbers or e-mail addresses, thus maintaining confidentiality. The professional, however, loses control over client records since they are stored on the server of a company and decisions about the use of records rest with the company. Even when a company has policies that promote ethical practice, there may be some confusion by professionals about the meaning and standard practice associated with legalistic disclaimers. In addition, research is needed to document the extent to which ethical practices such as checking credentials and providing identifying information for mandatory reporting take place in a timely and facilitative manner. The result, in this case study, shows some tension between the ability to meet professional ethics and the desire to provide a needed and valuable service. Further research is needed to examine both the company's perception of its obligation to abide by professional ethics and how professionals resolve their ethical concerns about online practice.

In conclusion, this case study suggests that innovative service models continue to develop and that careful consideration of ethical and legal obligations of practice in the context of new models is needed. Helping professionals will need to investigate the process and outcomes of these models and to develop standards of practice that both reward increased access and consumer choice while upholding the values of helping professionals. Finally, given the extent to which online practice is taking place, education programs in the helping professions should include content on etherapy practice and concerns in their curriculum.

REFERENCES

Ainsworth, M. (2001). The ABCs of Internet Therapy. Metanoia Web site. Retrieved November 27, 2007 from http://www.metanoia.org/imhs/directory.htm.

American Counseling Association (2005). ACA code of ethics. Retrieved April 7, 2007, from http://www.counseling.org/Resources/CodeOfEthics/TP/Home/CT2.aspx.

American Mental Health Counselors Association. (2000). Code of ethics. Retrieved February 15, 2008, from http://www.amhca.org/code/.

American Psychological Association. (1997). *APA statement on services by telephone, teleconferencing, & Internet*. Retrieved April 7, 2007, from http://www.apa.org/ethics/stmnt01.html.

Andersson, G., Strömgren, T., Ström, L., & Lyttkens, L. (2002). Randomized controlled trial of Internet-based cognitive behavior therapy for distress associated with tinnitus. *Psychosomatic Medicine, 64*, 810–816.

Barak, A. (2004). Internet counseling. In C. E. Spielberger (ed.), *Encyclopedia of applied psychology* (pp. 369–378). San Diego: Academic Press.

Barnett, J. E., & Scheetz, K. (2003). Technological advances and telehealth: Ethics, law, and the practice of psychotherapy. *Psychotherapy: Theory, Research, Practice, Training, 40*(1/2), 86–93.

Benderly, B. L. (2005). The promise of etherapy. *Scientific American Mind, 16*(4), 72–77.

Clinical Social Work Federation. (2001). *CSWF position paper on Internet text-based therapy*. Retrieved April 7, 2007, from http://www.cswf.org/www/therapy.html.

Carlbring, P., Furmark, T., Steczkó, J., Ekselius, L., & Andersson, G. (2006). An open study of Internet-based bibliotherapy with minimal therapist contact via email for social phobia. *Clinical Psychologist, 10*, 30–38.

Finn, J. (2006). An exploratory study of email use by direct service social workers. *Journal of Technology in Human Services, 24*, 1–20.

Finn, J., & Banach, M. (2002). Risk management in online human services practice. *Journal of Technology and Human Services, 20*(1/2), 133–154.

Finn, J., & Holden, G. (Eds.) (2000). *Human services online: A new arena for service delivery*. Binghamton, NY: The Haworth Press.

Freeny, M. (2001). Better than being there. *Psychotherapy Networker*. March/April, 31–39, 70.

Furher, A. (2008). Personal email communication, March 4, 2008.

Grohol, J. M. (2004). Online counseling: A historical perspective. In R. Kraus, J. Zack, & G. Stricker (Eds.), *Online counseling: A handbook for mental health professionals* (pp. 51–68). San Diego, CA: Elsevier Academic Press.

Hirai, M., & Clum, G. A. (2006). A meta-analytic study of self-help interventions for anxiety problems. *Behavior Therapy, 37*, 99–111.

Horrigan J., & Rainie, L. (2006). *The Internet's major role in life's major moments*. PEW Internet and American Life Project. Retrieved October 23, 2006, from http://www.pewinternet.org/.

Hsiung, R. C. (Ed.) (2002). *Etherapy: Case studies, guiding principles, and the clinical potential of the Internet*. New York: Norton.

International Society for Mental Health Online. (2000). *Suggested principles for the online provision of mental health services* (Vol. 3.11). Retrieved April 7, 2007, from http://www.ismho.org/suggestions.html.

Kraus, R., Stricker, G., &Zack, J. (2003). *Online counseling: A handbook for mental health professionals*. San Diego: Academic Press/Elsevier Science & Technology Books.

Krysik, J. L., & Finn, J. (2007). *Research for effective social work practice*. New York: McGraw Hill.

Lavallee, A. (2006, April 25). Etherapy: More people are turning to instant messaging and online therapy for a range of mental health issues because they're fast and anonymous. CRC Health Group. Retrieved February 28, 2008, from http://www.crchealth.com/press-releases-2006/060425-etherapy.asp.

Lenhart, M., Madden, M., & Hitlin, P. (2005). Teens and technology. Washington, DC: The Pew Internet & American Life Project. Retrieved November 30, 2005, from http://www.pewinternet.org/pdfs/PIP_Teens_Tech_July2005web.pdf.

Mallen, M. J., Vogel, D. L., & Rochlen, A. B. (2005). The practical aspects of online counselling: Ethics, training, technology, and competency. *The Counseling Psychologist, 33*, 776–818.

Mallen, M. J., Vogel, D. L, Rochlen, A. B., Day, S. X. (2005). Online counseling: Reviewing the literature from a counseling psychology framework. *Counseling Psychologist, 33*(6), 819–871.

Manhaul-Baugus, M. (2001). Etherapy: Practical, ethical, and legal issues. *Cyberpsychology and Behavior, 4*(5), 551–563.

Mitchell, D. L., & Murphy, L. J. (2004). Email rules! Organizations and individuals creating ethical excellence in telemental-health. In J. Bloom & G. Walz (Eds.), *Cybercounseling and cyberlearning: An ENCORE* (pp. 203–217). Alexandria, VA: CAPS Press and American Counseling Association.

Mulhauser, G. (2006). One million words of online counselling and online therapy. Counseling Resource. Retrieved February 28, 2008, from http://counsellingresource.com/features/2006/12/04/one-million/.

Newman, M. G. (2004). Technology in psychotherapy: An introduction. *Journal of Clinical Psychology, 60*(2), 141–145.

Ragusea, A. S. & Vandecreek, L. (2003). Suggestions for the ethical practice of online psychotherapy. *Psychotherapy: Theory, research, practice, training, 40*, 94–102.

Rochlen, A. B., Zack, J. S., & Speyer, C. (2004). Online therapy: Review of relevant definitions, debates, and current empirical support. *Journal of Clinical Psychology, 60*, 269–283.

Spek, V., Cuijpers, P., Nyklícek, I., Riper, H., Keyzer, J., & Pop, V. (2007). Internet-based cognitive behaviour therapy for symptoms of depression and anxiety: A meta-analysis. *Psychological Medicine, 37*, 319–328.

Suler, J. (2004). The psychology of text relationships. In R. Kraus, J. Zack, & G. Stricker (Eds.), *Online counseling: A handbook for mental health professionals* (pp. 19–50). London: Elsevier, Inc.

Tate, D. F., & Zabinski, M. F. (2004). Computer and internet applications for psychological treatment: Update for clinicians. *JCLP/In Session, 60*(2), 209–220.

Wantland, D. J., Portillo, C. J., Holzemer, W. L., Slaughter, R., & McGhee, E. M. (2004). The effectiveness of web-based vs. non-web-based interventions: A meta-analysis of behavioral change outcomes. *Journal of Medical Internet Research, 6*(4:e4). Retrieved December 15, 2006, from http://www.jmir.org/2004/4/e40/.

Zelvin, E., & Speyer, C. M. (2003). Online counseling skills, part I: Treatment strategies for conducting counseling online. In R. Kraus, et al. (Eds.), *Online counseling: A handbook for mental health professionals* (pp. 163–180). San Diego, CA: Elsevier Academic Press.

Ethical Issues in the Provision
of Online Mental Health Services
(Etherapy)

Donna M. Midkiff
W. Joseph Wyatt

The rapid emergence of information technology over the past decade has led it to become an integral component of day-to-day living (Barak, 1999; Newman, 2004; Tate & Zabinski, 2004). Mental health service providers such as those who practice clinical social work, psychology, psychiatry, and counseling had modestly joined this trend toward the end of the 1980s (Barak, 1999; Zgodzinski, 1996).

The Internet as a medium for the delivery of mental health treatment and information today is becoming increasingly widespread (Alleman, 2002; Benderly, 2005; Finn, 2002, 2006; Finn & Holden, 2000; Newman, 2004; Rotondi et al., 2005; Tate & Zabinski, 2004).

As the technology developed, mental health care providers began to offer their services online. The pace of ethical and legal and regulatory bodies in establishing guidelines for online mental health services has lagged behind the rapid advancement of the technology for delivery of therapy over the Internet (Barak, 1999; Frankel, 2000; Maheu, 2001; Rosik & Brown, 2001). Not surprisingly, within the professions there is ongoing concern regarding both the ethics and effectiveness of Internet therapy. A survey of several hundred central Pennsylvania social workers whose primary responsibility was direct services found that only 17.8 percent agreed that it is "ethical to provide ongoing Internet therapy." This may have been because 73.5 percent of them disagreed with the statement, "E-mail is generally an effective means for social workers to provide therapeutic services to clients" (Finn, 2006).

Several major mental health organizations have devised ethical guidelines for etherapy. The National Association of Social Workers (NASW, 2000); American Counseling Association [ACA] (1999); American Mental Health Counselors Association [AMHCA] (2000); International Society for Mental Health Online, [ISMHO] (2000); and the National Board for Certified Counselors [NBCC] (2001) all have issued ethical guidelines for online treatment. Earlier the Ethics Committee of the American Psychological Association issued a statement regarding services by telephone, teleconferencing, and Internet (Ethics Committee of the American Psychological Association, 1997). That statement contained no new etherapy-specific standards but pointed out that, although there were no ethics rules prohibiting such services, psychologists are to follow the applicable ethical standards. As these associations have taken pause to issue such ethical standards, it appears to be clear that there are significant areas of concern that need to be addressed in the risk management of the provision of online mental health services (Finn & Banach, 2002).

Some issues appear to be more problematic than others when one attempts to transpose them from in-person therapy to etherapy. Our selection of these is intuitive based on our experiences as full-time therapists as well as on the first author's experience with the Internet and the second author's experience as a trainer of therapists. This paper will address several ethical issues with the purpose of providing e-therapists with an outline of issues, precepts, and suggestions that will better insure that clients receive optimal care that is consistent with ethical standards. We will address several issues, including informed consent, boundaries of competence, cultural competence, bases for scientific and professional judgment, avoidance of harm, protection of client privacy, avoidance of false or deceptive statements, Internet forums, use of testimonials, solicitation of clients, and therapists' fees. In addition, we will describe potential legal pitfalls, with particular attention to the matter of licensure jurisdiction when etherapy crosses state lines.

FORMS PACKET

Informed consent, including the development of a "forms packet" is vital if therapy is to proceed ethically, whether in-person or etherapy. The online therapeutic provider should develop a comprehensive informed consent process and documentation. This packet should include, but is not limited to, a presession intake form, informed consent document, cultural values, and privacy policy. The presession intake form is consistent with outpatient practice of collecting data on the client's presenting signs and symptoms. A relatively comprehensive form is most useful and should include the primary symptoms of most major mental health disorders (e.g., depression, anxiety, substance abuse, etc.). The potential online client is instructed at the initial contact on how to complete the forms packet. He or she should submit all of the information to the provider prior to any agreement to work with the client.

Informed Consent

As with any therapy, online clients must sign an informed consent form. This process can be achieved in two ways. The individual may sign and fax the information to the therapist. A second option, one consistent with the nature of the virtual milieu, is to incorporate electronic signatures into the consent package. The Digital Signatures Act, passed in 1999, was formed to "require the adoption and utilization of digital signatures by Federal agencies and to encourage the use of digital signatures in private sector electronic transactions." Text signatures are now considered to be legal representations of individuals' signatures and therefore are as legally binding as pen and paper signatures. Many virtual service sites, with service broadly defined as anything from purchasing and downloading MP3s to registering an account on eBay, require the click of a box affirming that one has read and accepts the terms and conditions of the service. The action is considered legally binding. Given that this is a routine operation with most online service providers, it would likely be considered acceptable in the provision of online therapies as well. However, the added component of having the clients sign/type their names adds a perceptual layer to their commitment to the process. Consequently, this should strengthen the service provider's risk management position.

Boundaries of Competence

While it is a given that the therapist's speaking competence is paramount within the in-person session, written verbal competence on the part of the clinician is particularly relevant in the delivery of most (exceptions such as distance video/audio treatment are becoming fairly common)behavioral e-health services (Maheu, 2001). Verbal skill in face-to-face therapy does not necessarily translate into skill in written communication, especially interactive text-based communication that involves a series of interpersonal interpretations within each exchange (Childress, 2000). Conversely, written word skill does not automatically translate to well-spoken style when face to face. It is reasonable that the online clinician demonstrate, perhaps to a sub-committee of the state's licensing board (as with any claimed competence), through either formal methods (continuing education units [CEUs], course work) or informal methods (published written work, solicitation of collegial review, etc.) his or her abilities to communicate emotion and contextual intent solely through the written word. At this time, no such requirements are in place.

A related issue is how one achieves status as a reviewer of another's online written competence. There are no clear answers to this question. However, it is likely that within any given state there would be several answers to a licensing board's call for those requesting expert status in the area of online written communication competence. Such a board would then do well to be informed by those from other disciplines, including perhaps those in the areas of language arts and communication studies, as it works to establish criteria by which to designate expert status in written communication.

Cultural Competence

As with face-to-face therapy, cultural competence is a relevant issue. The therapist's familiarity with colloquial expressions, idioms, and local variations of word usage is important, given the many potential locations of their identified clients. Knowledge of the individual's age, ethnicity, and religious beliefs often allows for cultural awareness that may be quite valuable in treatment. It is also important that the client indicate fluency in the therapist's language. However, it is debatable as to whether clients should be required to provide racial or other information that could give rise to complaints of a therapist's bias. This could be addressed in the assessment component as well as included in the forms packet on a form titled "Cultural Values." It should be clear that etherapy presents some challenges in the area of cultural competency. For example, in face-to-face treatment a client's ethnic status may be relatively clear if the client enters the therapy room wearing jewelry or clothing that provides clues to such information. A client wearing a Star of David pendant is likely to be Jewish; one wearing a cross, Christian. Online therapy may have to proceed minus such potentially interesting information. Thus, one must be cognizant of the absence of important visual cues and what those cues could have brought to the session while at the same time developing compensatory strategies that assist in learning more about the client. For example, the e-therapist may ask additional questions at assessment or may inquire more frequently as to the client's present thoughts and feelings, or he or she may make use of readily available emoticons.

Assessment and Diagnosis

Competence in the areas of assessment, diagnosis, and treatment is also of significant concern (Rosik & Brown, 2001; Shapiro & Schulman, 1996). Given that face-to-face assessment works against the convenience nature of online therapy, the online therapist should be sensitive to nuances that are absent when it comes to online assessment. For example, there are distinctions of affect, clothing, hygiene, and other aspects of appearance that may provide valuable information in assessing the type and severity of pathology during a face-to-face mental status examination. These elements are lost with text-based online assessment (Gollings & Paxton, 2006; Skarderud, 2003). Internet video, where available, would eliminate most of these concerns, but not all. For example, body odor, pupil dilation, and glassy eyes would not be evident, even with better quality video, assuming that a wide angle view containing more than just the client's face appears on the screen. To deal with this issue, one could opt to not provide online services without an initial face-to-face meeting, or to include video conferencing at the onset of services or even ask for a picture of the client. At a minimum, and with heightened awareness of online-only limitations, a therapist should assure that an extensive initial assessment is conducted. As with all assessment, the goal is to determine the client's mental health treatment needs and whether, as with face-to-face treatment, the etherapy modality is appropriate. If not, the therapist must consider offering available alternatives and make referrals as needed

Clearly, ethical and practical competence presents new challenges for the online therapist. Although we have delineated a number of the major issues and offered suggestions, it is evident that a great deal remains to be done if the competency standards of etherapy are to approach those of face-to-face therapy. These efforts are the responsibility of national associations, state licensing boards, and the academic community. From a national level, the climate must be communicated that online therapy exists, is growing, and requires attention. Ethical guidelines are produced there. At the state level, licensing boards are obligated to add this area of expertise to their competency standards, and progressive curriculum development is needed from the academic community.

BASIS FOR SCIENTIFIC PROFESSIONAL JUDGMENT

The provision of online therapeutic interventions has a promising future, especially for technologies of a cognitive and behavioral nature (Gollings & Paxton, 2006; Hopps, Pepin, & Boisvert, 2003; Lange, Van de Ven, & Shreiken, 2003; Seligman, Steen, Park, &

Peterson, 2005; Tate, Jackvony, & Wing, 2003; Tate, Wing, & Winett, 2001; White et al., 2004). The online clinician should be sensitive to, and demonstrate knowledge of, several issues related to etherapy. First, just as the face-to-face therapist, the e-therapist must possess knowledge of proven effective online treatment strategies, their scopes, and their limitations. This should be clearly spelled out and included in the forms packet, likely under a heading of "Professional Responsibility." As in face-to-face therapy, competence is essential, and there must be no assumption that general therapeutic competence automatically translates to etherapy competence.

Second, a clinician not only should be knowledgeable in the study and practice of psychotherapy, he or she should also possess proficiency in the uses of computer technology. He or she should have an understanding of the computer and its relationship to the Internet. An online therapist should be proficient in the area of e-mail programs (e.g., send, receive, attachments, cc, bcc, dating of messages, flagging prioritization, HTML links, etc.). To be skilled with e-mail programming, or the principles of sending a document, is an essential time management tool. For example, a therapist may wish to send a document to the patient that will help him or her keep a diary of emotions. If, using chat mode, the therapist struggles to both find that document in the computer's memory and then discover how to attach and send it to the client, the time involved in those tasks probably has intruded significantly on the therapeutic interaction. An online therapist should be capable of maintaining a conversation while simultaneously sending the document.

The online clinician should be familiar with chat room environments and forums, including understanding the role of avatars, emoticons, and backgrounds. These tools are virtual means of communication, substitutes in the absence of face-to-face visual cues. In a forum, avatars are used as a means of self-expression or identity expression. An avatar is a picture or icon, often the size of a desktop icon, that serves as a means of communication. One individual might represent herself as a daisy while another identifies with a skull and crossbones. Although an avatar is not thought of as a statement of the whole person, it does, however, communicate a potentially useful bit of information about a person's self-identification.

Emoticons are *emotional icons* used to communicate specific feelings. When expressing a feeling in words, the writer may include a still or animated emoticon. For example, a client might express sadness in words, and then add as a degree of additional expression an icon with a frowning face, or a frowning face with one tear, or an animated face crying significantly. Thus, emoticons may be quite helpful in the communication process by visually representing varying degrees of feeling.

Proficiency in these skills could be demonstrated by a review of the therapist's experience, relevant coursework, or other training. State licensing boards could develop such standards, and they could devise and administer an exam to ensure that any licensed therapist who wishes to engage in etherapy indeed possesses these proficiencies.

A clinician should also have basic understanding of web development and hosting plans, in part to better utilize resources that enhance confidentiality and privacy. Not only is the online therapist ethically bound by confidentiality (e.g., keeping information that an individual has disclosed in a relationship of trust), the therapist must also protect the client's privacy, which means taking measures to stop information about the client from becoming known to people other than those chosen by the client.

MAINTENCE OF PRIVACY

It is understandable that clients and therapists alike are concerned that once their information is transmitted into cyberspace it may fall before the eyes of those for whom it was never intended. Today's technology provides virtual program development and the ability to incorporate secure sockets layers (SSL) and encryption technologies for Internet therapy and e-mail programs into the website. It is important that traditional chat or e-mail programs be upgraded to incorporate encryption technologies. Encryption provides security (prevention of those other than the intended target from viewing the information) while information is in transit or in storage by converting plain text to cipher text. Decryption refers to the reversal of this process. The SSL is suggested for the use of payment transactions, forums, virtual reality therapeutic environments, or any instance in which conversation is carried on or stored.

> The protocol supports server and client authentication and is application independent, which means that protocols like HTTP, FTP and Telnet may be layered on top of it transparently. The SSL protocol is able to negotiate encryption keys as well as authenticate the server before data are exchanged by the

higher-level application. It maintains the security and integrity of the transmission channel by using encryption, authentication and message authentication codes. (Report of the Technical Working Group on Telemedicine Standardization, 2003)

Together, SSL and encryption services insure security for the therapist and the client in the electronic transfer of information. HIPPA (Health Insurance Portability and Accountability Act of 1996, 1998) regulations are also helpful in guiding the online practitioner with respect to maximizing electronic security. The online therapist should be knowledgeable about the applicable regulations and demonstrate that knowledge to the potential client. This can be noted in the forms packet—"Privacy Practices." For example, HIPPA requires a password-protected computer as well as a timed "log out" on any computer used in mental health treatment facilities. This helps to prevent an unauthorized individual from accessing client information. Automatic virus filtering, spam filtering, and spyware removal are also required (SafetySend, 1996. Whether an individual practitioner chooses to offer etherapy only or decides to build a website that incorporates etherapy with other resources such as forums, utilization of SSL and encryption services is a must if one is to assure that the client's privacy and confidentiality are maintained.

It is also essential for the online therapist to educate the client as to measures that could be taken to increase security at the client's end of the computer. Examples include installing firewalls, using encrypted e-mail software, being aware of anyone in the client's household who may have access to the computer, and trying to limit or restrict that access. However, ultimately, the potential for a breech of privacy remains, just as it remains for material kept in a manila folder in a locked office. Thus, the therapist must remain up-to-date on current technological standards with regard to encryption and the like. The website homepage should include a link to a page that explains the nature of the site's SSL and encryption technology (e.g., privacy policy), HIPPA regulations, and the limits to confidentiality as they are typically addressed in face-to-face therapy.

The e-therapist should be aware of and abide by the limits to confidentiality in all states in which his or her clients reside. Most states provide exceptions to confidentiality when the client is thought to be a danger to either himself or herself or to others, or when a child, infirm person, or otherwise incompetent person is suspected to be a victim of abuse or neglect. For example, in our state of West Virginia, those who provide therapeutic services are mandated by law to report abuse or neglect, even if it is only suspected. Taking into consideration the absence of federal or international standards for abuse or neglect reporting, the most sensible approach for the online therapist is to be knowledgeable regarding the reporting laws and child protective services procedures in the states and/or countries where both the practitioner and client reside (Riemersma & Leslie, 1999; Rosik & Brown, 2001). This information is readily available on most states' websites or by calling any state's department of health and human resources and asking for reporting requirements.

Some online etherapy providers do not offer services to individuals under the age of 18 due to the added complexities (e.g., verification of age, verification of parent or guardian consent) of providing mental health services to children. Nevertheless, validation of identity is an essential component of informed consent. Given the anonymity of the web, validating identities can be difficult. A potential solution is to require photo identification and/or a signature declaration regarding personal demographics. Other intuitive suggestions include a more subjective approach such as looking for trends of dishonesty. This can be accomplished by cross-checking Internet protocol (IP) addresses with the stated address given at assessment. Each machine connected to the Internet has an address known as an Internet proto-col address (IP address). The IP address takes the form of four numbers separated by dots, for example: 123.45.67.890. One may purchase software that employs a noninvasive approach to collection of data such as country, region, city, postal code, and area from which a visitor's message originates. For example, consider that a cli-ent has signed an informed consent to treatment indicating that she is from Texas, but each time you meet online, her computer "pings" from Europe. In such a situation the software has given the online therapist reason to suspect dishonesty. That should trigger a plan of action (i.e., require additional proof of identity). Geographic dis-honesty can be particularly problematic when there is an emergency, or in matters of suspected abuse or neglect.

It is important to make arrangements in the client's local area so that one may address emergency and crisis situations that may arise (Barnett & Sheetz, 2003; Childress, 2000). For example, having access to emergency contact numbers in the client's location is an important measure to ensure that crises are adequately addressed. This information, collected from the client at assessment, should include numbers for a personal emergency contact as well as the direct numbers to the local fire and police departments and location of the local hospital emergency room.

Clearly, protection of etherapy clients is in some ways more cumbersome than is protection of clients who are seen face to face. Thus, our attention to the protections listed throughout this paper brings to light an irony of etherapy. Specifically, when provided in an ethical, legal, and prudent manner, online therapy may bring about a net loss of convenience, and perhaps even added costs, to the e-therapist.

It is important to inform clients of the measures being taken to ensure that the standard technologies are in place to protect their privacy. The same cautions should be provided as with face-to-face therapy. Moreover, the online therapist should also provide advance notice as to when technologies will be down for repair and also should offer backup strategies for unexpected crashes or electrical outages. For example, the website should offer instruction (whom to call, phone numbers, etc.) in the event of a power outage in the client's local area or in a time of emergency that occurs when the website is unavailable. Since power will not be available, these instructions should be kept in hard copy by the client and therapist.

AVOIDANCE OF HARM

To "do no harm" is the first and most oft-quoted principle when it comes to the provision of health care (Shapiro & Schulman, 1996). As with all health care interventions, the evaluation of potential harm must be balanced against potential benefits. The simple presence of risk does not necessarily preclude the use of an intervention that is sufficiently justified by the potential benefits (Childress, 2000). However, expectations are that a therapist will maintain a full understanding of the nature of the risks and will inform clients of those risks. The forms packet's "Informed Consent" document should include statements that are consistent with the research regarding the risks, benefits, and scope of research with regard to efficacy of the interventions. A model statement of benefits and risks follows:

Potential Benefits of Etherapy

There are potential unique benefits to receiving mental health services online. These may include: (1) being able to send and receive messages at any time of day or night; (2) never having to leave messages with intermediaries; (3) avoidance of voice mail and "telephone tag"; (4) being able to take virtually unlimited time to compose one's message and to reflect on the therapist's messages; (5) automatic maintenance of a record of communications; (6) cost savings, in some cases, as compared to face-to-face therapy; (7) feeling less inhibited about self-disclosure; (8) convenient scheduling; and (9) enjoyment of the comfort of one's own private space (Benderly, 2005; Barnett & Scheetz, 2003; Childress, 2000; Grohol, 1999).

Potential Risks of Etherapy

There also are potential risks or disadvantages to receiving mental health services online: (1) messages may be lost in cyberspace or otherwise may not be received; (2) breach of confidentiality by hackers or at the level of the Internet service provider is possible, though this is highly unlikely given our encryption services; (3) e-mails may not be received if they are sent to the wrong address (which might also breach confidentiality); (4) confidentiality could be breached at either end by others with access to the e-mail account or the computer, although therapists allow no one access to patient communications other than the therapist (Manhaul-Baugus, 2001; Rosik & Brown, 2001; Frankel, 2000; *Hunt v. Disciplinary Board*, 1980).

It would be prudent if this and other sections of the website were reviewed by at least one (and preferably two or three) therapists who are experienced in clinical practice and who are known to have special interest in ethical issues as a means to optimize accuracy of information dissemination. We suggest that a qualifying statement be included on the website's homepage to read, "The risks/benefits of techniques used here have been reviewed by a panel of experts in the field. For more information contact —."

AVOIDANCE OF FALSE OR DECEPTIVE STATEMENTS

In recent years it has become more common to see print and even television advertisements for in-person therapy, even though some therapists continue to frown on advertising because they feel it subtracts from the dignity of the profession. However, e-therapists will in many, if not most, cases construct website homepages that will function as advertisements. These will be viewed as a prelude to possible online therapy in many instances. Thus, it would be wise for the website to be reviewed for accuracy and clarity by one or more professionals who are familiar with the therapist's training and experience prior to placing the site online. This may best be done by review of a hard copy of the proposed content rather than by online review of a website that is under construction. As was the case with the first author, information about her website fell into the hands of those not targeted, at a time when the site was under construction and services were not yet being offered to potential clients. Hard copy development would most probably have prevented that unfortunate occurrence. An alternative would include clear wording that the website is "under construction," as a cautionary measure to prevent any misrepresentation of the information.

FORUMS

Internet therapeutic forums are common supportive services offered online. The premise behind these forums is to provide a peer-to-peer supportive environment for those who seek individuals with common experiences. It is not uncommon for the administrator or moderator of these forums to be a therapist, although the activities in the forum should be noted as helpful information only and, in our opinion, terms such as *therapy* or *treatment* should be avoided in describing this resource. Moderators may offer question-and-answer sections, such as "ask the therapist," or offer support for participation in the forum, and so on. Forum users should be required to complete an acknowledgement that they understand and accept these premises.

Given the likelihood that without structure certain misuse or abuse could occur in a forum, it is important for standards to be set and effectively communicated. In line with the ethical standards, some ground rules are suggested. First, forums may be more easily managed if they are issue specific rather than general. Although there is justification for general forums, there is concern that they contain risk of disputes among members as to what constitutes acceptable topics for discussion (as with any process group, based on our combined nearly 20 years of experience as full-time therapists), which may be especially difficult to resolve when not face to face. Second, the forum administrator or moderator must make it clear that a forum is not a substitute for mental health treatment. Third, the moderator must state the terms under which one may participate in the forum. Ordinarily these terms would include that the established topic (e.g., smoking cessation, child conduct, etc.) be adhered to, that verbal style be respectful, and that uninvited solicitation of other services by participants or by outside vendors is prohibited. Similarly, the terms of the forum should state that those who fail to follow the standards will be barred from the forum by the administrator. Forums present an example of the importance of technical proficiency—the administrator should be capable of blocking IP addresses and user names by navigating the forum administration panel (e.g., ban control, permissions, rank, word censors, styles, pruning, etc.). The bottom line for forum moderation is the development of rules, requiring that participants agree to abide by those rules, daily oversight to insure that those rules are being followed, and the ability to administer specified consequences if they are not.

TESTIMONIALS

In the face-to-face context, use of client testimonials has found minimal acceptance, as the practice is seen by many as beneath the dignity of the profession and because testimonials may carry the perception that clients have felt pressured to provide them. However, there are, and will continue to be, therapists who make use of testimonial advertising anyway. Very likely it is unwise to use testimonials on a website, except under very specific conditions. Identities must be protected, testimonials must be spontaneous, and permission must be obtained in writing and kept on file by the website owner. E-therapists may well find it quite tempting to use testimonials because they may do so (on their websites' homepages) at no additional cost to themselves and because clients are necessarily providing written statements from which it may be tempting to cull testimonial "sound bites." Despite those factors, we continue to advise against the use of client testimonials.

IN-PERSON SOLICITATION

Whether e-communication is best thought of as "in-person" is a matter of some discussion. Usually we think of in-person as "in the flesh" or appearing personally. However, assuming that in some sense, sending an e-mail may have the feel of a virtual knock on the door, the therapist would tend to be protected against complaints of solicitation if no overture is ever initiated by the therapist. A rule of thumb: no first contact by the therapist.

A related area of concern is the potential vulnerability of forum members to a therapist who also provides etherapy. Unlike face-to-face group therapy members, most forum members would not necessarily be considered clients in treatment. As such, they should never be solicited by the owner/therapist to become clients, although they should receive confidential direction regarding therapeutic alternatives should the therapist/moderator become aware that the client is dangerous or otherwise may benefit from therapy. Should a forum member inquire, the owner/therapist should follow standard precautions to ensure that the client's best interests are served. The online therapist may query as to the individual's primary concern and offer suggestions with viable treatment options (e.g. face-to-face psychotherapy, online therapy, psychiatric consult, etc.).

FEES AND FINANCIAL ARRANGMENTS

In general, the secure sockets layers (SSL) and encryption technologies that are employed with any online purchase will likewise protect both client and therapist. It is wise that a link to "fees" be prominent on the therapist's homepage. The fee amounts, any discounts, and an insurance disclaimer should be located at that link and clearly stated. Billing methods and payment procedures should be articulated there as well. A potential client should have read and agreed to the fee arrangement prior to the onset of therapy, as with face-to-face practice. Fees are not standardized. An individual might research other online therapists' fee structures in order to gain some insight. However, we have noted in our experience that fees typically range anywhere from $35 to $135 for a 45 minute etherapy session. Presently most health insurances do not cover etherapy sessions. Thus, etherapy is mostly a cash-based service and, given the novelty of etherapy, we recommend that it be offered at the lower end of the prevailing fee schedules.

SOME OBSERVATIONS ON LEAGAL JURISDICTION

While the vision of a global Internet community has a great deal to offer in the health care service arena, a number of legal sensitivities must be faced. In particular, jurisdictional questions have become increasingly complex with the explosion of Internet usage and technology (Frankel, 2000; Rosik & Brown, 2001). Some suggest that cyberspace does not belong to a single state or country but to a whole range of geographical topographies with diverse legal concepts, making regulation extremely difficult (Frankel, 2000, Markoff, 1995). A consumer traveling the information superhighway has been likened to the consumer driving the interstate highway (Stofle, 1996). No one argues that the physician who prescribes a 10-day course of antibiotics to prevent infection in an auto accident victim should be licensed to practice medicine in states to which the patient may travel on leaving the emergency room. Similarly, Internet treatment may cross state lines to the patient's benefit and development of enforceable state-only licensure requirements would appear to be filled with difficulty.

Traditionally, the licensure of health professionals is a function performed at the state level. Etherapy raises interesting questions. Should licensure laws in the therapist's state or the client's state apply? If the answer is the latter, how would such laws be enforced? Would, for example, Pennsylvania licensing boards for clinical social workers or psychologists attempt to sanction a therapist whose Internet practice is physically located in Oregon but whose client is in Pennsylvania? If so, would that necessarily be in the client's best interest?

Laws governing individual health care providers are enacted through state legislative action, with authority to implement the practice acts delegated to the respective state licensing boards (Rosik & Brown, 2001; Center for Telemedicine Law, 2003). In 1996 the Federation of State Medical Boards took the lead in addressing the issue of jurisdiction by adapting state licensure requirements to accommodate practice across state lines (Rosik & Brown, 2001). They published "A Model Act to Regulate the Practice of Medicine Across State Lines." Section II (Definitions) of the Model Act states:

> It is important to view the practice of medicine as occurring in the location of the patient in order that the full resources of

the state would be available for the protection of that patient. The same standard of care, already in existence in thepatient's home state, would be required of all individuals practicing medicine within that jurisdiction.... (p. 2)

There are even more conservative approaches. California law now states that only those therapists licensed in California can provide online therapy to residents of California (Frankel, 2000; Rosik & Brown, 2001; Stofle, 1996), although it is unclear how California authorities might undertake legal sanctions against e-therapists located in another state, or even in another country. In contrast to the evident intent of the California etherapy law, and by analogy to medical practice, a patient may routinely drive across state lines to obtain a physician's care. In such a case, the state in which the physician is located governs the practice. By analogy, a client who "travels" via the Internet to obtain therapy in another state seems quite similar. Thus, it is arguable whether the client's care is best governed by the state in which the therapist is located or by the state in which the client is located.

Current law in our state (West Virginia) has no prohibition against the provision of online mental health services across state lines, as exists in California. However, state laws are diverse and courts have ruled that a either a fee paid or repeated therapist-client communication constitutes a therapeutic relationship. Until clarifying laws/policies emerge, the online therapist must proceed cautiously when crossing state lines (*Hunt v. Disciplinary Board*, 1980; Rosik & Brown, 2001).

One option is to acquire licensure in every state in which an etherapy client resides. However, that restriction is likely problematic for several reasons, including that it may well deny services to individuals who have found one's website and responded to it favorably. This calls to mind the way that a potential client may respond favorably to a Yellow Pages ad or to an appearance in public by a therapist. What brought about the favorable response may have been some vague quality that prompted the client's inquiry. A refusal, even with a referral, may delay services or cause the client to become discouraged about the prospects of treatment entirely.

Another problem with requiring "every-state" licensure is that it is not practical, at least at present. Such a requirement would serve as a de facto requirement that etherapy be limited to one, or perhaps two or three, states for the majority of therapists. In addition, a law such as California's probably unduly restricts clients' access to therapists who possess expertise in treatment of specific disorders. For example, a potential client whose problem is trichotillomania may find expert treatment online and out-of-state while no affordable face-to-face expert exists within a hundred miles of the client's home or even online (to the client's knowledge) elsewhere in California. In such a case, it is conceivable that the California law is overly restrictive and inconsistent with the principle of protecting the public. Such a scenario may appear unlikely in a state such as California where surely there are several experts for every disorder. In contrast, low-population density states such as Montana, the Dakotas, or West Virginia present a different picture. There, online therapy may be the only practical solution for individuals in need of specific therapeutic expertise, and that expertise may be found out of state.

Given the previous, some suggested alternatives to the restrictive California law are considered. One of these is to require that a client be connected to a qualified therapist in his or her home state if the e-therapist is out-of-state. This could be accomplished if the e-thera-pist requires that the client have a face-to-face visit to a local therapist prior to the start of etherapy and at given intervals, such as following every fifth session. This suggestion raises a number of issues, how-ever. The local therapist must be comfortable in the backup role. The e-therapist and the backup must also deal with issues of payment, liability insurance, availability to the client, and therapeutic techniques. An ancillary issue is whether the local therapist may also be an e-therapist. An online network of providers (governed and regulated by standards accepted by the mental health communities) may facilitate that process. The issues should, however, be solvable. They are somewhat similar to the issues that arise when an on-call physician covers a practice when the primary physician is unavail-able. The on-call physician has no special expectation of seeing a given patient but nevertheless is available to the patient on an agreed-on basis. A complicating factor is the client's desire for gradual disclosure, a phenomenon common enough in face-to-face therapy that one may assume it for many, if not most, clients who are involved etherapy. Resolution of that problem is well beyond the scope of this paper. However, we trust that it is a difficulty that will receive ongoing attention as etherapy becomes more common.

A risky alternative to the restrictive nature of the California law is for the therapist to determine that he or she meets the requirements of the practice law in the client's state, without actually seeking licensure in that state. For example, assume the therapist's state and the client's state requirements for psychology licensure are that the therapist have a doctoral degree in clinical psychology from an APA accredited program and have completed a one-year internship. Assume as well that the therapist must have obtained a score of 140 on the national licensing exam and have passed an oral exam. Then the online therapist might consider it "safe" to conduct etherapy with that client. As with many issues involving online services, licensing regulations vary state to state, and therefore an assumed "reciprocity" should match accordingly if it is to be thought of as a "due diligence" effort. Nevertheless, such a standard not only invites a risky test in the courts but is quite vague and, thus, is not highly suitable. We are presently unaware of lower court tests, but it is safe to assume that they are coming. Thus, the therapy professions would be well served to deal with the possibility in a preventive fashion.

National minimum standards for etherapy across state lines ought to be established. Federal legislation should be informed by the various guilds (NASW, APA, etc.) and the standards already devised by organized medicine. In the final analysis, it is unlikely that a restrictive law such as that in California can or should be the model, given that it is virtually unenforceable, as etherapy continues to cross state lines. Although those who strongly prefer state control may disagree, our suggestion is that the state law in which the therapist is physically located should apply, and that there be no "across state lines" restriction. Furthermore, perhaps a national examination could be used for those states that do not have licensure for some professions.

CONCLUSION

Although there are thoughtful and principled positions from various sides of the issues of etherapy, it remains clear that the Internet and etherapy have established a sense of permanence in our lives. The legal and ethical issues of online therapy are here to stay, and they contain the potential for wrongful outcomes, as with face-to-face therapy, if not adequately addressed. We think it is important to echo the sentiment, "If the ethical therapist is not online, who is?" (Stofle, 1996).

Frankel (2000) writes effectively as to the need for such caution. While visiting in the East African country of Malawi, a friend cautioned him while walking one morning to watch out for the poisonous snake nicknamed "The Third Man Death." The snake earned its name because the first passerby would awaken it, the second would irritate it, and the third person would be bitten and killed by it. Despite the emergence and pace of dot.com mental health practices, there are several barriers yet to be addressed in order to protect the public, the profession, and the practitioner from harm. It may not be the first or second e-client who suffers; rather, harm may come about because potential hazards are either unknown to the "passerby" or have not been addressed by the client's guild.

The most pressing barriers include the lack of case law, lack of federal regulations, and the patchwork of professional guidelines for online mental health practitioners. It is our intent here to contribute to the debate with this review and discussion of several perspectives on etherapy and its ethical and legal concerns. In order to adequately and expeditiously address the issues articulated here, practitioners working within professions that lack legal, regulatory, or ethical guidelines are encouraged to continue this discussion. Additional helpful measures may include contacting Congress, state licensing boards, malpractice carriers, and professional associations regarding the need for written, clearly defined standards of acceptable practice (Maheu, 2001). Beyond all of this, the national nature of e-services demands that professional organizations devise works-in-progress standards that inform both their members and Congress, and that those organizations encourage Congress to establish thoughtful and equitable e-practice federal law.

There is yet a final issue that must not be avoided. It is the training of e-therapists by graduate programs. It would be unwise, we feel, for higher education departments to learn, after the fact, that many of their graduates were engaging in etherapy minus formal training. Thus, we recommend that the optimal outcome will occur if therapists-in-training are, at a minimum, allowed the option of receiving etherapy academic instruction under close supervision prior to entering the field as fledgling therapists. The pedagogy of such training should certainly be the focus of future research.

REFERENCES

Alleman, J. R. (2002). Online counseling: The Internet and mental health treatment. *Psychotherapy: Theory/Research/Practice/Training, 39*(2), 199–209.

American Counseling Association. (1999). *ACA Code of Ethics Technology Standards.* Retrieved June 17, 2006, from http://www.counseling.org/Resources/CodeOfEthics/TP/Home/CT2.aspx.

American Mental Health Counselors Association. (2000). *Code of Ethics.* Retrieved June 17, 2006, from http://www.amhca.org/code/.

Barak, Z. (1999). Psychological applications on the Internet: A discipline on the threshold of a new millennium. *Applied and Preventive Psychology, 8,* 231–245.

Barnett, J. E., & Scheetz, K. (2003). Technological advances and telehealth: Ethics, law, and the practice of psychotherapy. *Psychotherapy: Theory, Research, Practice, Training, 40*(1/2), 86–93.

Benderly, B. L. (2005). The promise of etherapy. *Scientific American Mind, 16*(4), 72–77.

Center for Telemedicine Law (2003). Telemedicine licensure report. Washington, DC: Center for Telemedicine Law.

Childress, C. A. (2000). Ethical issues in providing online psychotherapeutic interventions. *Journal of Medical Internet Research, 2*(1), e5. < URL:http://www.jmir.org/2000/1/:e5.

The Digital Signature Act (1999). Library of Congress, HR 1572 IH. Retrieved July 13, 2006, from, http://www.techlawjournal.com/cong106/digsig/hr1572ih.htm.

Ethics Committee of the American Psychological Association. (1997). *APA statement on services by telephone, teleconferencing, and Internet.* Retrieved June 17, 2006, from http://apa.org/ethics/stmnt01.html.

Finn, J., & Banach, M. (2002). Risk management in online human services practice. *Journal of Technology and Human Services, 20*(1/2), 133–154.

Finn, J. (2002). MSW student perception of the ethics and efficacy of online therapy. *Journal of Social Work Education, 38,* 403–420.

Finn, J. (2006). An exploratory study of email use by direct service social workers. *Journal of Technology in Human Services, 24,* 1–20.

Finn, J., & Holden, G. (Eds.) (2000). *Human services online: A new arena for service delivery.* Binghamton, NY: The Haworth Press.

Frankel, S. A. (2000). Watch out for the "Third Man Death." Retrieved June 22, 2006, from http://www.psychboard.ca.gov/pubs/12_2000.pdf.

Gollings, E. K., & Paxton, S. J., (2006). Comparison of Internet and face-to-face delivery of a group body image and disordered eating intervention for women: A pilot study. *Eating Disorders, 14,* 1–15.

Grohol, J. M. (1999). *Best practices in etherapy: Definition and scope of etherapy.* Retrieved June 17, 2006, from http://www.ismho.org/issues/9902.htm.

Health Insurance Portability and Accountability Act of 1996, Publ. L. No. 104–191, 110 Stat. 1998.

Hopps, S. L., Pepin, M., & Boisvert, J. M. (2003). The effectiveness of cognitive-behavioral group therapy for loneliness via inter-relay-chat among people with physical disabilities. *Psychotherapy: Theory, Research, Practice, Training, 40*, 136–147.

Hunt v. Disciplinary Board, 381 S. 2d 52 (Ala. 1980).

International Society for Mental Health Online. (2000). *Suggested principals for the online provision of mental health services.* Retrieved June 18, 2005, from http://www.ismho.org/suggestions.html.

Lange, A., van de Ven, J. P., & Shrieken, B. (2003). Interapy: Treatment of post-traumatic stress via the Internet. *Cognitive Behaviour Therapy, 32*(3), 110–124.

Maheu, M. M. (2001). Practicing psychotherapy on the Internet: Risk management challenges and opportunities. *Register Report, 27*, 23–28.

Manhaul-Baugus, M. (2001). Etherapy: Practical, ethical, and legal issues. *Cyberpsychology and Behavior, 4*(5), 551–563.

Markoff, J. (1995). Online service blocks access to topics called pornographic. *New York Times*, December 29.

NASW (National Association of Social Workers) (2000). *The National Association of Social Workers Code of Ethics.* Washington, DC: NASW Press.

National Board for Certified Counselors. (2001). *The practice of Internet counseling.* Retrieved June 17, 2006, from http://www.nbcc.org/webethics2.

Newman, M. G. (2004). Technology in psychotherapy: An introduction. *Journal of Clinical Psychology, 60*(2), 141–145.

Riemersma M., & Leslie, R. S., (1999). Therapy counseling over the Internet: Innovation or unnecessary risk. *The California Therapist, 11*(6), 33–36.

Report of the Technical Working Group on Telemedicine Standardization. (2003) *Recommended guidelines and standards for practice of telemedicine in India.* Retrieved June 20, 2006, from http://www.mit.gov.in/telemedicine/Report%20of%20TWG%20on%20Telemed%20Standardisation.pdf.

Rosik, C. H., & Brown, R. (2001). Professional use of the Internet: Legal and ethical issues in a member care environment. *Journal of Psychology and Theology, 2*, 106–120.

Rotondi, A. J., Haas, G. L., Anderson, C. M., Newhill, C. E., Spring, M. B., Ganguli, et al. (2005). A clinical trial to test the feasibility of a telehealth psychoeducational intervention for persons with schizophrenia and their families: Intervention and 3-month findings. *Rehabilitation Psychology, 50*(4), 325–336.

SafetySend. (1996). HIPPA compliance requirements (1996). Retrieved July 13, 2006, from http://www.safetysend.com/HIPPA-Requirements.htm.

Seligman, M., Steen, T. A., Park, N., & Peterson, C. (2005). Positive psychology progress: Empirical validation of interventions. *American Psychologist, 60*(5), 410–421.

Shapiro, D. E., & Schulman, C. E. (1996). Ethical and legal issues in e-mail therapy. *Ethics and Behavior, 6*, 107–124.

Skarderud, F. (2003). Shame in cyberspace. Relationships without faces: The E-media and eating disorders. *European Eating Disorders Review, 11*, 155–169.

Stofle, G. S. (1996). Thoughts about online psychotherapy: Ethical and practical considerations. Retrieved June 21, 2006, from http://www.members.aol.com/stofle/index.htm.

Tate, D. F., & Zabinski, M. F. (2004). Computer and Internet applications for psychological treatment: Update for clinicians. *JCLP/In Session, 60*(2), 209–220.

Tate, D. F., Jackvony, E. J., & Wing, R. R. (2003). Effects of Internet behavioral counseling on weight loss in adults at risk for type 2 diabetes: A randomized trial. *Journal of the American Medical Association, 289,* 1172–1177.

Tate, D. F., Wing, R. R., & Winett, R. A. (2001). Using Internet technology to deliver a behavioral weight loss program. *Journal of the American Medical Association, 285,* 1172–1177.

White, M. A., et al. (2004). Mediators of weight loss in a family-based intervention presented over the Internet. *Obesity Research 12*(7), 1050–1059.

Zgodzinski, D. (1996). Cybertherapy. *Internet World, 96,* 50–53.

How Sturdy is that Digital Couch? Legal Considerations for Mental Health Professionals Who Deliver Clinical Services Via the Internet

Jason S. Zack

Just as nearly every other service has been transplanted to the Internet, so too have mental health professionals begun to explore how they may harness the power of e-mail, instant messaging, and the World Wide Web to serve their clients. Indeed, for more than a decade, a vanguard of psychologists, psychiatrists, social workers, mental health counselors, and family therapists have been providing clinical services to a wide range of clients. Proponents of online counseling tout its convenience and also its sometimes lower costs and the disinhibiting, facilitating effects of computer-mediated communication (Rochlen, Zack, & Speyer, 2004; Grohol, 2003). Consumers of online counseling services may be existing clients who have moved away or are unable to come to their therapist's office for some reason (e.g., work, travel, infirmity), or they may have discovered their online counselor in a web search. They may be mental health veterans or clients seeking help for the first time. They may be individuals who live in rural areas where mental health professionals are in short supply, lacking specialized therapeutic skills, or too familiar for comfort. They may be persons for whom online counseling offers a less-threatening alternative to "seeing a shrink." They may be accessing their providers from across town, or across the globe.

Despite promising process and outcome research (Mallen, 2003), many mental health professionals remain reluctant to enter the online fray because they perceive many legal and ethical concerns (Ragusea & Vandecreek, 2003). In short, therapists wonder if online counseling is legally "okay," under what circumstances, and with what sorts of clients. This paper reviews the key legal issues and the state of the law as it pertains to online counseling with clients located in the United States (regardless of where the provider resides). It is not meant to offer, nor should it be considered, legal advice. Rather, it is intended to provide a starting point for mental health professionals, their legal counsel, and any organizations or agencies that may be wondering about the legal ramifications of providing mental health services via the Internet.[1]

The first section of this article explains why the law matters, arguing that existing law clearly applies to online counseling activities. The second section addresses the question of whose laws apply and how they might be enforced. Finally, the third section surveys specific duties and legal issues that are particularly relevant to online counseling.

SCOPE OF PRACTICE: THE LAW MATTERS

At the time of this writing, there appears to be no case law precedent specifically involving online mental health services, but this does not mean that the law simply doesn't apply. When any novel situation arises in the law, courts interpret existing statutes and analogize from rules adopted in other contexts. Because online mental health counseling shares many of the same features of traditional counseling approaches, judges are unlikely to simply throw up their hands and say "anything goes."

Any discussion of legal issues must begin with a comparison of the scope of the law and the scope of the activity to which it ostensibly applies. Terminology appears to be important with regard to online mental health services and the law. Some suggest that what professionals call their services (e.g., online therapy, cybertherapy, etherapy, e-counseling, online counseling, life coaching, etc.) might affect their legal responsibilities (e.g., Grohol, 1999).[2] In one sense, they may be correct. There are a variety of terms to describe health services delivered at a distance (e.g., telehealth, telemedicine, e-health, cybermedicine, etc.), each having their own subtle distinctions (Fleisher & Dechene, 2004). On the other hand, because most statutes define professional practice terminology based on the specific activities conducted, the term a provider adopts for his or her service is irrelevant in the eyes of the law. Thus, it is disingenuous to simply assert that online counseling is not "real" counseling (e.g., Manhal-Baugus, 2001; Ainsworth, n.d.). The differences between online psychotherapy and "etherapy" are not self-evident in view of the practice definitions on the books, and one cannot simply assert that because there are no statutes or case law specifically invoking the term *etherapy* that the law for psychotherapy and personal counseling do not apply. The applicability of any given law will depend on exactly what the provider is *doing*. A court will ask what services the provider offered, and compare them to the relevant statutes. What the provider called his or her services is unlikely to matter. For example, in Delaware, "marriage and family services":

> [I]ncludes the diagnosis and treatment of mental and emotional disorders, whether cognitive, affective, or behavioral, within the context of interpersonal relationships, including marriage and family systems, and involves the professional application of

psychotherapy, assessment instruments, counseling, consultation, treatment planning, and supervision in the delivery of services to individuals, couples and families. (Del. Code Ann. Tit. 24, § 3051)

Thus, a Delaware-licensed marriage and family therapist may offer "life coaching," but it is hard to see that the term would make the law irrelevant if the life coaching involves counseling or consultation, which it almost certainly would. Likewise, omitting one of the example activities (e.g., treating but not diagnosing mental and emotional disorders) would not make the statute inapplicable.

In most cases, it will probably not suffice to claim that "etherapy" is somehow different or "less than" other, more traditional forms of psychological services. Just as "it is hard to argue that activities, which can be seen as treatment or diagnosis, even though electronically delivered, do not constitute the practice of medicine" (Blum, 2003, p. 422), it will be hard to argue that mental health evaluation and counseling services provided via the Internet do not constitute psychotherapy or counseling or consulting or any of the myriad terms that state laws define as the "practice" of the various mental health professions.

In fact, some states have already enacted statutes clarifying that psychotherapy includes distance-based services. For example, Arizona's behavioral health statute states:

> [u]nprofessional conduct includes the following, whether occurring in this state or elsewhere: ... Failing to comply with the laws of the appropriate licensing or credentialing authority to provide *behavioral health* services *by electronic means* in all governmental jurisdictions where the client receiving these services resides. (Ariz. Rev. Stat. Ann. § 32-3251 [12][dd] (2006)) (emphasis added)

Then, "Practice of Behavioral Health" is defined as:

> the practice of marriage and family therapy, *professional counseling*, social work and substance abuse counseling. ... " (Ariz. Rev. Stat. Ann. § 32–3251 [6] (2006)) (emphasis added)

Furthermore, "Professional Counseling" is broadly defined to mean:

> [T]he professional application of mental health, psychological and human development theories, principles and techniques to:
>
> (a) Facilitate human development and adjustment throughout the human life span.
> (b) Assess and facilitate career development.
> (c) Treat interpersonal relationship issues and nervous, mental and emotional disorders that are cognitive, affective or behavioral.
> (d) Manage symptoms of mental illness.
> (e) Assess, appraise, evaluate, diagnose and treat individuals, couples, families and groups through the use of psychotherapy. (Ariz. Rev. Stat. Ann. § 32-3251 [8] (2006))

Thus, in Arizona, online counseling is explicitly covered under the general statutory scheme for professional counseling. Other states have adopted similar statutes. In Minnesota:

> "Practice of social work" means working to maintain, restore, or improve behavioral, cognitive, emotional, mental, or social functioning of clients, in a manner that applies accepted professional social work knowledge, skills, and values, including the person-in-environment perspective, by providing in person or through telephone, video conferencing, or *electronic means* one or more of the social work services described in [the statute, which includes services typically offered by social workers offering online counseling]. (Minn. Stat. Ann. § 148D.010 Subd. 9 (2006)) (emphasis added)

WHOSE LAWS APPLY, AND HOW?

It is fine to know that states regulate what online counselors do, but whose laws apply? For example, if a therapist is based in one state, and the client is in another, the provider may wonder: (1) Where must I be licensed? (2) Should I worry if violate a law in the client's state? and (3) Where can I be sued? What if the client or therapist receives/conducts mental health services from multiple locations (e.g., from a summer home)? In this section, I review what has been called "perhaps the largest of all legal impediments to be overcome" in online counseling: the question of how to address the legal problem of being in two places at once (Sammons & DeLeon, 2003, p. xxviii).

The General Statutory and Regulatory Legal Scheme

Like everyone, online counselors practicing in the United States need to be aware of federal laws, state laws (including statutes and common law), and regulations (rules promulgated and enforced by both federal and state agencies).

Federal law. The federal government (i.e., Congress) creates laws under the powers granted to it in the U.S. Constitution. For example, Congress has the authority to pass laws related to telehealth and other businesses that potentially involve interstate commerce (broadly construed) under authority granted in the Commerce Clause (U.S. Const., art. I, § 8). Federal law will also determine rules related to federally funded programs and services created under Congress's authority to spend to promote the general welfare of the United States (U.S. Const., art. I, § 8). Agencies, part of the executive branch of the government, are responsible for enforcing laws passed by Congress and for promulgating their own rules within the scope of their authority. Agencies responsible for health care service delivery fall under the Department of Health and Human Services (http://www.hhs.gov) (U.S. Department of Health and Human Services, 2003). The Health Resources and Services Administration (HRSA), a division of HHS, administers telehealth and telemedicine projects (Health Resources and Services Administration, n.d.).

State law. Most laws related to health care service delivery, however, are enacted by the individual states, which regulate professions under the "police power" left to them under the Tenth Amendment. States establish licensure requirements for mental health professionals and create specialized agencies to oversee professions—generally with the authority to enact rules necessary to enforce the statutes passed by the state legislatures. The regulations passed by those agencies (e.g., a state's board of psychology) are laws that are just as valid and important to follow as state statutes. State laws may cover anything that is not preempted or otherwise disallowed by federal law (including the Constitution) (Sullivan & Gunther, 2004). State law not only determines what are criminal offenses (enforced by state and local law enforcement agencies), but also creates private causes of action—rights of private parties to sue for violation of duties established by the state.

State law includes more than just what is enacted by state legislatures, however. State courts generally recognize a variety of common law (judge-made) causes of action as well. Although there is similarity in most states' approaches to common law, states may differ when it comes to establishing rules as to what plaintiffs must show to make out a claim against a defendant and what defenses are available to defendants to avoid those claims. Thus, it is important for online counselors (and any mental health professionals) to know the exact rules that govern the practice of their profession in the state(s) where they practice.

Procedure

State actions. If an online counselor violates a statute or regulation (e.g., by practicing without a license or revealing a client's confidential information), he or she may be subject to criminal charges or civil sanctions brought by state or federal prosecutors or state professional boards. The matter would then be adjudicated by a court or agency tribunal (e.g., a hearing before a state board of psychology). Prosecutors and agencies vary in the extent to which they pursue alleged offenders. Enforcement patterns may change over time in response to political agendas, levels of complaints filed, relative danger to the public, or a high-profile news event. Penalties are established by statute or agency regulation, and may range from reprimand, to license suspension, to fines, to imprisonment.

Private actions. If an aggrieved online counseling client (or other party) seeks a remedy available to him or her under the relevant law, the plaintiff may file a civil lawsuit against a counselor in state court for any cause of action he or she wishes (under state law or federal law). An aggrieved client may also file a civil lawsuit in federal court in certain circumstances. The question of which state's law would apply is complicated and beyond the scope of this article, but generally in negligence cases "the rights and liabilities of the parties... are determined by the local law of the state which, with respect to the issue, has the most significant relationship to the occurrence and the parties..." taking into account "(a) the place where the injury occurred, (b) the place where the conduct causing the injury occurred, (c) the domicil [sic], residence, nationality, place of incorporation and place of business of the parties, and (d) the place where the relationship, if any, between the parties is centered." Rest. 2d Conflict of Laws § 145 (1971). This could be problematic for Internet counseling cases, where the location of the harm and the location of the cause of the harm seem evenly split between the client's state and the counselor's state.

Personal Jurisdiction in Internet Civil Law Suits

A court must be able to assert personal jurisdiction over a party to a lawsuit in order to try the case. A plaintiff can always sue a defendant in the state where the defendant resides, but plaintiffs often prefer to sue in their home state because it is easier to litigate where they live. Online counselors should know that they are probably amenable to lawsuits filed in their clients' states.

The analysis of whether a state can exercise personal jurisdiction over a nonresident defendant involves two steps. First, the court must determine whether the state's "long-arm" statute authorizes the suit. Long-arm statutes usually authorize actions against defendants for actions related to, among other things, business conducted in the state, contracts executed in the state, real estate held in the state, and torts that harm residents of the state. Second, the court must determine whether the exercise of jurisdiction comports with constitutional constraints—that is, whether the defendant had sufficient *minimal contacts* with the state and exercising jurisdiction would not "offend traditional notions of fair play and substantial justice." *International Shoe Company v. Washington* (1945). Under the constitutional analysis:

> Courts may exercise *general jurisdiction* over nonresidents when their contacts with the forum state are so "substantial... continuous and systematic" that they should expect to be within the jurisdiction of its courts on any claim. Alternatively, under a lower threshold, courts may exercise *specific jurisdiction* over nonresidents when they have "purposefully availed [themselves] of forum benefits" and the claim "arises out of" their contacts with the forum state. The "purposeful availment" requirement for specific jurisdiction may be satisfied in intentional tort cases, under the so-called *effects test*, which is used to determine whether the defendant's conduct is aimed at, or has a significant

effect in, the forum state (Halkett, 2003, p. 21) (emphasis added).[3]

The law is still evolving with regard to how courts resolve jurisdiction in civil cases involving the Internet, especially with regard to harm allegedly caused by information placed on (and retrieved from) a website that is available to anyone in the world (Kaye, 2000/2007). Cases vary as to what sort of Internet interactions represent sufficient minimum contacts to justify jurisdiction, although there are some general rules. For example, "interactive" websites typically lead to a finding of personal jurisdiction, whereas "passive" sites do not (*Zippo Manufacturing Company v. Zippo Dot Com, Inc.*, 1997). This analysis has been adopted by a number of courts (Halkett, 2003). Thus, even in the absence of a client-therapist relationship, an online counselor's website alone could expose him or her to lawsuits in other states, especially if the site offers more than a static "online brochure."

However, the cases most likely to be brought (tort claims) would probably base jurisdiction on traditional notions of "minimum contacts," focusing on the harm that allegedly occurred to the client in the state where the lawsuit is brought. When harm results from interstate transactions, personal jurisdiction is generally appropriate in either the defendant's state of residence or the state where the alleged harm occurred to the plaintiff. For example, Pennsylvania law authorizes jurisdiction over nonresidents "causing harm or tortious injury by an act or omission in this Commonwealth" *or* "causing harm or tortious injury in this Commonwealth by an act or omission *outside* this Commonwealth" (42 Pa. Cons. Stat. Ann. § 5322[a] [3]-[a][4]) (emphasis added).

Enforcement of Default Judgments

If the provider's attorney is 100 percent convinced that there is no ground for asserting personal jurisdiction, then she or he might simply choose not to appear; but in that case, a default judgment would be entered against the therapist after a hearing to determine damages (Hazard et al., 2005). The judgment could then be enforced against the therapist in any state in the country, under the Full Faith and Credit Clause (U.S. Const., art. IV, § 1; Hazard et al., 2005). At that point, the therapist could litigate the issue of whether the out-of-state court had jurisdiction (a "collateral attack"), but would be precluded from raising any substantive issues (Hazard et al., 2005). In other words, if the home-state court rules that jurisdiction was proper, then the therapist is out of luck. If there is any doubt about jurisdiction (to be expected in any online counseling case), most states will allow the therapist's attorney to make a "special appearance" in the out-of-state court solely for the purpose of contesting jurisdiction (Hazard et al., 2005). Thus online therapists should be aware that, even if they believe jurisdiction in the client's state is improper, simply the possibility that it is proper means the therapist should be prepared to be haled into court in the client's state, at least for the purpose of disputing jurisdiction.

Contractual Provisions for Forum Selection and Choice of Law

In order to avoid disputes about jurisdiction, online counselors may ask their clients to sign comprehensive contracts at the outset of their work together, whereby the client acknowledges that any disputes will be settled under the law of and/or litigated in the provider's state. Such "forum selection" clauses generally enjoy presumptive validity (17 A Am. Jur. 2d *Contracts* § 259 (2007)), but are not airtight. Forum selection clauses may be overridden if:

> application of the law of the chosen state would be contrary to a fundamental policy of a state which has a materially greater interest than the chosen state in the determination of the particular issue and which ... would be the state of the applicable law in the absence of an effective choice of law by the parties. (Rest. [2d] of Conflict of Laws § 187 (2006))

Beyond that, some states do not recognize forum selection clauses or merely use them to inform the court's decision whether to claim jurisdiction over the matter (17 A Am. Jur. 2d *Contracts* § 259 (2007)). Thus, it may be difficult to enforce such clauses if the client's state has laws protecting consumers from negligent online counseling but the therapist's state does not (17 A Am. Jur. 2d *Contracts* § 263 (2007)). Finally, as with any contract, a plaintiff may dispute the agreement with the ordinary contract defenses such as fraud, duress, undue influence, and unconscionability.

LEGAL ISSUES PARTICULARLY RELEVANT TO ONLINE COUNSELORS

Licensure

Licensure is often one of the first concerns that mental health professionals raise when contemplating offering services online. Most states regulate the practice of mental health counseling, in all of its forms, although the states vary in their definitions (Fleisher & Dechene, 2004, § 1.02[2][a]). State practice laws generally require that anyone providing mental health services to residents of that state be licensed. New York law, for example, states that:

> Only a person licensed or otherwise authorized under this article shall be authorized to practice psychology or to use the title "psychologist" or to describe his or her services by use of the words "psychologist," "psychology" or "psychological" in connection with his or her practice. (N.Y. Educ. Law § 7601; McKinney, 2007)

The statute further defines "practice" to include "counseling, psychotherapy, marital or family therapy, psychoanalysis, and other psychological interventions, including verbal, behavioral, or other appropriate means as defined in regulations promulgated by the commissioner."

Indeed, most states restrict unlicensed individuals from practicing anything that even *looks* like mental health counseling, typically exempting particular occupations such as clergy, or professions that are regulated elsewhere in the statutes, such as nursing. In Florida, the "Practice of Psychology" is defined as:

> [T]he observations, description, evaluation, interpretation, and modification of human behavior, by the use of scientific and applied psychological principles, methods, and procedures, for the purpose of describing, preventing, alleviating, or eliminating symptomatic, maladaptive, or undesired behavior and of enhancing interpersonal behavioral health and mental or psychological health. The ethical practice of psychology includes, but is not limited to, psychological testing and the evaluation or assessment of personal characteristics such as intelligence, personality, abilities, interests, aptitudes, and neuropsychological functioning,

including evaluation of mental competency to manage one's affairs and to participate in legal proceedings; *counseling*, psychoanalysis, *all forms of psychotherapy*, sex therapy, hypnosis, biofeedback, and behavioral analysis and therapy; psychoeducational evaluation, *therapy*, *remediation*, and *consultation;* and *use of psychological methods* to diagnose and treat mental, nervous, psychological, marital, or emotional disorders, illness, or disability, alcoholism and substance abuse, and disorders of habit or conduct, as well as the psychological aspects of physical illness, accident, injury, or disability, including neuropsychological evaluation, diagnosis, prognosis, etiology, and treatment. (Fla. Stat. 490.003[4]) (emphasis added)

Clearly such a comprehensive definition encompasses just about anything a psychologist is likely to do with a client on or off the Internet (and practice definitions of other specialties and the term *psychotherapy* tend to be equally broad). The definitional statute goes on to specify that psychological services may be offered "without regard to place of service" (Fla. Stat. § 490.003[4][a]). The statute says nothing about an office, a couch, or talking.

Thus, state governments: (1) regulate the practice of mental health services and (2) require anyone providing such services to state residents to be licensed. Before the rise of telehealth, these two concepts were a unity, but now they may function to require licensure in both the therapist's state and in the client's state.

Many states offer an exemption for professionals who are licensed in another state and are practicing only temporarily. Depending on how the exemption is written, there may be latitude for occasional or limited work with clients in that state. For example, New York's statute allows for:

[T]he representation as a psychologist and the rendering of services as such in this state for a temporary period of a person who resides outside the state of New York and who engages in practice as a psychologist and conducts the major part of his practice as such outside this state, provided such person has filed with the department evidence that he has been licensed or certified in another state or has been admitted to the examination in this state . . . Such temporary period shall not exceed ten consecutive business days in any period of ninety consecutive days or in the aggregate exceed more than fifteen business days in any such ninety-day period. (N.Y. Educ. Law § 7605[8]; McKinney, 2007)

Other states may not require filing proof of licensure, and practitioners could have tremendous latitude, especially for e-mail therapy, if laws are written to allow a certain number of hours per month by unlicensed or elsewhere-licensed individuals (Koocher & Morray, 2000). Online counselors should be thoroughly familiar with the licensure restrictions and exemptions, both in their states of licensure as well as in the states in which their clients are located. This puts a burden on practitioners who wish to provide services across state lines (especially those who offer services to individuals to and from many different states), but unfortunately this is the law in the absence of national licensure laws or lenient reciprocity rules.

It is worth noting that the federal government has expressed some interest in promoting telehealth by addressing the licensure issue. In 2004, Sen. John Edwards introduced a bill entitled the "Telehealth Improvement Act of 2004" (S. 2325, 2004) requiring that "[w]ithin 1 year of the date of enactment . . . the Secretary [of HHS] shall convene a conference of State licensing boards, local telehealth projects, health care practitioners, and patient advocates to promote interstate licensure for telehealth projects" (Fleisher & Dechene, 2004; § 1.02[2][b][iii]). In December 2006 a similar bill, the "Telehealth and Medically Underserved and Advancement Act of 2006," (H.R. 6394, 2006) was introduced in the House of Representatives. Unfortunately, both bills died in committee.

Unlike contract clauses that may work to contractually limit the client-therapist relationship, concomitant duties, and choice of law for civil disputes, it is the *state* that determines whether a license is required for various occupations and their practices. Contracts are made between private parties, and it is unlikely to make a difference to the state whether a client clicks an agreement acknowledging that the counseling takes place in the counselor's state (i.e., that the client is virtually traveling to the counselor's office).

Legal Duties

Psychotherapists have many duties to their clients, duties defined by statute or under common law doctrine (25 Am. Jur. Proof of Facts

3d 117, 2007). Violation of these duties may be grounds for a civil lawsuit (e.g., for malpractice) against the professional. The duties most often implicated in online counseling may be grouped into the general categories of competence, consent, and confidentiality.

Competence and the standard of care. The breach of a legal duty potentially results in liability for negligence. Just as in face-to-face (FTF) therapy, an online mental health professional will be liable for negligence if (1) a professional-patient relationship exists, (2) the professional breached a legal duty imposed by virtue of that relationship, (3) the breach of that duty caused injury to the client, and (4) the client suffered damages as a result of that injury. (57 A Am. Jur. 2d Negligence § 71.) The specific cause of action (malpractice, wrongful death, etc.) will depend on the exact circumstances of the case and the exact duties will vary for each type of suit, but these are the general elements of negligence. In other words, the "basic liability issues" are no different from those in FTF settings (Sammons & DeLeon, 2003; Rice, 1997). "In negligence cases, the duty is always the same, to conform to the legal standard of reasonable conduct in light of the apparent risk" (*Darling v. Charleston Community Hospital*, 1965, p. 257). In the medical context, the standard is generally "what a reasonable physician in the same specialty would do in a similar circumstance, regardless of where the care was provided" (Johnson, 2003; Rannefeld, 2004). However, it has been noted that, unlike FTF mental health counseling, "standards of care for distance service provision have not been firmly established" (Sammons & DeLeon, 2003, p. xxix). Litigation will be necessary to flesh out the standards of care for online counseling. For example, how much effort must a counselor go through in order to provide for the client's safety in the event she or he believes the client is a danger to himself or herself or to others? Could the duty be less than (or different from) that established for FTF counselors (Koocher & Morray, 2000)? Online counselors might argue that the benefits of making services available to clients via the Internet weigh in favor of relaxing the burden on them to act in an emergency. Conversely, a state might argue that the safety of its citizens is paramount, and if online counselors cannot meet their duties in a time of crisis, then such services should not be allowed.

At the most basic level, however, all mental health providers have an ethical duty to provide competent care (e.g., American Counseling

Association, 2005; § C.2). Legal duties can be informed by ethics codes, and a key question in litigation will be, "what entails competence when it comes to online counseling?" Simply being a competent FTF counselor may not suffice. Online counselors are wise to engage in some sort of professional training (continuing education, or self-training) so that they may make a showing that they have made reasonable efforts to acquire the level of skill required to be considered competent in the field of online counseling. A number of experienced online mental health professionals have begun to offer such training and certification classes (e.g., www.etherapytraining. org, www.kateanthony.co.uk, and www.counsellingresource.com). Many authors have written about the special skills necessary to be effective in text-based communications (e.g., Zelvin & Speyer, 2003; Stofle & Chechele, 2003).

Consent. Mental health professionals should be well acquainted with the concept of informed consent. The current legal standard is that health care providers must give their patients any information that would materially impact patients' decisions whether or not to undergo the treatment offered to them (25 Am. Jur. Proof of Facts 3d. 117 § 8 (2007)). If something goes wrong in the treatment, the professional may be sued for malpractice on the grounds that the client was not properly informed of the risks (25 Am. Jur. Proof of Facts 3d. 117 § 8 (2007)). In any mental health treatment, clients should be made aware of the risks of undergoing the treatment (e.g., limitations, the chance they will get worse). Online counselors need to inform their clients of the additional risks due to the online medium that might impact their decision whether or not to engage in online counseling versus FTF counseling (Berger, 2003; Dreezen, 2004). These might include the risk that their confidential information might be inadvertently disclosed (see discussion infra), the risk that technical difficulties might cut off the communication in the middle of a session (for synchronous modalities), the risk that misunderstandings might occur due to limitations inherent in text-based communications, or the risk that the counselor might not be able to intervene in the event of an emergency. Health care professionals offering innovative therapies or experimental treatments must disclose that the treatment is new, and "should always disclose the existence of the standard practice alternative" (15 Am. Jur. Proof of Facts 2d 711 (2006)). Likewise, online counselors should disclose that their services are still part of a developing field for which there is not yet a comprehensive body of efficacy research as compared with traditional therapeutic modalities. In sum, because "many jurisdictions recognize a presumption of valid and informed consent in situations where a written consent to treatment is executed by the patient and where the consent meets the criteria established within both the medical community and the legal arena where the operation or treatment occurs," wise online counselors will draft a comprehensive written consent form and make sure that their clients understand the risks specific to this treatment modality (25 Am. Jur. Proof of Facts 3d 117 (2007)).[4]

Confidentiality: Privacy and disclosure. The general duties related to keeping clients' information private need not be elaborated extensively here, but, next to licensure and competence, concerns about confidentiality are probably the most often cited concerns in connection with online counseling. In most states, mental health professionals have a legal duty to protect their clients' confidential information. For example, under Colorado law:

> A [mental health] licensee, school psychologist, registrant, or unlicensed psychotherapist shall not disclose, without the consent of the client, any confidential communications made by the client, or advice given thereon, in the course of professional employment; nor shall a licensee's, school psychologist's, registrant's, or unlicensed psychotherapist's employee or associate, whether clerical or professional, disclose any knowledge of said communications acquired in such capacity; nor shall any person who has participated in any therapy conducted under the supervision of a licensee, school psychologist, registrant, or unlicensed psychotherapist, including, but not limited to, group therapy sessions, disclose any knowledge gained during the course of such therapy without the consent of the person to whom the knowledge relates. (Colo. Rev. Stat. Ann. § 12-43-218[1])

Unauthorized disclosure may lead to a private cause of action (Spielberg, 1999; *Gracey v. Eaker*, 2002). Obtaining informed consent as to the potential privacy risks of online counseling (e.g., lost or stolen computers, prying eyes, etc.), discussed supra, may help defend the provider against potential client arguments that they believed their information was 100 percent secure, but in any event, online counselors should take care to protect their e-mail communications with clients (Zack, 2003). As with clinical competence, the standard of care for protecting confidentiality has yet to be established. A court would try to determine what is reasonable, given the risks to the client, standard industry practice, and technological feasibility.

HIPAA. Under federal regulations promulgated pursuant to the Health Insurance Portability and Accountability Act (HIPAA), a person who knowingly "discloses individually identifiable health information to another person" may be fined up to $50,000, imprisoned up to a year, or both (42 U.S.C. § 1320d-6). Because HIPAA applies to any providers who do any electronic billing to third-party sources for services rendered, virtually all mental health professionals must be HIPAA compliant, with exemption only for those who "have no interface . . . with any insurance carrier, hospital, managed care company, state or federal program, or other third-party payer that currently or in the future may require some form of electronic transaction" (American Psychological Association Insurance Trust, n.d.). Online counselors should be particularly aware of HIPAA because of the increased volume in electronic transactions and the increased use of electronically stored private health information in the etherapy modality . The American Psychological Association Insurance Trust has assembled an informative and comprehensive guide on HIPAA for mental health professionals (American Psychological Association Insurance Trust, 2002).

Duty to Warn. As mental health professionals are aware, the law in many states mandates that professionals have a legal obligation to break confidentiality in certain circumstances, such as when the client is in imminent danger of harming himself or herself or someone else. In some states it will be sufficient to notify the appropriate authorities, but in other cases it is necessary to warn an endangered third party. Kentucky, for example, requires that (among other things, and with certain exceptions) mental health professionals make "reasonable efforts . . . to communicate" an "actual threat of physical violence" to a "clearly identified or reasonably identifiable victim" and to "notify the police department closest to the patient's and the victim's residence of the threat of violence" (Ky. Rev. Stat. Ann. § 202 A.400[1]-[2]).

If the online counselor resides in a state, or is working with a client in a state where such reports or warnings are required, the counselor may subject to criminal penalties or a civil lawsuit (e.g., wrongful death) should a client harm himself or herself or someone else (assuming the counselor was in a position to know the danger). In many states, mental health professionals also have a duty to report any knowledge of abuse (to children and/or the elderly). For example, California mandates that mental health professionals report suspected child abuse or neglect "to any police department or sheriff's department, not including a school district police or security department, county probation department, if designated by the county to receive mandated reports, or the county welfare department" (Cal. Penal Code § 11165.9).

FTF therapists take care to inform clients about limits of confidentiality at the outset of work with clients, and online counselors should have a similar discussion. Online counselors are at a significant disadvantage, however, when it comes to their ability to take action when their clients are geographically distant. It is especially difficult for counselors who are willing to work with clients who choose to remain anonymous. Clients may sign agreements acknowledging the counselor's limitations that might make it harder for them to bring a civil suit, but those agreements may not affect the rights of a third-party victim or family member who decides to bring a claim. Such agreements would also not shield providers from professional or civil sanctions by state authorities. Working with anonymous clients might create other risks as well—if there is no way to authenticate the client's identity at the outset of a session or at the beginning of treatment, then the therapist runs the risk of disclosing confidential information to the wrong individual (e.g., a hostile spouse).

Maintenance of records. Mental health professionals are ethically (and often legally) obligated to maintain records of their work with clients, documenting observations, actions, and treatment plans (e.g., American Counseling Association, 2005, § A.1.b). In one sense, online counselors are at an advantage, because they have the capacity to store transcripts of every session with their clients via chat logs or e-mails. Chances are that clients will be maintaining this information too. In fact, this is considered one of the benefits of online counseling, since the client has the opportunity to go back and review the interactions with their counselors and reflect on what transpired (Speyer & Zack, 2003). Professionals should be aware that the entirety of their interaction with a client may be used as evidence in a lawsuit brought by the client. In other words, counselors used to having some latitude in the sorts of things they say in FTF sessions are well advised to avoid saying (writing) anything that they would not feel comfortable with a judge or jury hearing. Every session should be treated as though it is being recorded. Like many aspects of online counseling, this may be a benefit and a curse, given that clients always receive a copy, and the therapist has no control over how that copy is used. As mentioned previously, online counselors should make special efforts to protect their records, using the many technological solutions available to them today (Zack, 2003).

Business Issues

Most online counselors will be offering services in exchange for some sort of fee, and a variety of remuneration structures are available to providers. In the simplest formulation, online counselors charge clients directly for individual sessions, or session packages (e.g., four e-mail exchanges for $100). Payments may be received by personal check, or through online credit card processing services. Other online counselors join popular online counseling services, such as HelpHorizons.com or OnlineClinics.com (n.d.), that offer secure communications technology platforms and ancillary services such as client scheduling, record keeping, and payment processing. Counselors using both options are also beginning to bill their online therapy services to third-party payers. Aside from the application of HIPAA, discussed supra, there are several legal issues related to the way that online counselors structure their business.

Thank you for your patients: Referral fees. Online counselors who join practice groups or who use technology service platforms should evaluate their terms carefully before deciding which service to use. Unlike other industries that allow a variety of incentives to generate business, the health care industry is heavily restricted, and certain business practices are illegal (Bodenger & Raphaely, 2002). Online counselors should be aware that, if federal funds are involved, fee-splitting arrangements are potentially violations of the federal anti-kickback statute, 42 U.S.C.A. § 1320a-7b(b). Such arrangements may violate state anti-kickback rules as well. For example, under California law:

> [T]he offer, delivery, receipt, or acceptance by any person licensed [in the healing arts] of any rebate, refund, commission, preference, patronage dividend, discount, or other consideration, whether in the form of money or otherwise, as compensation or inducement for referring patients, clients, or customers to any person, irrespective of any membership, proprietary interest or co-ownership in or with any person to whom these patients, clients, or customers are referred is unlawful. (Cal. Bus. & Prof. Code § 650[a])

Because services *other than* the referral of patients may be allowable so long as the fees are commensurate with the value of the services provided, a platform provider structured to charge a "technology fee" may be safer option. And monthly "virtual office" fees, not based on number or length of transactions, are even better (avoid situations in which the platform's revenue is at all connected with the amount of business they generate for the clinician). In any event, it is important for online counselors to confer with legal counsel if there are any doubts as to the propriety of the platform's fee structure (Bordeau, 1996/2007). In reviewing agreements with platform providers, online counselors should ask:

> 1) Is a party in a position to receive patient referrals or to refer patients to another party to the arrangement in question; 2) does the referral source receive anything of value?; 3) who is the referral source?; 4) what is the purpose of the remuneration?; 5) how to determine remuneration? (Boedenger & Raphaely, 2002, p. 127)

Third-party payments. Some advocates of online counseling have long argued that the practice would be fully accepted and flourish once insurance companies paid for it. Indeed, traditional third-party payers appear to be looking more closely at online counseling services. Some employee assistance programs have reported great success in implementing online counseling services for covered employees (Zack, 2002). Private health insurers may be the next to follow. According to the American Medical Association, Current

Procedural Terminology (CPT) code 0074 T is now available for "[o]nline evaluation and management service, per encounter, provided by a physician, using the Internet or similar electronic communications network, in response to a patient's request, established patient" (American Medical Association, 2004). Online counseling advocates assert that this code may be used to bill insurance companies for Internet therapy sessions (Grohol, 2006; OnlineClinics.com). It should be noted, however, that the code definition refers to "established patients." Providers submitting claims to third-party payers must ensure that the service for which they are billing conforms to the service that was provided, or they may be liable for insurance fraud, or penalties under the federal False Claims Act (1994, if it applies. In any event, online counselors should check with the third-party payer to determine whether their services are reimbursable, and how they should be reported, carefully documenting the conversation in case of any future disputes. Unless directed otherwise by the payer, billing online counseling services as standard "individual psychotherapy" sessions may be a risky move leading to mandated remuneration or stiff penalties.

Finally, although it is unclear how many online counseling clients are eligible, federal regulations indicate that Medicare Part B will pay for telehealth services, including individual psychotherapy, under certain conditions, but only if the psychotherapy is "furnished by an interactive telecommunications system," specifically defined as to exclude e-mail and text-based modalities (HHS Rule on Telehealth Services for Medicare Part B, 42 C.F.R. § 410.78 (2005)).

Website Issues

Intellectual property. Online counselors should take care in their use of copyrighted materials, both in their clinical work and in the development of their web presence (McMenamin, 2003). Mental health professionals should be aware that sending an article to a client or reproducing it on a website without permission may be a violation of the author's exclusive rights to reproduction and publication under the Copyright Act (1976). There appears to be no legal problem with hyperlinking to content on other sites, so long as the linked material is not itself known to be infringing, and it is made clear that the linked material is not associated with the counselor's website (Dockins, 2005; Pokotilow & Gornish, 2005). There are exceptions for "fair use," of course, but in the context of a commercial endeavor

such as online counseling, and where the work is substantially repro-
duced with little if any transformation, fair use would probably not
apply were the use to be challenged by the copyright holder (Nimmer,
2006). It therefore behooves online counselors to ensure that
they have permission to use the materials on which they rely in their
practice.

Advertising. Online counselors must be accurate in the representations they make on their websites and group service provider profiles.
Many states consider false or misleading statements to be examples of
unprofessional conduct. For example, under Arizona law:

> "Unprofessional conduct" includes the following, whether
> occurring in this state or elsewhere: ... Any false, fraudulent or
> deceptive statement connected with the practice of behavioral
> health, including false or misleading advertising by the licensee
> or the licensee's staff or a representative compensated by the
> licensee. (Ariz. Rev. Stat. Ann. § 32-3251[12][d] (2007))

Note that the statute prohibits misleading ads by licensees
anywhere. Mental health professionals should take care to accurately
represent the skills they truly possess and the services they offer, and
should be clear about where they are licensed or certified to practice.
For example, the pronouncement "Available 24/7!" could be
problematic if the provider does not actually monitor incoming contacts 24 hours a day. They must also avoid making any promises or
guarantees about the effectiveness of their services.

CONCLUSION

As we have seen, a variety of state and federal laws apply to the
delivery of mental health services via the Internet, and a number of
concerns arise that simply are not present in traditional FTF psychotherapy. Furthermore, numerous issues, such as those involving
jurisdiction and licensure, are as yet unresolved, and are likely to
remain that way until courts have had an opportunity to rule or
legislatures have decided to enact statutes. This in itself is relevant
to online counselors because it means that, should they find themselves involved in litigation, it has the potential to be particularly

time-consuming and expensive. Whether a therapist needs to be licensed in both his or her home state and his or her client's state is an open question, though it appears that dual licensure may be strictly necessary until telehealth licensure portability is established. Counselors who choose to work with clients in other states where they are not licensed may risk criminal charges, or board sanctions at the least.

As for protection from client lawsuits, the wisest legal course for clinicians is to act responsibly. Professionals will be most protected if they presume that the laws of traditional FTF counseling apply, both for their home jurisdiction and their client's jurisdiction. When therapists start work with someone in another state, they should become familiar with the legal standards of that state for mental health professionals and err on the side of the laws that are most protective of their clients. If a duty is impossible or particularly burdensome, the therapist should make best efforts to comply—not simply assume that a particular responsibility is simply inapplicable. Following any guidelines promulgated by state boards or professional organizations is a good place to start, as those may be used as evidence of the standard of care in a negligence suit. For example, recommendations for online practice have been published by the American Counseling Association (2005), the Clinical Social Work Federation (2001), the American Psychological Association (1997), and the International Society for Mental Health Online (2000).

It would be shortsighted to suggest that the best or only course of action is to avoid online mental health service delivery at all costs. "To abandon or ignore e-health because of risk considerations is to throw the baby out with the bathwater" (McMenamin, 2003, p. 56). There is a need for such service, as legislatures (state and federal) have begun to realize: they have offered bills and enacted online-service-related laws, if only to fund pilot projects. It has been said, "technology is a sprinter and the law is a marathon runner" (credited to A. K. T. Rex). If this is the case then tech-savvy counselors should always be prepared to have the law plod along behind them, but those who may benefit from their services will appreciate their efforts. The most important thing for trailblazers to remember is that the law has developed in an attempt to balance competing interests in a logical and fair way. Online counselors should look to existing laws for FTF counseling as guides for proper practice, not fear them as obstacles to providing effective service in the twenty-first century.

ACKNOWLEDGEMENT

The author is grateful to Judith Allen, PhD, Luis Suarez, Esq., and Professor Kristin J. Madison, PhD, JD, for their helpful feedback on early drafts of this article.

NOTES

1. This article is limited to legal issues that arise specifically out of the practice of *online* mental health counseling. For comprehensive information on legal issues related to mental health counseling, readers are urged to consult more general texts (e.g., Reisner et al., 2004; Swenson, 1997; Stromberg et al., 1988).

2. I arbitrarily refer to online mental health services by different terms, partly for variety, but primarily to emphasize that, under most state laws, there is no real difference whether a mental health provider describes his or her work as "counseling" or "therapy," or whether they deliver services to "clients" or "patients."

3. Interested readers may wish to consult these well-known Supreme Court cases laying out the basic constitutional contours of personal jurisdiction: *International Shoe Company v. Washington* (1945) (requiring minimum contacts with the forum state); *World-Wide Volkswagen v. Woodson* (1980) (requiring reasonable anticipation of being haled into court in the forum state); *Burger King v. Rudzewicz* (1985) (requiring purposeful direction of activities toward the forum state); and *Asahi Metal Industry Company v. Super. Ct. of Cal., Solano County* (1987) (requiring that it be reasonable and fair to assert jurisdiction so as not to violate the due process clause of the Fourteenth Amendment, considering, among other things, (1) the burden on the defendant, and (2) the interests of the plaintiff and the forum state in asserting jurisdiction).

4. Note that the Electronic Signatures in Global and National Commerce Act, which took effect in October 2000, provides that:

> [W]ith respect to any transaction in or affecting interstate or foreign commerce, a signature, contract, or other record relating to such transaction may not be denied legal effect, validity, or enforceability solely because it is in electronic form, and that a contract relating to such transaction may not be denied legal effect, validity, or enforceability solely because an electronic signature or electronic record was used in its formation. (Zitter, 2006)

REFERENCES

Ainsworth, M., (n.d.). ABCs of "Internet therapy." Retrieved March 16, 2007, from http://www.metanoia.org/imhs/.

American Counseling Association. (2005). ACA code of ethics. Retrieved April 7, 2007, from http://www.counseling.org/Resources/CodeOfEthics/TP/Home/CT2.aspx.

American Medical Association. (2004). CPT code/relative value search. Retrieved April 7, 2007, from https://catalog.ama-assn.org/Catalog/cpt/cpt_search_result.jsp?_requestid = 11926.

American Psychological Association. (1997). APA statement on services by telephone, teleconferencing, & Internet. Retrieved April 7, 2007, from http://www.apa.org/ethics/stmnt01.html.

American Psychological Association Insurance Trust. (n.d.). HIPAA for psychologists—Questions & answers. Retrieved April 7, 2007, from http://apait.org/apait/resources/hipaa/faq.aspx.

American Psychological Association Insurance Trust. (2002). Getting ready for HIPAA: What you need to know now: A primer for psychologists. Retrieved April 7, 2007, from http://www.apait.org/apait/download.aspx?item=hipaa_booklet.

Asahi Metal Industry Company v. Super. Ct. of Cal., Solano County, 480 U.S. 102 (1987).

Berger, K. (2003). Informed consent: Information or knowledge. *Medicine & Law, 22*, 743–750.

Blum, J. D. (2003). Internet medicine & the evolving legal status of the physician-patient relationship. *Journal of Legal Medicine, 24*, 413–455.

Bodenger, G. W., & Raphaely, R. C. (2002). Fraud & abuse: Overview of business & legal issues. In B. Bennett (ed.) *E-health business & transactional law* (pp. 113–142). Washington, DC: American Bar Association.

Bordeau, J. A. (1996/2007). Illegal remuneration under Medicare anti-kickback statute. 132 A.L.R. Fed. 601.

Burger King v. Rudzewicz, 471 U.S. 462 (1985).

Clinical Social Work Federation (2001). *CSWF position paper on Internet text-based therapy*. Retrieved April 7, 2007, from http://www.cswf.org/www/therapy.html.

Copyright Act, 17 U.S.C. $106 (1976).

Darling v. Charleston Cmty. Hosp., 211 N.E.2d 253 (Ill. 1965).

Dockins, M. (2005). Comment, Internet links: The good, the bad, the tortious, and a two-part test. *University of Toledo Law Review, 36*, 367–404.

Dreezen, I. (2004). Telemedicine & informed consent. *Medicine & Law, 23*, 541–549.

False Claims Act, 31 U.S.C. $3729 (1982).

Fleisher, L. D. & Dechene, J. C. (2004). *Telemedicine & e-health law*. New York: Law Journal Press.

Gracey v. Eaker, 837 So.2d 348 (Fla. 2002).

Grohol, J. M. (1999, October 31). Best practices in etherapy: Legal & licensing issues. PsychCentral. Retrieved April 7, 2007, from http://psychcentral.com/best/best4.htm.

Grohol, J. M. (2003). Online counseling: A historical perspective. In R. Kraus, et al. (eds.), *Online counseling: A handbook for mental health professionals* (pp. 51–68). San Diego, CA: Elsevier Academic Press.

Grohol, J. M. (2006, January 25). CPT code for online counseling. *World of Psychology*. Retrieved April 7, 2007, from http://psychcentral.com/blog/archives/2006/01/25/cpt-code-for-online-counseling/.

Halkett, K. A. (2003, May). Determining personal jurisdiction in Internet-related litigation, *L.A. Lawyer*, 21–28.

Hazard, G. C., Jr., et al. (2005). *Pleading & procedure: State & federal cases & materials* (9th ed.). New York: Foundation Press.

Health Resources and Services Administration (n.d.). *Telehealth grantee directory.* Retrieved April 7, 2007, from http://www.hrsa.gov/telehealth/grantee.htm.

International Shoe Company v. Washington, 326 U.S. 310 (1945).

International Society for Mental Health Online (2000). *Suggested principles for the online provision of mental health services* (vol. 3.11). Retrieved April 7, 2007, from http://www.ismho.org/suggestions.html.

Johnson, L. J. (2003, January 10). Malpractice consult: Legal risks of telemedicine. *Medical Economics, 80*, 101. Retrieved April 7, 2007, from http://www.memag.com/memag/article/articleDetail.jsp?id=111223.

Kaye, R. E. (2000/2007). Internet web site activities of nonresident person or corporation as conferring personal jurisdiction under long-arm statutes & due process clause. 81 A.L.R.5th 41.

Koocher, G. P. & Morray, E. (2000). Regulation of telepsychology: A survey of state attorneys general. *Professional Psychology: Research & Practice, 31*, 503–508.

Mallen, M. J. (2003). Online counseling research. In R. Kraus, et al. (eds.), *Online counseling: A handbook for mental health professionals* (pp. 69–89). San Diego, CA: Elsevier Academic Press.

Manhal-Baugus, M. (2001). E-therapy: Practical, ethical, and legal issues. *Cyberpsychology & Behavior, 4*, 551–563.

McMenamin, J. (2003). Risks of e-health. In S. Callens (Ed.), *E-health & the law* (pp. 45–56). The Hague, the Netherlands: Kluwer Law Int'l.

Nimmer, D. (Ed.) (2006). The defense of fair use. In *Nimmer on Copyright* (Vol. 4–13, $ 13.05). New York: Matthew Bender & Co.

OnlineClinics.com (n.d.). CPT code 0074T allows healthcare consults online. Retrieved April 7, 2007, from http://www.onlineclinics.com/pages/content.asp?iglobalid=44.

Pokotilow, M. D. & Gornish, D. (2005). Internet linking & framing issues. American Law Institute—American Bar Association Continuing Education, April 21–22. *Internet Law for the Practical Lawyer*, 31–49.

Ragusea, A. S. & Vandecreek, L. (2003). Suggestions for the ethical practice of online psychotherapy. *Psychotherapy: Theory, research, practice, training, 40*, 94–102.

Rannefeld, L. (2004). The doctor will e-mail you now: Physicians' use of telemedicine to treat patients over the Internet. *Journal of Law & Health, 19*, 75–105.

Reisner, R., et al. (2004). *Law & the mental health system: Civil & criminal aspects* (4th ed.). St. Paul, MN: Thompson-West.

Rice, B. (1997). Will telemedicine get you sued? *Medical Economics, 74*, 56.

Rochlen, A. B., Zack, J. S. & Speyer, C. (2004). Online therapy: Review of relevant definitions, debates, & current empirical support. *Journal of Clinical Psychology, 60*, 269–283.

Sammons, M. T., & DeLeon, P. J. (2003). Foreword, whither online counseling: Conceptualizing the challenges & promises of distance mental health service provision. In R. Kraus, et al. (eds.), *Online counseling: A handbook for mental health professionals* (pp. xxi–xxxvi). San Diego, CA: Elsevier Academic Press.

Speyer, C. M., & Zack, J. S. (2003). Online counseling: Beyond the pros & cons. *Psychologica, 23*, 11–14.

Spielberg, A. R. (1999). Online without a net: Physician-patient communication by electronic mail. *American Journal of Law & Medicine, 25*, 267–295.

Stofle, G. S., & Chechele, P. J. (2003). Online counseling skills, part II: In-session skills. In R. Kraus, et al. (eds.), *Online counseling: A handbook for mental health professionals* (pp. 181–196). San Diego, CA: Elsevier Academic Press.

Stromberg, C. D., et al. (1988). *The psychologist's legal handbook*. Washington, DC: National Register of Health Service Providers in Psychology.

Swenson, L. C. (1997). *Psychology & law for the helping professions* (2nd ed.). Pacific Grove, CA: Brooks/Cole.

Sullivan, K. M., & Gunther, G. (2004) *Constitutional law* (15th ed.). New York: Foundation Press.

Telehealth Improvement Act of 2004. S. 2325, 108th Cong. (2004).

Telehealth and Medically Underserved and Advancement Act of 2006. H.R. 6394, 109th Cong. (2006).

U. S. Department of Health and Human Services (2003). General overview of standards for privacy of individually identifiable health information [45 CFR Part 160 and Subparts A and E of Part 164]. Retrieved April 7, 2007, from http://www.hhs.gov/ocr/hipaa/guidelines/overview.pdf.

World-Wide Volkswagen v. Woodson, 444 U.S. 286 (1980).

Zack, J. S. (2002, August). Online counseling and EAP work. Invited lecture to the South Florida Chapter of the Employee Assistance Professionals Association. Fort Lauderdale, Florida.

Zack, J. S. (2003). Technology of online counseling. In R. Kraus, et al. (eds.), *Online counseling: A handbook for mental health professionals* (pp. 93–121). San Diego, CA: Elsevier Academic Press.

Zelvin, E. & Speyer, C. M. (2003). Online counseling skills, part I: Treatment strategies for conducting counseling online. In R. Kraus, et al. (eds.), *Online counseling: A handbook for mental health professionals* (pp. 163–180). San Diego, CA: Elsevier Academic Press.

Zippo Manufacturing Company v. Zippo Dot Com, Inc., 952 F. Supp. 1119 (W.D. Pa. 1997).

Zitter, J. M. (2006). *Construction and application of electronic signatures in global and national commerce act (E-Sign Act)*, 15 U.S.C.A. $\$\$$ 7001 to 7006, 2006 A.L.R. Fed. 2d

Best Practices in Online Therapy

Jo-Anne M. Abbott
Britt Klein
Lisa Ciechomski

Internet-based therapy (*etherapy*) is a relatively new but burgeoning means of delivering mental health services. Etherapy typically involves the interaction between a consumer and a therapist (e-therapist) via the Internet (Castelnuovo, Gaggioli, Mantovani, & Riva, 2003; Rochlen, Zach, & Speyer, 2004) and incorporates the use of a structured, web-based treatment program for consumers to access in conjunction with e-therapist assistance. The interaction between the e-therapist and consumer frequently occurs via time-delayed means of communication, such as by e-mail, but can sometimes include simultaneous communication, such as chat-based text exchanges, videoconferencing, and virtual reality technology (Grohol, 2004; Mallen, Vogel, & Rochlen, 2005; Rochlen et al., 2004).

It is important, however, to appreciate the difference between etherapy and other types of mental health services offered via the Internet. The different types of services offered are outlined in Table 1 and include etherapy, e-counseling, mental health information websites, self-guided treatment, support groups, and online mental health screening and assessments (Castelnuovo et al., 2003; Manhal-Baugus, 2001; Rochlen et al., 2004; Ybarra & Eaton, 2005). In particular, etherapy is often confused with e-counseling despite, in our conceptualization, these being two quite different treatmentmodalities.

E-counseling generally involves the provision of advice and support via textual communications relayed back and forth between a therapist and consumer, usually in real time, and it rarely includes a structured "treatment" program; rather it mimics the face-to-face supportive counseling approach for assistance with generic psychological issues. Etherapy, as applied by our programs on the other hand, usually incorporates e-mail communication between the therapist and consumer, with directive treatment-oriented communications, and the addition of an Internet-based treatment program for the treatment of specific disorders. Internet-based treatment programs frequently incorporate cognitive-behavior therapy principles, are structured, and have an evidence base. Internet-based treatment programs usually also incorporate rigorous assessment

TABLE 1. Types of Mental Health Services Provided on the Internet

Type of Internet Mental Health Service	Definition	Examples of Service
Etherapy	Communication between the therapist and consumer (usually delayed communication via e-mail), with directive treatment-oriented communications and the addition of an Internet-based treatment program for the treatment of specific disorders (current authors' definition).	Panic Online Step 2: http://www.swinburne.edu.au/lss/swinpsyche/etherapy/ Tinnitus distress program: https://medsys.uas.se/tinntreat/ (in Swedish, but see Anderson et al. 2002 for a discussion of this program).
E-counseling	Provision of advice and support via textual communications relayed back and forth between a therapist and consumer, usually in real time (e.g., chat-based communication), and rarely including a structured "treatment" program (current authors' definition).	Turning Point Alcohol and Drug Centre: http://www.counsellingonline.org.au/en/ Relationship Help Online: http://www.relationshiphelponline.com.au/
Mental health information websites	Websites that provide information (usually text-based) such as self-help suggestions, resources for further help, and referrals. They do not involve treatment or therapist interaction (Ybarra & Eaton, 2005).	PTSD Online Step 1: www.ptsd-online.org Anxiety Panic Hub: http://www.panicattacks.com.au/index.html
Self-guided treatment program websites	Internet-based treatment programs without consumer and therapist interaction (Ybarra & Eaton, 2005).	E-couch: http://ecouch.anu.edu.au/welcome MoodGym: www.moodgym.anu.edu.au

(Continued)

TABLE 1. Types of Mental Health Services Provided on the Internet
(continued)

Type of Internet Mental Health Service	Definition	Examples of Service
Online support groups	A means for persons with a mental health issue to communicate with one another (either in real-time or time-delayed, e.g., by discussion forums, e-mail, or chat rooms) without the aid of a therapist (although often moderated to ensure the appropriate use of the group) (Castelnuovo et al., 2003).	Find the Light: www.findthelight.net/ The Online PPD Support Group: http:// www.ppdsupportpage.com/ (for postpartum mood disorder support)
Online mental health screening and assessments	Online websites where consumers can fill in screening questionnaires to obtain an indication of their physical or mental health status (Ybarra & Eaton, 2005).	SMH Screening: https://www. mentalhealthscreening. org/screening/welcome.asp Drinker's Check-up: http:// www.drinkerscheckup.com/

procedures prior to commencement of treatment to ensure that the consumer has the clinical disorder that the program treats.

This article highlights important issues in best practice in the delivery of etherapy. The examples provided of the implementation of best-practice principles are largely based on the clinical and research work of members of the Swinburne University of Technology Etherapy Unit, which is comprised of a team of psychologists. The Etherapy Unit develops and evaluates Internet-based interventions for physical and mental health conditions, and delivers education and training programs for students and health professionals (http://www.swinburne.edu.au/lss/swinpsyche/etherapy). In particular, some team members are recognized internationally for their Panic Online program, which has been rigorously tested through five randomized controlled trials. Panic Online has been found to be efficacious in helping clinically diagnosed people with panic disorder (with or without agoraphobia) and negative affect (Klein, Richards, & Austin, 2006; Klein &

Richards, 2001; Richards, Klein, & Austin, 2006). Other etherapy programs being delivered by the Etherapy Unit help people cope with posttraumatic stress disorder (www.ptsd-online.org) and tinnitus distress (http://tinnitusassistonline.med.monash.edu.au/screening/), understand how lifestyle factors can affect heart health (http://med.-monash.edu/mentalhealth/paceheart), and facilitate positive mental health (e.g., http://epw.janison.com/registration/). Most of these programs are currently being evaluated in research studies, are largely based on time-delayed communication via e-mail between therapist and consumer, and incorporate several multimedia channels (e.g., text, graphical, audio, and video).

Etherapy offers numerous benefits to consumers, including the potential to contact a therapist at their own convenience rather than by appointment, reduced cost compared to face-to-face therapy, increased perception of anonymity, and accessibility for isolated or stigmatized groups (Castelnuovo et al., 2003; Griffiths, Lindenmeyer, Powell, Lowe, & Throgood, 2006; Manhal-Baugus, 2001; Rochlen et al., 2004). Many consumers of our programs have reported that the convenience of not having to leave their home for treatment was an important factor when registering their interest. Our programs have been offered at no charge (as these trials were funded by the NH&MRC, beyondblue, Australian Rotary Health Research Fund, BP Australia, and the Australian Institute of Sport), which is also appealing to participants. Overall, preliminary research (e.g., Klein et al., 2006; Mihalopoulos et al., 2005) indicates that etherapy is less expensive than face-to-face therapy. Importantly for many Australians living in regional and rural areas, our programs have increased accessibility, as many participants were previously unable to access appropriate mental health services close to where they resided.

Etherapy programs have been found to be effective for treating a range of psychological disorders, including panic disorder (e.g., Carlbring et al., 2005; Klein et al., 2006), tinnitus distress (Andersson, Strömgren, Ström, & Lyttkens, 2002), depression (Andersson et al., 2005), headaches (Ström, Pettersson, & Andersson, 2000), posttraumatic stress symptoms (Lange, van de Ven, & Schrieken, 2003), and body image concerns (Winzelberg et al., 2000). However, as with any new field of professional practice, it is necessary to be cognizant of the potential risks, limitations, and challenges that etherapy can present. These include the lack of visual and auditory communication aids, restricted ability to verify the client's identity, security issues in ensuring the confidentiality of online information exchanges, and ensuring therapists are competent in the use of this relatively new medium (Childress, 2000; International Society for Mental Health Online, n.d.a; Mallen et al., 2005; Manhal-Baugus, 2001; Rochlen et al., 2004; Suler, 2001). This paper will discuss these challenges. Awareness of these issues will enable e-therapists to work within best practice guidelines and to enhance the credibility of the field.

THE SUITABILITY OF A POTENTIAL CONSUMER FOR ETHERAPY

In offering etherapy services, it is important to recognize that individuals with some mental health problems may be less suited to etherapy than face-to-face therapy (Australian Psychological Society, 2004). This may include individuals with psychiatric disorders in which they experience distortions of reality, suicidal ideation, are currently a victim of violence or sexual abuse, or are experiencing a high rate of secondary, comorbid psychiatric disturbance (Australian Psychological Society, 2004; Mallen et al. 2005; Manhal-Baugus, 2001; Rochlen et al., 2004; Suler, 2001). Thorough and rigorous clinical assessments are required to ensure that individuals with these types of problems are identified and referred appropriately by the e-therapists. Our team has, in most cases, verified the suitability of a potential consumer through a structured telephone interview of approximately 90 minutes (Klein et al., 2006). It is important to note, however, that many participants in our trials presented with a variety of secondary clinical conditions (e.g., depression, dysthymia, social anxiety disorder, generalized anxiety disorder, specific phobia, etc.) at preassessment. Results indicate that participants' secondary condition symptoms also improved after they completed the program (e.g., Klein et al., 2006).

Individuals with limited computer experience and knowledge may also be less suited to online therapy (Suler, 2001). In this regard, it is advisable to ask potential consumers whether they can access a computer and the Internet and, if required, whether they can obtain technical assistance (Mallen et al., 2005; Suler, 2001). In earlier Panic Online trials, some participants experienced information technology difficulties, largely due to a lack of skill; however, we found that with the provision of adequate support from the project manager and/or allocated e-therapist, this obstacle was easily overcome (Richards, Klein, & Calbring, 2003). Anecdotally, issues relating to a lack of computer skills, experience, and anxiety have become less common over the past five years.

A more important issue is how well the consumer is able to read and write in text-based communication, especially those with a different cultural background than the e-therapist (Mallen et al., 2005; Suler, 2001). The written material placed in etherapy programs should be set at a maximum reading level of year 8 (or age 14) as a means to increase the accessibility of etherapy to those with limited reading and writing skills. Interestingly though, we did not find that successful treatment outcome was related to education level on any post-assessment variable (Richards et al., 2003). These variables included measures of panic disorder symptomatology, agoraphobia, depression, anxiety, and stress.

It is also necessary for e-therapists to monitor consumers for potential barriers to continuing with etherapy. For example, a consumer may need to be referred on due to the development of suicidal ideation or clinical depression. In our Etherapy Unit, it is mandatory that the contact details of the participant and their general practitioner are provided. Furthermore, in instances where a participant failed to respond to the e-therapist's e-mails, the e-therapist would then telephone the participant to ensure that he or she was safe. During our trials, this procedure was used in approximately 5 percent of cases. The most commonly reported reason for lack of participant response was that they had been "extremely busy" and had not checked their e-mails or had had information technology difficulties (e.g., ISP was offline). In our trials we waited, on average, approximately two weeks before contacting a participant, but this depended on factors such as the length of the trial, the condition being treated, the participant's preassessment presentation (e.g., if more severe, we would contact them earlier), and what the participant expressed when we last communicated with them.

MAINTAINING CONFIDENTIALITY AND SECURITY

Care needs to be taken that e-mails and other sources of consumer information are kept confidential and secure. This largely relates to human error, for example, making sure that one does not send an e-mail to the wrong recipient (Childress, 2000; Grohol, 1999), ensuring that other people using the e-therapist's computer cannot access their e-mail account and that the consumer's e-mail address is a private one. There is also potential for confidential information to be more easily forwarded on to an unauthorized person, both at the e-therapist's and consumer's end. For example, a consumer could forward on to a friend an e-mail targeted specifically for them (Australian Psychological Society, 2004; Childress, 2000). In addition, the server used must be secure, incorporating password protection facilities, firewalls, data encryption, and/or web anonymity services to increase security (Australian Psychological Society, 2004; Mallen et al., 2005).

An example of the use of encryption programs is in our team's PTSD Online program, for which we use Secure Shell software (SSH), which is network security protocol, which encrypts data sent from the sender's computer and decrypts it on the receiver's computer. It also provides authentication, requiring a person to provide digital proof of their identity if they log onto an account from a remote computer (Barrett, Silverman, & Byrnes, 2005). Both participants and therapists access their e-mail through the program website itself rather than via their usual e-mail accounts. Another option is that e-therapists could encourage consumers to use encryption services such as Hushmail, which is a free web-based e-mail service using encryption via open PGP ("pretty good privacy") standard algorithms ("Hushmail Evaluation," 2002).

INFORMED CONSENT

It is vital to communicate sufficient information for consumers to be able to provide their informed consent to take part in etherapy treatment. While an advantage of etherapy can be the potential for consumers to remain more anonymous in comparison to face-to-face therapy, there is also the potential for consumers to relay misleading information; for example, in relation to their age. This can make it difficult to know whether parental consent is required. However, with our etherapy studies, a rigorous face-to-face or telephone-based structured clinical interview is conducted (Klein et al., 2006; Klein & Richards, 2001; Richards et al., 2006). Therefore, if information were to be provided that was potentially misleading, this would be more readily identified during the structured clinical interview phase. Since commencing our etherapy treatment trials, we have not encountered misleading participant information as an issue. If an e-therapist had doubts about a person's age—for example, if working with young adults—they could require a copy of proof-of-age identification, although we have not found it necessary to ask for this.

Consumers should also be informed prior to conducting any therapy about the e-therapist's qualifications, potential risks and benefits of online therapy, the limits of confidentiality, possible safeguards, and what they can expect from the therapy and the e-therapist (Australian Psychological Society, 2004; Suler, 2001). In terms of the maintenance of professional boundaries, appropriate guidelines regarding the frequency of e-therapist contact and amount of information provided to the consumer needs to be made clear from the very beginning. (Australian Psychological Society, 2004; Suler, 2004). For example, at the beginning of treatment, our tinnitus distress program specifies a set of requirements for the consumer and e-therapist to adhere to. This includes requirements that the consumer and e-therapist check their e-mails every three days and respond as quickly as possible, and that the e-therapist answer questions on e-mail and respond to diary entries. This online information also addresses potential challenges, such as the consumer ensuring they have adequate computer skills and avoiding misunderstandings.

TRAINING OF E-THERAPISTS

E-therapists need to be adequately trained and supervised and be able to communicate their knowledge via text to consumers. This includes training in the technology and in communicating via a computer, particularly via text-based methods (International Society for Mental Health Online n.d.b; Childress, 2000; Mallen et al., 2005). Therapist skills in providing treatment via the Internet include the ability to communicate empathy via text (Childress, 2000; Mallen et al., 2005) as well as positive reinforcement and encouragement. For example, where participants in the Panic Online program reported annoyance and frustration about having panic attacks, an e-therapist would respond with something such as:

> I sense your frustration with yourself over having panic attacks. Please remember that learning the skills for reducing panic

symptoms takes time and daily practice. Let's look at what has gone well for you this week. You've reported that you did not have a panic attack when you went into a shopping centre. Well done!

E-therapists also require training in the ethics of providing etherapy and in the ability to communicate potential risks to consumers (Childress, 2000). Methods of training could include e-therapists using the technologies in supervision sessions (Mallen et al., 2005) and incorporating etherapy curriculum into therapist training and professional development programs. Our Etherapy Unit has written etherapy curriculum for postgraduate psychology courses and aims to commence the delivery of this curriculum in 2008. Supervision of e-therapists in our programs has incorporated a range of strategies, including the trainee e-therapist becoming familiar with the program and practicing skills and techniques using "dummy" participants, observing the work of experienced e-therapists, and ongoing clinical supervision (i.e., face to face and via Skype or e-mail) when practicing.

Although etherapy is not extensively regulated, it is increasingly becoming part of ethical codes, such as those of the Australian Psychological Society (2004); American Psychological Association (1997, 2002); American Counseling Association (2005); National Board for Certified Counselors (U.S.) (n.d.); and the International Society for Mental Health Online (International Society for Mental Health Online, n.d.a; Grohol, 2004; Mallen et al., 2005; Manhal-Baugus, 2001). It is likely that this area will become more tightly regulated once this type of therapy becomes common practice.

COMMUNICATING VIA THE INTERNET

There are a number of issues regarding communicating via the Internet that need to be considered for best practice delivery. Since the e-therapist and consumer are more removed from one another than they would be if working face-to-face (International Society for Mental Health Online, n.d.b), consumers may require greater motivation and self-management ability to successfully engage in and complete etherapy treatment. Although we have not achieved a 100 percent completion rate in any of our trials, we have found that many participants were motivated and completed the treatment program successfully. More specifically, the attrition rates of our etherapy programs has been as low as 5 percent, compared to 28 percent attrition for those taking part in an information-only program and 17 percent attrition for those utilizing a print-based self-help program (Klein et al., 2006). However, more work is required to identify the factors that increase motivation, treatment adherence, and completion.

Consumer self-management and motivation may be increased through the incorporation of graphics, pictures, video, and audio files into the treatment material and by setting exercises and homework activities (International Society for Mental Health Online, n.d.b; Manhal-Baugus, 2001). In addition, etherapy treatment programs are generally well structured and guidelines are provided so the consumer is aware of what should be done (e.g., week by week). Our etherapy programs incorporate a variety of multimedia modalities and specify homework exercises as a means to increase participant engagement and treatment adherence. For example, audio files can be downloaded to practice relaxation techniques, and self-monitoring forms can also be downloaded for recording panic attack symptoms over the course of the program.

The e-therapist also plays a large role in increasing motivation, enhancing consumer self-management practices and treatment adherence. Research studies are starting to demonstrate that the inclusion of an e-therapist does enhance treatment outcome. More specifically, in a recent meta-analysis of anxiety and depression Internet interventions, Spek and colleagues (2007), found that Internet interventions involving some level of e-therapist support obtained larger treatment effect sizes than those that were purely, or primarily, self-help. However, it is still unknown how much therapist assistance is actually required for beneficial outcomes, and, in addition, what the predictors of completion and noncompletion are. These are currently two major areas of investigation for our team.

It has been suggested that the loss of visual and auditory feedback between therapist and consumer may affect ease of communication and can lead to greater potential for miscommunication (Australian Psychological Society, 2004; Childress, 2000; Manhal-Baugus, 2001; Rochlen et al., 2004) and negatively impact therapist helping alliance (i.e., the strength of the working relationship between the participant and therapist, Klein et al., 2006). In our etherapy studies, e-therapists usually discuss the possibility that miscommunications may arise, as text-based communications in comparison to verbal communications can be more confined. Participants are also encouraged to inform their e-therapist of any misunderstandings or concerns that they may have, should this transpire. By acting quickly, the e-therapist could then clear up any miscommunications or concerns. We have also required that e-therapists respond to consumers' e-mails within one to three days, which also ensures speedy resolution of misunderstandings. We have found misunderstandings to be very rare.

In terms of the establishment of a therapeutic helping alliance when using etherapy, we have not found this relationship to be compromised. In our randomized, controlled trials that compared either face-to-face therapy (Kiropoulos et al., under review) or telephone-based therapy (Klein et al., 2006) to Panic Online, therapist alliance scores have been comparable, in that participants reported being equally (and highly) satisfied with their working relationship with their therapist in all different treatment delivery modes. We propose that one reason for these comparable levels of therapeutic alliance is that etherapy allows for more frequent contact with the therapist than face-to-face therapy and thereby increases continuity of care. In our trials, the frequency of contact varied depending on the participants' responsiveness to etherapy, but it was usually at least once a week. For example, in one trial of the Panic Online program, e-therapists sent on average 16 e-mails and received 13 over a six week period (Klein et al., 2006).

A virtually unexplored area in etherapy to date is whether the same theories of therapeutic change can be applied to etherapy as for face-to-face therapy (Manhal-Baugus, 2001). Although face-to-face therapy and etherapy share several commonalties (e.g., the provision of structured, evidence-based treatment information, and therapist guidance and support to increase consumer understanding and motivation to complete required homework tasks), both delivery methods also vary on other important elements, largely the lack of "real time" verbal dialogue and visual cues inherent in face-to-face therapy. Based on our experiences with Panic Online in particular, we suggest that etherapy compensates for this loss of direct contact by taking advantage of several other features.

The main features of etherapy involve consumers communicating their experiences, asking and responding to e-therapist questions in textual form and the associated recursive nature of engaging in this type of a task. Consumers are also able to revisit all the treatment communications from their e-therapist in their own time, which is thought to reinforce treatment information learning more readily than by exposure to the "once off" verbal exchanges with face-to-face therapists. As mentioned previously, consumers also experience more frequent contact with their therapist, albeit briefer, which increases the continuity of therapist-consumer contact.

These unique etherapy features provide consumers with greater opportunities to learn and reflect over the treatment information, via both the etherapy e-mails and the web-based treatment program, which also stimulates a higher level of cognitive functioning (i.e., assimilation, processing, elaboration, integration, and differentiation), thereby enhancing treatment learning. As face-to-face therapy communications are verbal and immediate and etherapy communications are commonly textual and delayed, treatment learning is reinforced in different ways and at different intensities. We believe that it is in these differences that etherapy has an advantage and that these features promote effective treatment learning and successful behavior change.

Future research needs to expand on methods of increasing the ability of the consumer to engage with the etherapy program. For example, we will be investigating what combination of interactive web-based components increase motivation and improve treatment outcome (e.g., interactive exercises to complete online and offline, journal keeping, personalized tailoring of information and the use of webcams, blogs, chat rooms, and message posting). In addition, we will also look at other information technology devices such as the use of virtual reality technology and mobile Internet/e-mail messaging tools.

CONCLUSION

This report has highlighted a number of important issues that need to be taken into account when providing etherapy to consumers. These include ensuring that potential consumers are suited to e-therapy and understand what is involved, taking steps to protect the security and confidentiality of consumer information, providing adequate training and supervision to e-therapists, and developing methods to enhance the ability of consumers and therapists to communicate effectively via the Internet. Future research is needed as to ways to further enhance the ability of consumers to engage with e-therapy programs. Based on our experiences with several Internet-based treatment programs and related outcome studies, we firmly believe that over the next decade, etherapy will become just one other consumer option in the delivery of evidence-based treatment for clinical mental health disorders.

ACKNOWLEDGEMENT

The authors would like to thank the following organizations for making our research trials of our programs possible: Australian Rotary Health Research Fund, NH & MRC and beyondblue, BP Australia, the Australian Institute of Sport, the University of Ballarat, and Monash University. We thank all of the participants and general practitioners who have been involved in the programs.

We would also like to acknowledge the contributions of those who have been involved with Panic Online over the past 10 years: the late Jeff Richards (the primary chief investigator on the Panic Online trials), Alan Penhall, Dr. Marlies Alvarenga, Tony Archbold, Gwenda Cannard, Dr. David Austin, Joe Bolza, Dr. Marcia Pope, Dr. Felicity Smith, Dr. Craig Stapleton, Dr. Ciaran Pier, Peter Schattner, Dr. David Pearce, Dr. Tori Wade, Dr. Litza Kiropoulos, Jo Mitchell, Dr. Kathryn Gilson, Kerrie Shandley, Katy Symons, Mal Boyle, and Leon Piterman.

REFERENCES

American Counseling Association (2005). ACA code of ethics. Retrieved May 27, 2007, from http://www.counseling.org/Files/FD.ashx?guid=cf94c260-c96a-4c63-9f52-309547d60d0f.

American Psychological Association (1997). APA statement on services by telephone, teleconferencing, and Internet. Retrieved July 31, 2007, from http://www.apa.org/ethics/stmnt01.html.

American Psychological Association (2002). Ethical principles of psychologists and code of conduct. Retrieved July 31, 2007, from http://www.apa.org/ethics/code2002.html.

Andersson, G., Bergström, J., Holländare, F., Carlbring, P., Kaldo, V., & Ekselius, L. (2005). Internet-based self-help for depression: Randomised controlled trial. *The British Journal of Psychiatry, 187,* 456–461.

Andersson, G., Strömgren, T., Ström, L., & Lyttkens, L. (2002). Randomized controlled trial of Internet based cognitive behaviour therapy for distress with tinnitus. *Psychosomatic Medicine, 64,* 810–816.

Australian Psychological Society (2004). APS ethical guidelines: Guidelines for providing psychological services and products on the Internet. Retrieved November 29, 2006, from www.psychology.org.au.

Barrett, D.J., Silverman, R.E., & Byrnes, R.G. (2005). *SSH, the secure shell: The definitive guide.* Cambridge: O'Reiley.

Carlbring, P., Nilsson-Ihrfelt, E., Waara, J., Kollenstam, C., Buhrman, M., Kaldo, V, et al. (2005). Treatment of panic disorder: Live therapy vs. self-help via the Internet. *Behaviour Research and Therapy, 43,* 1321–1333.

Castelnuovo, G., Gaggioli, A., Mantovani, F., & Riva, G. (2003). From psychotherapy to etherapy: The integration of traditional techniques and new communication tools in clinical settings. *CyberPsychology & Behavior, 6,* 375–382.

Childress, C.A. (2000). Ethical issues in providing online psychotherapeutic interventions. *Journal of Medical Internet Research, 2.* Retrieved from http://jmir.org/2000//e5/.

Griffiths, F., Lindenmeyer, A., Powell, J., Lowe, P., & Throgood, M. (2006). Why are health care interventions delivered over the Internet? A systematic review of the published literature. *Journal of Medical Internet Research, 8.* Retrieved from www.jmir.org/2006/2/e10/.

Grohol, J. M. (1999). Psych central. Best practices in etherapy. Confidentiality and privacy. Retrieved January 8, 2007, from www.psychcentral.com/best/best2.htm.

Grohol, J. M. (2004). Online counselling: A historical perspective. In R. Kraus, J. Zack, & G. Stricker (Eds.), *Online counselling: A handbook for mental health professionals* (pp. 51–68). London: Elsevier, Inc.

Hushmail (email software) evaluation. (2002, May). *PC Magazine* 21(9). Retrieved July 2007 from Thomson Gale database.

International Society for Mental Health Online, Clinical Case Study Group (n.d.a). Assessing a person's suitability for online therapy. Retrieved November 29, 2006, from www.ismho.org/casestudy/ccsgas.htm.

International Society for Mental Health Online, Clinical Case Study Group (n.d.b). Myths and realities of online clinical work. Retrieved November 29, 2006, from www.ismho.org/casestudy/myths.htm.

Kiropoulos, L., Klein, B., Austin, J. W., Gilson, K., Pier, C., Mitchell, J., & Ciechomski, L. (in press). Is Internet-based CBT for panic disorder and agoraphobia as effective as face-to-face? *Journal of Anxiety Disorders.*

Klein, B., & Richards, J.C. (2001). A brief Internet-based treatment for panic disorder. *Behavioural and Cognitive Psychotherapy, 29,* 113–117.

Klein, B., Richards, J. C., & Austin, D. W. (2006). Efficacy of Internet therapy for panic disorder. *Journal of Behavior Therapy and Experimental Psychiatry, 37,* 213–238.

Lange, A., van de Ven, J. P., & Schrieken, B. (2003). Interapy: Treatment of post-traumatic stress via the Internet. *Cognitive Behaviour Therapy, 32,* 110–124.

Mallen, M.J., Vogel, D.L., & Rochlen, A.B. (2005). The practical aspects of online counselling: Ethics, training, technology, and competency. *The Counseling Psychologist, 33,* 776–818.

Manhal-Baugus, M. (2001). Etherapy: Practical, ethical, and legal issues. *CyberPsychology & Behavior, 4,* 551–563.

Mihalopoulos, C., Kiropoulos, L., Shih, S., Gunn, J., Blashki, G., & Meadows, G. (2005). Exploratory economic analyses of two primary mental health care pathways: Issues for sustainability. *Medical Journal of Australia, 183*, s73-s76.

National Board for Certified Counselors. (2007). The practice of Internet counselling. Retrieved July 31 from http://www.nbcc.org/webethics2.

Richards, J. C., Klein, B., & Austin, D. W. (2006). Internet cognitive behavioural therapy for panic disorder: Does the inclusion of stress management information improve end-state functioning? *Clinical Psychologist, 10*, 2–15.

Richards, J., Klein, B., & Carlbring, P. (2003). Internet-based treatment for panic disorder. *Cognitive Behaviour Therapy, 32*, 125–135.

Rochlen, A. B., Zach, J .S., & Speyer, C. (2004). Online therapy: Review of relevant definitions, debates, and current empirical support. *Journal of Clinical Psychology, 60*, 269–283.

Spek, V., Cuijpers, P., Nyklicek, I., Riper, H., Keyzer, J. & Pop, V. (2007). Internet-based cognitive behaviour therapy for symptoms of depression and anxiety: A meta-analysis. *Psychological Medicine, 37*, 319–328.

Ström, L., Pettersson, R., & Andersson, G. (2000). A controlled trial of self-help treatment of recurrent headache conducted via the Internet. *Journal of Consulting and Clinical Psychology, 68*, 722–727.

Suler, J. (2001). Assessing a person's suitability for online therapy: The IMHO Clinical Case Study Group. *CyberPsychology and Behavior, 4*, 675–679.

Suler, J. (2004). The psychology of text relationships. In R. Kraus, J. Zack, & G. Stricker (Eds.), *Online counseling: A handbook for mental health professionals* (p. 19–50). London: Elsevier, Inc.

Winzelberg, A. J., Eppstein, D., Eldredge, K.L, Wilfley, D., Dasmahapatra, R., Dev, P. et al. (2000). Effectiveness of an Internet-based program for reducing risk factors for eating disorders. *Journal of Consulting and Clinical Psychology, 68*, 346–350.

Ybarra, M.L., & Eaton, W.W. (2005). Internet-based mental health interventions. *Mental Health Services Research, 7*, 75–87.

Grounding Online Prevention Interventions in Theory: Guidelines from a Review of Selected Theories and Research

Brian Wuder Peng
Dick Schoech

The literature on developing prevention interventions has consistently suggested that interventions grounded in theory tend to have a stronger impact (Amaro et al., 2001; Dryfoos, 1996; Mihalic, Fagan, Irwin, Ballard, & Elliott, 2004; Skiba, Monroe, & Wodarski, 2004). A theoretical model is important because it can guide the design, development, implementation, and evaluation of the online intervention. For example, content, dosage, fidelity, settings, subjects, and the training of implementers are all influenced by the theoretical model on which an online intervention is based. While online applications are increasing, linking information technology (IT)–based interventions with theory has been difficult. One key difficulty has been the lack of consensus on a theoretical model to drive online prevention interventions. In contrast, some IT–supported interventions are based on a clear theoretical model; for example, virtual reality interventions for phobias are typically based on exposure therapy (Hoffman, n.d.). Theoretical models for grounding all phases of online interventions, that is, design, development, implementation, dissemination, and evaluation, have not yet been established.

This article reviews theories related to online prevention interventions. The focus will be on prevention interventions for youth because youth are IT savvy and quick to use interventions built on the wide range of technology available on the Internet. This review does not try to be comprehensive, but seeks to pull together major theories from the field of psychotherapy, social work, health promotion, gaming, and innovation dissemination that have potential for grounding the design, development, implementation, and evaluation of online prevention programs. Theories reviewed are: (1) health belief model, (2) theory of planned behavior and reasoned action, (3) social cognitive and social learning theory, (4) cognitive-behavioral theory, (5) motivational models, (6) game theory, (7) resiliency theory, (8) transtheoretical model, (9) ecological perspective, and

(10) diffusion of innovation theory. While prevention is the primary focus, some theories and applications reviewed are also applicable to treatment. Treatment, as distinguished from prevention, involves a problem/strengths assessment, diagnosis, and formal intervention plan.

Studies were reviewed to illustrate how these 10 theories have been used in online interventions. The goal of this review is to help researchers and IT developers better understand the pros and cons of various theories and how they can be used for grounding the design, development, implementation, and evaluation of online prevention application. Unfortunately, the theories guiding the design of online interventions are seldom specified, so they must be deduced from intervention evaluations. The theory used to design an intervention, however, may not be the same theory used to evaluate the intervention. After reviewing relevant studies, two integrated theoretical models for grounding interventions are presented along with guidelines suggested by the review.

THEORIES AND RESEARCH RELEVANT TO ONLINE INTERVENTIONS

The 10 theories reviewed present a systematic way of looking at concepts and their interrelationship in order to explain what makes prevention effective. After describing the theories, research will be cited to illustrate the theory's use and to examine its strengths and weaknesses for underpinning online interventions. In reviews such as this, definitions and concepts often must be summarized and generalizations made. For example, some of the theories might be classified as models or perspectives, or vice versa. Many theories are overlapping, with each using similar concepts in slightly different ways. Some theories are not used alone but are combined with other theories when used in online interventions. The attempt is not to standardize theoretical concepts and nomenclature but to explore the usefulness of theories for online interventions.

Health Belief Model

The Health belief model (HBM) considers people as using a value balancing mechanism to consider health-related factors before acting out a behavior. HBM addresses the individual's perceptions of the threat posed by a health problem (susceptibility, severity), the benefits of avoiding the threat, and factors influencing the decision to act such as barriers, cues to action, and self-efficacy (Glanz & Rimer, 2005). A study by Lin, Simoni, and Zemon (2005) found that HBM constructs, including perceived severity, perceived susceptibility, perceived benefits, self-efficacy, and perceived barriers, reliably predicted the risky sexual behavior of 144 Taiwanese students in the United States. Self-efficacy, defined as a person's belief in how capable he or she could perform a certain behavior, was the strongest predictor of the factors within the HBM.

Online applications using a pure HBM are infrequently found. A British application called SMS Teen-Text Line used HBM concepts in a project where a general practitioner gave clinical advice to youth and initiated intakes via mobile text messages (Buckley, 2005). Text messaging topics included the risk of unplanned teenage pregnancy with the reassurance of a confidential, nonjudgmental service for teenagers' pregnancy consultations. The outcome of first contact was usually either fast-tracking of an appointment or referral to another agency. The success of using the Text Line could not be measured because no baseline data were collected. Nonetheless, HBM concepts, such as perceived severity or benefits, were perceived to be beneficial when connecting to high-risk youth via online mobile phone technology.

Theories of Planned Behavior and Reasoned Action

According to the theory of reasoned action (TRA), behavioral intention is influenced by the degree to which persons positively or negatively value a behavior (attitudes) and by beliefs about whether individuals who are important to the person approve or disapprove of the behavior (subjective norm). Theory of planned behavior (TPB) includes an additional construct: people's perceptions of their ability to change their behavior (perceived behavioral control). Both TPB and TRA assume that behavioral intention, or one's readiness to perform a behavior, is the most important determinant of actually performing a behavior (Ajzen, 2002). The TPB and TRA assume that all other factors (e.g., culture, knowledge, or environmental factors) operate through the models' constructs, and independently do not explain the likelihood that a person will behave a certain way. For example, increased knowledge might make one a more intelligent user rather than prevent abuse. While increased knowledge is not a major construct in TPB or TRA, it is often cited as a measure of prevention program effectiveness, possibly because increases in knowledge can be quickly produced and easily measured.

Some research supports the use of TPB in online interventions. Alcohol 101 is a CD-ROM program that helps college students make wise decisions about drinking. The program uses a variety of interactive features such as games, videos of high-risk drinking scenarios, a blood alcohol concentration (BAC) estimator, and information about impaired driving and high-risk sexual behavior. Reis, Riley, Lokman, and Baer (2000) found that students who received Alcohol 101 gained significantly more knowledge and had greater intent to use safe strategies at parties than those in an alternative education group and in a no-treatment control. Intent was measured by three factors: self-efficacy, attitudes and related expectations regarding the consequences of alcohol consumption, and peer norms. No behavioral outcomes were reported.

Some studies focus on just one or two of the constructs of TPB/TRA model. For example, after reviewing the literature, Neighbors, Larimer, and Lewis (2004) concluded that subjective norms were a key factor influencing college student drinking behavior and that norms could be influenced using e-mail or web pages. They tested whether alcohol consumption could be reduced by a computer-delivered normative feedback intervention that was personalized to reveal discrepancies between individual behavior, perceived typical student behavior, and actual typical student behavior. Result showed that normative feedback was effective in changing perceived norms and reducing alcohol consumption at three- and six-month follow-up. In summary, the TPB/TRA suggest that online interventions for changing behavior can be evaluated by measuring behavioral intention, which is influenced by attitudes, norms, and perceived behavioral control. The TPB/TRA is supported by substantial research, and concrete guidance exists on constructing TPB/TRA measures (Francis et al., 2004; Ajzen, 2006a,b).

Social Cognitive and Social Learning Theories

Social learning theory (SLT) asserts that people learn from their own experiences and by observing the actions of others and the benefits of those actions (Glanz & Rimer, 2005). SLT was updated by social cognitive theory (SCT) in which behavior, cognition, and other personal factors, along with environmental influences operate as interacting determinants that influence one another bidirectionally (Bandura, 1989). Bandura considers that self-efficacy is the most important personal factor in changing behavior and is a ubiquitous variable in health behavior theories (Glanz & Rimer, 2005).

Consider this is an SCT-based Internet program consisting of six modules that reduce expectations concerning smoking and smoking prevalence (Buller et al., 2006). Buller and colleagues (2006) conducted a group-randomized pretest-posttest controlled study using sixth through ninth grade students in the United States (n = 1,234) and Australia (n = 2,077). Although the amount of program exposure was low, the study found a 30-day smoking prevalence reduction that was mediated by decreased subjective norms.

Another study by Duncan, Duncan, Beauchamp, Wells, and Ary (2000) gave stronger support to both SCT and TPB. They evaluated Refuse to Use, an interactive CD-ROM program designed to reduce adolescent substance use. The program uses video vignettes to teach refusal skills and socially acceptable responses to substance use situations, specifically offers of marijuana. Students learn refusal skills by seeing and vicariously experiencing each choice that is made (Villarruel et al., 2000). Significant changes were observed at posttest on (1) the adolescent's personal efficacy to refuse the offer of marijuana, (2) the adolescent's intention to refuse marijuana if offered, and (3) the adolescent's perceptions of the social norms associated with substance use and the importance of respecting another's decision to refuse a drug offer. Although this program did not specify its theoretical background, the skills learned seem based in social cognitive theory. However, the evaluation was based in TPB concepts of personal efficacy, social norms, attitude, and intention. Refuse to Use demonstrates that an online intervention may be based in several compatible theories, one to design the intervention and another to evaluate the intervention. In summary, SLT/SCT supports online prevention designs in which users interact with multimedia of real-life situations in order to influence TPB factors, especially perceived behavioral control, which is the same as self-efficacy.

Cognitive Behavior Theory (CBT)

Cognitive-behavior theory/therapy/treatment (CBT) is a combination of cognitive therapy and behavioral therapy. CBT "is a problem-focused approach designed to help people identify and change the dysfunctional beliefs, thoughts, and patterns of behavior that contribute to their problems. Its underlying principle is that thoughts influence emotions, which then influence behaviors" (Office of Juvenile Justice and Delinquency Prevention Model Programs Guide, 2007). CBT techniques include development of trust, normalizing, coping strategy enhancement, reality testing, and work with dysfunctional affective and behavioral reactions to psychotic symptoms (Turkington, Dudley, Warman, & Beck, 2006). Many well-researched applications are based on CBT, for example, COPE (Jones et al., 1999), FearFighter (Marks et al., 2003), and Beating the Blues (Proudfoot et al., 2004).

Bruning-Brown, Winzelberg, Abascal, and Taylor (2004) evaluated the effectiveness of Student Bodies, an Internet-delivered CBT eating disorder prevention program for adolescents along with a supplemental program for their parents. Student Bodies is a structured, eight-week, psychoeducational intervention which includes a bulletin board to discuss reactions and to exchange emotional support. It was hypothesized that students using the prevention program would adopt healthier body images, eating, and dietary practices, and would decrease their level of weight and shape concerns. It was hypothesized that parents would decrease critical behaviors and attitudes toward their daughters', their own, and others' weight and shape. During the intervention phase (baseline to post assessment), significant group differences were found on the Eating Disorder Examination–Questionnaire (EDE-Q) Restraint subscale and on the overall knowledge test. The 165 female teens who used the program reported significantly reduced eating restraint and had significantly greater increases in knowledge than did students in a comparison group. However, the significant differences were not maintained at follow-up. The 69 parents involved significantly decreased their critical attitudes toward weight and shape (Bruning-Brown et al., 2004). This study might have been the first intervention that attempted to change a student's family environment using online CBT, and the authors recommend the integration of student and parent prevention interventions.

Another web-based CBT application provided a 12-session program for panic disorder and agoraphobia (Farvolden, Denisoff, Selby, Bagby, & Rudy, 2005). Study results revealed an extremely high attrition rate with only 12 (1.03 percent) out of 1,161 registered users of the Panic Center completing the 12-week program. For those who remained in the program less than 12 weeks, statistically significant reductions ($p < .002$) were found in self-reported panic attack frequency and severity from a 2-week baseline to data at 3, 6, or 8 weeks. This study suggests that while online CBT-based self-help interventions can be effective, they may also be associated with high attrition. Combining CBT with theories that motivate at various stages of change might be useful in reducing the dropout rate.

Tate, Jackvony, & Wing (2006) compared a CBT individualized feedback systems delivered by computer to that delivered by a human counselor. One hundred ninety-two adults were randomized to 1 of 3 treatment groups: (1) no counseling (NC; $n = 67$); (2) computer-automated e-mail feedback (AF, $n = 61$); or (3) human e-mail counseling (HC, $n = 64$). The feedback algorithms used for the AF group were based on CBT, focusing on the weekly behavior change and suggesting behavioral strategies to improve adherence and weight loss (Tate et al., 2006). Retention was 82 percent at 3 months and 80 percent at 6 months for all 3 groups. This study provides support for the use of CBT-based self-management interventions that use automated, computer-tailored feedback to reduce attrition. In summary, CBT's focus on education and cognitive change approaches makes it useful for online interventions. To handle the high attrition that occurs in some online self-help interventions, CBT might be combined with motivational models and techniques.

Motivational Models

Motivational models of change suggest that biological, psychological, sociological, and spiritual factors, as well as "therapeutic partnership" are important to enhance client motivation for change. Motivational interviewing can be defined as a counseling style that is client-centered, intended to support individuals in resolving ambivalence, and that supports the client in seeing the discrepancy between his or her current behaviors and his orher larger goals and values (Walker, Roffman, Picciano, & Stephens, 2007). Motivational strategies, for example, may focus on the clients' strengths rather than their problems and use empathy rather than authority or power (Miller, 1999). Motivation-enhancing techniques are associated with increased participation in treatment as well as positive treatment outcomes. Walker and colleagues (2007) reviewed a series of studies using motivational enhancement therapy (MET) from various field settings and concluded that the motivational model seem to be more powerful than other theories in sustaining the effect of an intervention, but that different populations, at-risk behaviors, and stage of change may need very different motivational approaches.

The Drinker's Check-Up (DCU) is a software program based on the principles of brief motivational interventions for problem drinkers (Squires & Hester, 2004). It provides integrated assessment, feedback, and assistance with decision making for individuals experiencing problems with alcohol. A randomized control trial with 61 problem drinkers found DCU reduced user's drinking quantity and frequency by 50 percent with similar reductions in alcohol-related problems (Hester, Squires, & Delaney, 2005). Results were sustained through 12-month follow-up. In summary, motivational techniques can increase the effectiveness of online interventions, especially if they are customized to the user's situation and continually assess and increase user motivation throughout the intervention.

Game Theory

Many people are attracted to and engaged more deeply by information that is pictorial, interactive, challenging, and in motion (Foreman, n.d.). A game is a simulation that uses techniques such as interactivity, feedback, challenge, and competition to motivate, amuse, or entertain. Online, multiuser games can allow many players to interact either synchronously or asynchronously. Some games allow users to form communities of players who create new worlds and challenges. While the science and underlying theories of online game design are evolving, projects such as the Serious Games Initiative are moving games from the entertainment sector into the area of behavioral change (see http://www.seriousgames. org/). Games such as Generation Fit, which includes yoga, stretching, and balance exercises on the action-oriented Wii platform, are especially interesting because they offer an interface that requires physical interactivity rather than keyboarding skills and sitting in front of a computer.

Surveys suggest game players tend to be younger and male (Griffiths, Davies, & Chappell, 2004), although these distinctions are beginning to fade. Results also show that in general, the younger the player, the longer they spent each week playing (Griffiths et al.,

2004). Malone and Lepper (1987) investigated students who played computer games and identified seven key factors for creating an intrinsically motivating instructional environment: challenge, curiosity, control, fantasy, cooperation, competition, and recognition. In a series of computer-assisted instruction experiments, Lepper and Cordova (1992) demonstrated that computer games raise the efficiency of learning if they increase the intrinsic motivation and link the goals "winning the game" to "learning the material." Belanich, Orvis, and Sibley (2007) analyzed the questionnaires of 21 players of the "basic training" portion of a popular army game. The result showed that multimedia components such as graphic images and spoken text were recalled more accurately than printed text. Participants indicated that the following motivational factors influenced their likelihood to continue playing the game: challenge (not too hard and not too easy), realism (audiovisual realism and adhering to laws of nature), exploration (opportunity to discover new things), and control (manipulating the virtual environment through keyboard/mouse interface).

Several online human services prevention games exist, but evaluations have been limited. Reconstructors, a game to teach the neurobiology of substance abuse and research on club drugs, demonstrated significant knowledge gain across game episodes of middle school students (Miller, Moreno, Willcockson, Smith, & Mayes, 2006). However, as seen earlier when discussing TPB, knowledge increases are often not associated with behavior change.

Re-Mission, a video game/online community that allows youth with cancer to connect and share information demonstrated significant improvements in cancer-related self-efficacy, social quality of life, and cancer-specific knowledge in 375 youth with cancer at 34 medical centers. Participants who played Re-Mission maintained high levels of adherence to their prescribed medication regimens, had higher levels of chemotherapy in their blood, and took their antibiotics more consistently than those in the control group (Hope-Lab, 2006). Based on the successful results of Re-Mission, HopeLab is developing games to help youth with other chronic illnesses such as autism, depression, obesity, and sickle cell disease. In summary, game techniques can increase the success of online interventions by attracting users, enhancing motivation, and maximizing intervention exposure. Linking successful game characteristics with behavioral change theories is difficult but potentially rewarding.

Resiliency Theory

Resiliency is the ability to recover strength and spirit in both internal (self) and external (family, school, community, and peer relation) domains for a positive outcome to adversity (National Center on Education, Disability, and Juvenile Justice, 2006; Catalano & Hawkins, 1996; Search Institute, 2005). Risk factors are personal characteristics or environmental conditions scientifically established to increase the likelihood of problem behavior (Kirby & Fraser, 1997). Protective factors are personal characteristics or environmental conditions that interact with risk factors and that have been scientifically established to reduce the likelihood of problem behavior. For example, a family risk factor might be the lack of parental supervision, while a protective factor might be effective parenting skills. The resiliency framework indicates that no single factor is essential but rather multiple factors (both risk and protective) combine to shape behavior over the course of adolescent development (Development Services Group, 2007). Exposure to multiple risk factors in the absence of protective factors has a cumulative negative effect on behavior. The exposure to, and development of protective factors in youth serves to buffer risk factors, interrupts the processes through which risk factors operate, and prevents the initial occurrence of a risk factor (Hawkins, Catalano, & Miller 1992; National Institute on Drug Abuse, 2004). Many U.S. government departments suggest using risk and protective factors when designing prevention programs; for example, see the National Institute on Drug Abuse (http://www.drugabuse.gov/infofacts/lessons.html), the Substance Abuse and Mental Health Services Administration (http://bblocks.samhsa.gov/educators/lesson_plans/prevention_tools.aspx), the White House (http://guide.helpingamericasyouth.gov/programtool.cfm), and the Office of Juvenile Justice and Delinquency (http://www.dsgonline.com/mpg2.5/mpg_index.htm). In summary, resiliency theory is useful for designing programs and targeting an intervention. However, resiliency theory does not provide a model for evaluating behavior change because it involves multiple risk and protective factors and does not specify the interactions between these factors. Resiliency theory based interventions may need a compatible theory for their evaluation.

Transtheoretical Model

The transtheoretical model (TTM), or stages-of-change model, has its roots in smoking-cessation research (Prochaska & DiClemente, 1983). TTM proposes that people progress through six change stages: precontemplation, contemplation, preparation, action, maintenance, and termination (Prochaska & Norcross, 2001). At each stage, different interventions produce optimal progress, so interventions that are matched to the respective change stage are more effective. Spencer, Pagell, Hallion, and Adams (2002) reviewed 54 validation studies, 73 population studies, and 37 interventions. The evidence to support TTM to reduce tobacco use was strong, with supportive studies being more numerous and of a better design than non-supportive studies.

Based on TTM, Etter and Perneger (2001) randomly assigned 2,934 subjects into a computer-tailored smoking cessation program versus no intervention. The intervention group received computer-tailored e-mails for three months based on their stage of change, level of tobacco dependence, self-efficacy, and personal characteristics. Results showed that abstinence was 2.6 times greater in the intervention group than in the control group (5.8 percent versus 2.2 percent). The program was most effective in "precontemplators" who were not motivated to quit smoking at baseline (intervention 3.8 percent versus control, 0.8 percent; $P = .001$). Similar positive results were found with an intervention where personalized smoking cessation advice, support, and distraction were delivered to smokers' mobile phones (Rodgers et al., 2005). In summary, strong research exists for considering users' stage of change in any online behavioral change intervention.

Ecological Perspective

The key tenant of the ecological perspective is that individual behavior both shapes and is shaped by multiple levels of one's social environment. Research suggests that individually focused models will not be as successful in changing behavior as models that also focus on the family, peers, school, and the community (National Institute on Drug Abuse, 2005).

Combining the ecological perspective with resiliency theory, Marsiglia, Miles, Dustman, and Sills (2002) surveyed 2,125 Latino seventh graders as part of a school-based prevention intervention in the urban Southwest. Results demonstrated that youth's high degree of parental and school attachment was a protective factor against drug use. Another study tested ecological factors when predicting seven risk behaviors of abused adolescents (Perkins & Jones, 2004). The results show that peer group characteristics were the most commonly shared predictor for all seven risk behaviors, followed by positive school climate, religiosity, other adult support, family support, view of the future, and involvement in extracurricular activities. In summary, support for including family, peers, school, work, community and other environmental factors in interventions is high. However, few evaluative studies were found of online interventions based on the ecological perspective. Perhaps evaluations are lacking because incorporating multiple intervention levels may require a more complex evaluation design with lengthy pre-posttests in order for researchers to isolate the effect and interactions of each level.

Diffusion of Innovation Theory

Diffusion of innovation theory concerns the factors associated with the successful introduction of a new technology or behavior. When technology is involved, the term *technology acceptance model* is often used along with constructs such as perceived usefulness and ease of use (Adams, Nelson, & Todd, 1992). Rogers (2003) suggests that adoption of an innovation, such as a new process or tool, is determined by the nature of the innovation, the communication channels, and the receiver. Research concerning the nature of the innovation suggests innovations should be easily tried, reversible, advantageous, and consistent with the values, past experiences, and needs of the receiver. Research concerning communication channels suggests that behavior change processes where communication is clear, gradual, consistent, frequent, rewarded, and delivered over multiple channels will have a better chance of success. Research concerning the adoption units (individuals and others in their environment) suggests that behavior change will be more effective where the receiver system is cohesive (Kyriakidou et al., 2007). In summary, given the high attrition associated with online interventions, factors that increase use and acceptance should be considered in the design process.

INTEGRATION AND GUIDELINES FOR THE DEVELOPMENT OF ONLINE INTERVENTIONS

Each theory has its strengths and weakness in helping design, develop, implement, and evaluate online interventions. Resiliency theory points out factors that should be increased and reduced by an intervention. The ecological perspective suggests risk and protective factors need to be considered in a user's social networks (e.g., family, peers, school/workplace, and community). Cognitive-behavioral therapy offers a strong basis for the design of inter-vention components such as e-mail feedback. The transtheoretical model suggests designers target interventions to a user's current stage of change to increase their chance of success. Motivational and game theories provide techniques for making interventions fun and rewarding, thus reducing attrition, and increasing users' motivation to change. Diffusion theory focuses the developer on the importance of the values and characteristics of the user, innovation, and the communication channels in order to increase successful implementation, dissemination, and use. The theory of planned behavior provides a strong evaluation model where change factors and intentions can be measured rather than measuring actual behavior.

While each theory is useful, increasing the success of an online intervention by grounding it in multiple relevant theories can be a complex task. Glanz & Rimer (2005) developed the integrative model in Figure 1 for understanding, explaining, and evaluating an indivi-dual's dynamics during behavior change associated with an online interventions. However, the model does not address the user's change stage, which could be embedded in each variable. Nor does it include knowledge, which might be added as an individual variable. Environ-mental factors, such as those identified by ecological and diffusion models are not well integrated into the individually oriented model in Figure 1 and seem to be almost an afterthought.

Figure 2 presents the authors' attempt to integrate theories into a model that can guide online intervention design and development. Figure 2 suggests that online intervention developers approach beha-vior change from each of the corners of the triangle. Approaching behavior change from the top left corner makes one examine the protective and risk factors in users, their families, peers, schools,

FIGURE 1. An Integrated Theoretical Model Useful for Evaluation and Design

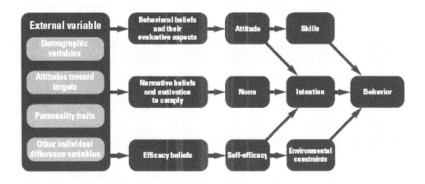

workplaces, and community. Approaching development from the bottom corner stresses that technology tools and gaming techniques be incorporated to ensure user acceptance and motivation to change. Approaching development from the right top corner suggests that models of behavior changes need to be combined with user' current

FIGURE 2. An Integrated Theoretical Model Useful for Online Intervention Design

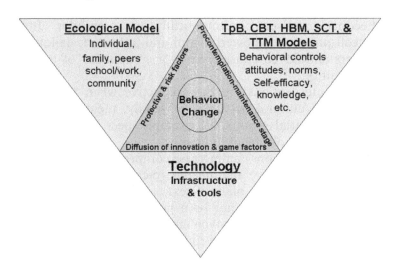

stage of change to increase effective behavior change. While Figure 2 focuses the developer on considering and integrating theories during the design and development phase, it does not provide an evaluative framework for online interventions.

Besides considering an integrated model for online program design, development, implementation, and evaluation, this review concludes with a list of guidelines. These should be considered only as preliminary suggestions derived from theory, the literature, or limited studies. They have not been validated by substantial research on various populations or for many different types of online intervention. Thus, the guidelines point to the need for much additional research as well as provide development advice.

1. Protective and risk factors for the individual, family, peers, school/work, and community should be considered as targets of any online intervention during the initial design phase. For example, examine the research on risk and protective factors at the U.S. government URLs presented earlier to explore the target of any online intervention.

2. Attrition rate can be a persistent problem with online interventions, although incorporating concepts and principles from game theory can lower the attrition rate. In addition, motivational and transtheoretical models suggests that success could be increased by tailoring motivational messages to a person during each stage of change.

3. Feedback delivered automatically via computer, Internet, or cell phone is a powerful tool and automatic tailored reinforcers should be considered as a component of any online intervention.

4. Online interventions are more effective when they build on social and cultural networks of family, mentors, peers, and other influential groups; for example, peer discussion groups and parent involvement in change.

5. Online interventions can increase comprehension and retention by using interactive multimedia (pictures, animation, video, voice, music, etc.) in place of text.

6. Knowledge gain may not be a good predictor of behavioral change and should be avoided as the sole measure of the success of an online intervention. In contrast, self-efficacy is consistently seen as a key predictor of behavior change.

7. Online interventions should be given the capacity to assess and monitor program exposure or dosage. There may be an optimum dosage level with any interventions where providing less than the dosage severely sacrifices the chance for success, and providing more than the optimum dosage is a waste of resources. User's stage of change and motivation level might be factors in determining optimum dosage.

8. Online interventions often tend to produce short-term effects, with long-term effects much more difficult to achieve. Evaluation designs should include 3, 6, and 12 month follow-up to ensure that significant effects do not fade with time.

9. While effectiveness studies should compare online with traditional approaches, online approaches that appeal to youth because they are highly interactive and have gamelike features may not have a traditional counterpart with which they can be compared.

10. Randomized controlled trial (RCT) or true experimental design has been deemed as a requisite for knowledge building. However, the RCT model works best with content that is structured, consistent, and repetitive over time. Interventions that take advantage of the interactive multimedia and game features of the Internet may not provide enough structure to ensure that each user consistently gets the same intervention and dosage. New evaluative models are needed for online interventions.

CONCLUSION

Many online interventions for behavior change have been developed and researched within the past 15 years, although substantial evaluative research is lacking. Online interventions are especially relevant for teens who are technologically savvy and who feel at home in an online environment. The literature suggests that applications grounded in theory have a greater chance for success. This review of 10 major theories and selected supporting research is summarized in two integrative models and 10 guidelines. As new technologies develop, such as mobile computing and smartphone, we have an increasing number of IT tools that need to be considered and grounded in theories and existing research in order to improve the effectiveness of online interventions.

REFERENCES

Adams, D. A., Nelson, R. R., & Todd, P. A. (1992). Perceived usefulness, ease of use, and usage of information technology: A replication. *MIS Quarterly, 16,* 227–247.

Ajzen, I. (2002). Perceived behavioral control, self-efficacy, locus of control, and the theory of planned behavior. *Journal of Applied Social Psychology, 32*(4), 665–683.

Ajzen, I. (2006a). *Constructing a TpB questionnaire: Conceptual and methodological considerations.* Retrieved October 16, 2007, from http://www.people.umass.edu/aizen/pdf/tpb.measurement.pdf.

Ajzen, I. (2006b). *Interactive TpB diagram.* Retrieved August 10, 2007, from http://www.people.umass.edu/aizen/tpb.diag.html.

Amaro, H., Blake, S. M., Schwartz P. M., et al. (2001). Developing theory-based substance abuse prevention programs for young adolescent girls. *Journal of Early Adolescence, 21*(3), 256–293.

Bandura, A. (1989). Social cognitive theory. In R. Vasta (Ed.), *Annals of Child Development* (Vol. 6; pp. 1–60). Greenwich, CT: JAI Press.

Belanich, J., Orvis, K. L., & Sibley, D. E. (2007). *PC-based game features that influence instruction and learner motivation.* Retrieved April 25, 2007, from http://www.aptima.biz/publications/2006-InPress_Belanich_Orvis_Sibley.pdf.

Bruning-Brown, J., Winzelberg, A. J., Abascal, L. B., & Taylor, C. B. (2004). An evaluation of an Internet-delivered eating disorder prevention program for adolescents and their parents. *Journal of Adolescent Health, 35*(4), 290–296.

Buckley, O. (2005). How I connected with teens by text messaging. *Pulse, 65*(39), 58–58.

Buller, D. B., Borland, R., Woodall, W. G., Hall, J. R., Hines, J. M., Burris-Woodall, P., et al. (2006). Randomized trials on consider this, a tailored, Internet-delivered smoking prevention program for adolescents. *Health Education & Behavior, 20*(10), 1–22.

Catalano, R. F., & Hawkins, J.D. (1996). The social development model: A theory of antisocial behavior. In J. D. Hawkins, A. Blumstein, & D. Farrington (Eds.) *Delinquency and crime: Current theories* (pp. 149–197) Cambridge, UK: Cambridge University Press.

Development Services Group. (2007). *Prevention. OJJDP Model Programs Guide Version 2.5.* Retrieved March 4, 2007, from http://www.dsgonline.com/mpg2.5/mpg_index.htm.

Dryfoos, J. G. (1996). Adolescents at risk: Shaping programs to fit the need. *Journal of Negro Education, 65*(1), 5.

Duncan, T. E., Duncan, S. C., Beauchamp, N., Wells, J., & Ary, D. V. (2000). Development and evaluation of an interactive CD-ROM refusal skills program to prevent youth substance use: "Refuse to use." *Journal of Behavioral Medicine, 23*(1), 59–72.

Etter, J. F., & Perneger, T. V. (2001). Effectiveness of a computer-tailored smoking cessation program: A randomized trial. *Archives of Internal Medicine, 161*(21), 2596–2601.

Farvolden, P., Denisoff, E., Selby, P., Bagby, R. M., & Rudy, L. (2005). Usage and longitudinal effectiveness of a web-based self-help cognitive behavioral therapy program for panic disorder. *Journal of Medical Internet Research, 7*(1), e7.

Foreman, J. (n.d.). *Learning with visualization.* Retrieved May 26, 2007, from http://www.convergemag.com/story.php?catid=231 & storyid=98168.

Francis, J. J., Eccles, M. P., Johnston, M., Walker, A., Grimshaw, J., Foy, R., et al. (2004). *Constructing questionnaires based on the theory of planned bahaviour: A manual for health service researchers.* Retrieved October 17, 2007, from http://www.rebeqi.org/ViewFile.aspx?itemID=212.

Glanz, K., & Rimer, B. K. (2005). *Theory at a glance: A guide for health promotion practice* (2nd ed.). Washington, DC: U.S. Department of Health and Human Services, Public Health Service, National Institutes of Health, National Cancer Institute.

Griffiths, M. D., Davies, M. N. O., & Chappell, D. (2004). Online computer gaming: A comparison of adolescent and adult gamers. *Journal of Adolescence, 27*(1), 87–96.

Hawkins, J. D., Catalano, R. F., & Miller, J. Y. (1992). Risk and protective factors for alcohol and other drug problems in adolescence and early adulthood: Implications for substance abuse prevention. *Psychological Bulletin, 112*(1), 64–105.

Hester, R. K., Squires, D. D., & Delaney, H. D. (2005). The Drinker's Check-Up: 12-month outcomes of a controlled clinical trial of a stand-alone software program for problem drinkers. *Journal of Substance Abuse Treatment, 28*(2), 159–169.

Hoffman, H. (n.d.). *VR therapy for spider phobia.* Retrieved August 15, 2007, from http://www.hitl.washington.edu/projects/exposure/.

HopeLab (2006). *Unprecedented research shows Re-Mission video game benefits young people with cancer.* Retrieved August 10, 2006, from http://www.hopelab.org/docs/Re-MissionPressRelease%20FINAL%2004%2003.pdf?f=/c/a/2006/05/22/BUG7BIU4EE1.DTL&hw=hopelab&sn=001&sc=1000.

Jones, R., Pearson, J., McGregor, S., Cawsey, A. J., Barrett, A., Craig, N., et al. (1999). Randomised trial of personalised computer based information for cancer patients. *British Medical Journal, 319*, 1241–1247.

Kirby, L. D., & Fraser, M. W. (1997). Risk and resilience in childhood: An ecological perspective. In M. W. Fraser (Ed.) *Risk and resilience in childhood: An ecological perspective* (2nd ed.; pp. 10–33). Washington, DC: NASW Press.

Kyriakidou, O., Bate, P., Peacock, R., Greenhalgh, T., MacFarlane, F., & Robert, G. (2007). *Diffusion of innovations in health service organisations: A systematic literature review.* Oxford, UK: Blackwell Publishing Limited.

Lepper, M. R., & Cordova, D. I. (1992). A desire to be taught: Instructional consequences of intrinsic motivation. *Motivation and Emotion, 16*(3), 187–208.

Lin, P., Simoni, J. M., & Zemon, V. (2005). The health belief model, sexual behaviors, and HIV risk among Taiwanese immigrants. *AIDS Education and Prevention, 17*(5), 469–483.

Malone, T. W., & Lepper, M. R. (1987). Making learning fun: A taxonomy of intrinsic motivations for learning. *Aptitude, Learning, and Instruction, 3*, 223–253.

Marks, I. M., Mataix-Cols, D., Kenwright, M., Cameron, R., Hirsch, S., & Gega, L, L. (2003). Pragmatic evaluation of computer-aided self-help for anxiety and depression. *British Journal of Psychiatry, 183*, 57–65.

Marsiglia, F. F., Miles, B. W., Dustman, P., & Sills, S. (2002). Ties that protect: An ecological perspective on Latino/a urban pre-adolescent drug use. *Journal of Ethnic & Cultural Diversity in Social Work, 11*(3/4), 191–220.

Mihalic, S., Fagan, A., Irwin, K., Ballard, D., & Elliott, D. (2004). *Blueprints for violence prevention (report)*. Washington, DC.: Office of Juvenile Justice and Delinquency Prevention (OJJDP).

Miller, L.M., Moreno, J., Willcockson, I., Smith, D., & Mayes, J., (2006). An online, interactive approach to teaching neuroscience to adolescents. *Cell Biology Education, 5*, 137–143.

Miller, W. R. (1999). Conceptualizing motivation and change. [Electronic version]. TIP35: Enhancing Motivation for Change in Substance Abuse Treatment. Retrieved October 16, 2006, from http://www.ncbi.nlm.nihi.gov/books/bv.fcgi?rid=hstat5.section.61626.

National Center on Education, Disability, and Juvenile Justice. (2006). *Prevention*. Retrieved March 4, 2007, from http://www.edjj.org/prevention/phcsc.html.

National Institute on Drug Abuse (NIDA). (2005, December 19). *2005 monitoring the future survey shows continued decline in drug use by students*. Retrieved May 26, 2006, from http://www.drugabuse.gov/newsroom/05/NR12-19a.html.

Neighbors, C., Larimer, M. E., & Lewis, M. A. (2004). Targeting misperceptions of descriptive drinking norms: Efficacy of a computer-delivered personalized normative feedback intervention. *Journal of Consulting and Clinical Psychology, 72*(3), 434–447.

Office of Juvenile Justice and Delinquency Prevention Model Programs Guide. (2007). *Cognitive behavioral treatment*. Retrieved August 15, 2007, from http://www.dsgonline.com/mpg2.5/cognitive_behavioral_treatment_prevention.htm.

Perkins, D. F., & Jones, K. R. (2004). Risk behaviors and resiliency within physically abused adolescents. *Child Abuse and Neglect, 28*(5), 547–563.

Prochaska, J. O., & DiClemente, C. C. (1983). Stages and processes of self-change of smoking: Toward an integrative model of change. *Journal of Consulting and Clinical Psychology, 51*(3), 390–395.

Prochaska, J. O., & Norcross, J. C. (2001). Stages of change. *Psychotherapy: Theory, Research and Practice, 38*(4), 443–448.

Proudfoot, J., Ryden, C., Everitt, B., Shapiro, D., Goldberg, D., Mann, A., et al. (2004) Clinical efficacy of computerised cognitive- behavioural therapy for anxiety and depression in primary care: Randomised controlled trial. *British Journal of Psychiatry, 185*, 46–54.

Reis, J., Riley, W., Lokman, L., & Baer, J. (2000). Interactive multimedia preventive alcohol education: A technology application in higher education. *Journal of Drug Education, 30*(4), 399–421.

Rodgers, A., Corbett, T., Bramley, D., Riddell, T., Wills, M., Lin, R. B., et al. (2005). Do u smoke after txt? Results of a randomised trial of smoking cessation using mobile phone text messaging. *Tobacco Control, 14*(4), 255–261.

Rogers, E. M. (2003). *Diffusion of innovation.* (5th ed.). New York: Free Press.

Search Institute (2005). *40 Developmental Assets.* Retrieved August 21, 2005, from http://www.search-institute.org/assets/40Assets.pdf.

Skiba, D., Monroe, J., & Wodarski, J. (2000). Adolescent substance use: Reviewing the effectiveness of prevention strategies. *Social Work, 49*(3). Retrieved June 5, 2004, from http://www.aed.org/ToolsandPublications/ upload/efarep.pdf.

Spencer, L., Pagell, F., Hallion, M. E., & Adams, T. B. (2002). Applying the trans-theoretical model to tobacco cessation and prevention: A review of literature. *American Journal of Health Promotion, 17*(1), 7–71.

Squires, D. D., & Hester, R. K. (2004). Using technical innovations in clinical practice: The Drinker's Check-Up software program. *Journal of Clinical Psychology, 60*(2), 159–169.

Tate, D. F., Jackvony, E. H., & Wing, R. R. (2006). A randomized trial comparing human e-mail counseling, computer-automated tailored counseling, and no counseling in an Internet weight loss program. *Archives of Internal Medicine, 166*(15), 1620–1625.

Turkington, D., Dudley, R., Warman, D. M., & Beck, A. T. (2006). Cognitive-behavioral therapy for schizophrenia: A review. *Focus, 4*(2), 223–233.

Villarruel, F. A., Faiver, R. T., Onaga, E., Youatt, J. P., Eppler, C., Carter, S., et al. (2000). Thirty-first annual national council on family relations media awards competition. *Family Relations, 49*(1), 107–114.

Walker, D. D., Roffman, R. A., Picciano, J. F., & Stephens, R. S. (2007). The check-up: In-person, computerized, and telephone adaptations of motivational enhancement treatment to elicit voluntary participation by the contemplator. *Substance Abuse Treatment, Prevention, and Policy, 2*(1), 2.

Design Imperatives to Enhance Evidence-Based Interventions with Persuasive Technology: A Case Scenario in Preventing Child Maltreatment

Walter LaMendola
Judy Krysik

The pervasive and growing use of web and wireless technologies suggests that there is a role for human service practitioners in the design of computer-based human service interventions. This article introduces such an emerging role by reviewing a class of interactive computer applications known as persuasive technologies. Persuasive technologies can be defined as interactive computer applications specifically created to change behaviors and attitudes (Fogg, 2003). The purpose of the review is to lay a foundation for thinking about the manner in which human service practitioners can collaboratively work with others already involved in persuasive technology design. We believe that such collaborative work will produce more effective human service interventions. The authors detail a few major differences in knowledge, method, and purpose among the various disciplines, but speculate that design steps already identified in the human services and the design sciences might be successfully staged together. The six design imperatives described in this article model one iteration of a process that begins with developing a shared understanding of the problem. The final imperative argues for continuous attention to ethics across all of the involved disciplines. The proposed design process provides an initial framework for optimizing persuasive technology application development in the human services.

The Eindhoven Institute of Technology hosted the first international conference on Persuasive Technology for Human Well-Being in 2006. The conference focused on persuasive technology applications that were designed to support access to services; to enhance physical, mental, or social well-being; and to support changes in human behavior and relationships (Ijsselsteijn, de Kort, Midden, Eggen, & van den Hoven, 2006). The study of the overlap between human well-being, persuasiveness, and technology is part of a developing, multidisciplinary field of knowledge called *captology*. *Captology* is a word social psychologist B. J. Fogg, Director of the Stanford University Persuasive Technology Lab, composed from the first four letters of the words "computers as persuasive technologies." Fogg coined the term to refer to the multidisciplinary study of interactive computer products created for the purpose of changing people's attitudes and behaviors (Fogg, 2003). Fogg names these products *persuasive technologies*. Persuasion, or how influence is exercised using communication, always involves attempts to change behavior or attitudes, and as such the practice of persuasion has "immense social consequences" (Dillard & Pfau, 2002, pp. x–xi).

Persuasive technology applications regularly found online that have relevance to human service professionals are diverse, such as social service websites, social support group blogs, and prevention initiatives. What is known as *etherapy* is another important persuasive technology application of relevance to human service professionals.

Clearly there has been acceleration in the use of Internet, web, and wireless services to deliver human service interventions. An increase in MEDLINE citations for web-based therapies has been reported from 13 in 1996 to 152 in 2002 (Wantland, Potillo, Holzemer, Slaughter, & McGhee, 2004). In addition, the 2006 report from the International Society for Research on Internet Interventions noted 25 randomized controlled trials of mental health interventions identified in the literature, with 10 more nearing publication (Ritterband, Andersson, Christensen, Carlbring, & Cuijpers, 2006).

CONCEPTS IN PERSUASIVE TECHNOLOGY

Computing technologies have advanced to a point where their interactivity can support the use of influential communications for behavioral change. Fogg (2003) has developed a useful typology that combines intentional persuasion practices with computing technologies that usually incorporate Internet, web, and wireless capabilities. Fogg's typology, the *functional triad*, includes computing technologies used as tools, medium, and social actors. Each of the three elements in the Fogg triad is discussed in the next section, with examples to illustrate. Often we find these three forms of persuasive use are mixed throughout an intervention. Our scenario presented later in this paper provides additional examples of how the mix of these forms might occur in practice.

Persuasive Tools

A computing technology is a *persuasive tool* when it is designed to potentially increase the capacity of a person to act or act differently (Fogg, 2003). There are numerous examples of the use of computing technologies as persuasive tools in the human services. For example, social service websites *tunnel* people to services by providing choices that they hope will allow the user to interactively find their way

TABLE 1. Seven Persuasive Tools

Persuasive Tools	Description
Conditioning	Reinforcement to shape or transform behaviors
Reduction	Reduces complex behavior to simple tasks
Self-monitoring	Tracking performance to help people to achieve outcomes
Suggestion	Offers suggestions at opportune moments
Surveillance	Observes others' behavior
Tailoring	Customized to factors relevant to the individual
Tunneling	Guides users through a process or experience

Note: These persuasive tools are described in Fogg (2003).

to the appropriate service (see, for example, http://www.utah.gov/residents/healthandss.html). *Tunneling* is one example of the seven types of persuasive tools described by Fogg (2003). Other persuasive tools are shown in Table 1.

The example of a web page for a rape crisis center shown in Figure 1 displays five of the seven persuasive tools listed in Table 1. There is information about the problem, and three ways to request assistance are offered to the visitor, one of which is available 24 hours per day, seven days per week. The visitor can *tunnel* into the choice that fits his or her preference. Yellow buttons indicate available assistance and suggest that the services will be tailored to fit individual needs, an example of *tailoring*. The process of obtaining immediate assistance is reduced to a single action, an example of *reduction*. Efforts to *condition*, that is, to shape or transform the behavior of the site visitor, include persuading the visitor to learn more about the problem by earning continuing education units (CEUs). One of the most important of the available tools in Table 1 is *suggestion*. An example of suggestion in Figure 1 is the question, "Need help now?" Here the help question is suggestive in the sense that it provides the opportunity for interaction. Suggestion is highly persuasive if it occurs at an opportune moment.

There are no surveillance or self monitoring tools on this site. An example of *surveillance* in this area would be an ankle bracelet that tracks the movements of the perpetrator. *Self-monitoring* might occur if the rape victim participated in periodic online anxiety assessments.

FIGURE 1. An Example of an Internet Service used as a Persuasive Tool

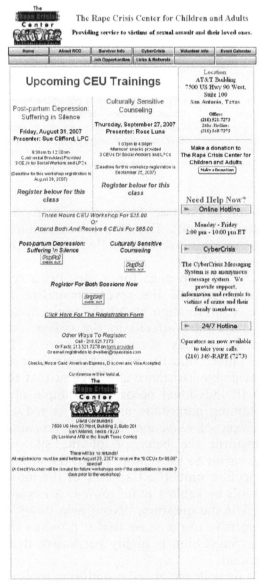

Persuasive Medium

When used as *persuasive medium*, computing technologies are organized to provide experience (Fogg, 2003). The experience may motivate reflection or rehearsal. An example of computing technologies as persuasive medium in the human services is the alcohol screening assessment shown in Figure 2. The site requests a few

FIGURE 2. An Example of an Internet Service Used as a Persuasive Medium

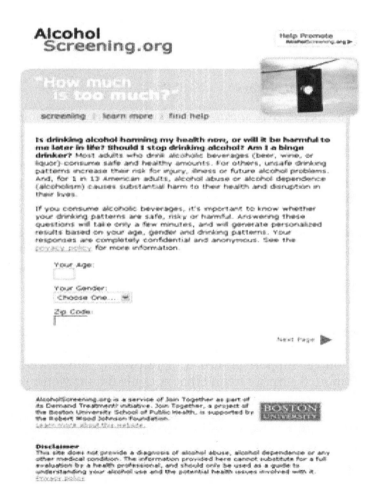

demographics such as age and gender and then leads the respondent through an assessment of his or her alcohol consumption and related behavior. The site completes the assessment by delivering specific indicators of probable consequence that may motivate reflection by the respondent. This allows the respondent to explore the cause-and-effect relationship between his or her behavior and the probable consequences in an anonymous and nonthreatening environment. The respondent can also rehearse the effects of increased or decreased consumption by completing the assessment multiple times.

Persuasive medium can also provide users with motivational vicarious experiences; for example, a career choice video. Some applications may assist with the rehearsal of a behavior, such as social work students who record and review client interviews to develop interviewing skills.

Persuasive Social Actors

Used as *persuasive social actors*, computing technologies are developed to respond to user interaction or to provide guidance or support (Fogg, 2003). Examples in the human services include an e-mail congratulations card that is sent to a user on the completion of an online treatment. These applications reward the user with positive feedback and provide social support earned through participation and interaction.

Participation and interaction are usually signaled by social cues. In the human services, many practitioners across the disciplines are especially skilled in observing social cues. Social cues are situational and contextual clues gathered from social situations that trigger understanding and behavior. Words and pictures have been shown to evoke social cues and simultaneously initiate both the mental processes and the expected behaviors that are derived from the meaning of the cue (Arbib, 2006). Alemi and colleagues (2007) in their study of online support groups with recovering substance abusing women reported surprise to find that not only did the women process available social cues, they "behaved as though they were face to face" (p. 9). Similar effects have been documented for some time in the computer sciences, most famously by Clifford Nass and his colleagues (Nass & Brave, 2005; Reeves & Nass, 1996). The variety of available social cues and examples of desired responses to them are shown in Table 2.

TABLE 2. Social Cue Categories, Modes, and Desired Responses

Categories of Social Cues	Mode	Examples of Desired Reaction
Physical	Images or videos of people, nature, or art	The computer application evokes an emotion in me
Psychological	Humor, sorrow, anger, thoughtfulness, comforting	I feel the computer application is empathetic to my needs
Language	Conversation, storytelling, dialogue, comment	I can listen, understand, and express myself
Social dynamics	Social distance, cooperation, recognition, responsiveness, reciprocity	The computer application is responsive to me
Roles	Coach, expert, player, teacher, friend, coach	The computer application shares expertise

Note: The categories of social cues in this table were adapted from Fogg (2003).

A physical cue, for instance, might be a scenic sunset on a meditation website. Often bodily images are used to cue users, such as the golfer on the AARP website. Psychological cues are shown on the Ripple Effects website in Figure 3, which deals with software for implementers of elementary and adolescent skills training. The photos in Figure 3 are intended to communicate specific feelings. In the software for Kids, there is a photo of a young student with a thoughtful look. Language is used as a social cue on the website with comments from users and consumers. The alert on the left side that announces a fix for potential installation problems is a social dynamic cue that indicates responsiveness. Below it is another social dynamic cue that relies on recognition, that is, an award for excellence with an official seal. One of the software products is titled the "Coach for Implementers." "Coach" is a role that evokes social cues; for instance, coaches are authority figures who use their expertise to assist and support individuals to win. The term *coach* is used purposively in this software product as a persuasive technique to influence how individuals perceive and relate to the software. By simply evoking the social cue of a role, a visitor to this site might be persuaded to believe that the Coach software is credible, trustworthy, and contains knowledge gained from experience.

The use of the social cues related to the "coach" role is also an example of the intersection of human service intervention theory

FIGURE 3. An Example of an Internet Service Used as a Social Actor

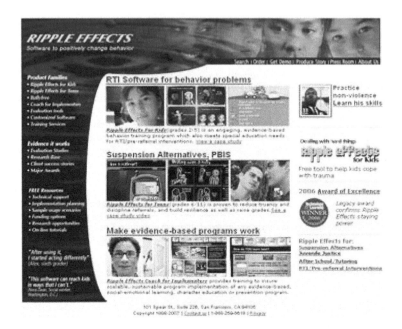

and persuasive technology design that was mentioned at the outset of this article. For example, a person who acts as "recovery coach" may offer services as a regular part of an online addiction recovery program. In traditional, face-to-face addictions programming, White (2006) has written about the qualities that distinguish the recovery coach (RC) role from other possible roles such as sponsor, peer guide, or professional addictions counselor. White points out that the role of RC needs further "definition and standards to assure its peer integrity...a model RC code of ethical conduct, and manualized, evidence-based RC service protocol" (p. 21). From the viewpoint of a technology designer, the term *recovery coach* could simply be used as a social cue to increase persuasiveness. In contrast, human service practitioners would recognize role differences that require attention in design, such as those drawn out by White (2006). Examples of this type indicate the need for specific content knowledge when involved with human service captology design.

Our interpretation of Fogg's (2003) conception of persuasive technology, with principles already familiar to human service practitioners, underpins our thinking about collaborative work with others already involved in persuasive technology design. Most human service writers have identified the potential advantages of Internet, web, and wireless enhanced human services as structural, such as increased access to human services, decreased cost, and improved coordination, or personal, including greater disclosure (see for example Parker-Oliver & Demiris, 2006). However, as we complete our description of persuasive technologies and move into the next section that prescribes design imperatives, it should be clear that this paper is focused on intervention effectiveness, grounded by the contribution of human service practice knowledge to ethical design.

DESIGN IMPERATIVES

As illustrated previously, the design of ethical and effective human service technology applications requires content knowledge and the purposeful integration of design concepts. Captology has highlighted the intersection of computing sciences and engineering with the social, cognitive, and behavioral sciences. What must also be drawn in are what Owen (1998) called the *design disciplines*. As human service practitioners, we are familiar with the intersection of social, cognitive, and behavioral sciences and to some extent we build our professions around their approach to knowledge building. While working with computer scientists and engineers is not the norm, those disciplines share much of the same approach to knowledge building as the behavioral sciences. However, it is when we are involved in design, regardless of discipline, that we become involved in a different way of thinking.

Herbert Simon (1996) called the design disciplines the Sciences of the Artificial, a body of knowledge about artificial objects and phenomena designed to bring about certain goals. He was particularly concerned with distinguishing between the sciences that deal with nature and natural events and those that *artificially* create the object of the science. For example, as a result of the design of a computer program that generates speech, all or part of the phenomena we hear is created as opposed to occurring naturally. Knowledge about *artificial speech* is generated and accumulated through writing the computer program, studying the effects of it, and rewriting the program. This type of design activity builds knowledge about artificial speech as it creates and refines it. Owen (1998) points out that the primary concern of the technology designer is probably the performance of the computer program, and not, for example, the psychological effects of exposure to it. Owen would point out that the technology designer is building knowledge about the generation of artificial speech by a computer program. In captological undertakings, it is most often the case that the primary focus of the technology goals of the project is design types of knowledge building activities. In contrast, the primary focus of the behavioral science goals of the project include context, content, use, and effects. It is the authors' contention that both activities are essential. In order to incorporate both successfully, a design process such as the one we have outlined in Figure 4 may be considered. In Figure 4 the steps of the technology design process, as adapted from Tankeda, Veerkamp, Tomiyama, and Yoshikawa (1990) are portrayed, as they might simultaneously be undertaken and merged with steps in the human service intervention continuous quality improvement process.

The six design imperatives we present in this section begin with a planned process for determining what technological adaptations or enhancements to pursue, they then briefly consider implementing and evaluating the pilot, and finish with ethical considerations. The Healthy Families America program is used as a limited scenario to illustrate how those with expertise in human services and those with expertise in technology might work together. The combined process defines and optimizes persuasive technology enhancements that can improve the existing evidence-based, face-to-face program.

Healthy Families America

HFA is a national model of home visitation that serves families identified as at-risk for child abuse and neglect by a two-stage screening and assessment process. Thus, HFA falls under the category of secondary prevention. In Arizona, the HFA program is available to prospective parents during pregnancy and within three months postpartum and can serve families for up to five years after birth. The three goals of the program are (1) to prevent child abuse and neglect, (2) improve child health and development, and (3) promote positive parent-child interaction. Home visiting for new families is usually once a week for one hour and can be more frequent with

FIGURE 4. The Combined Human Service Intervention and Technology Design Process

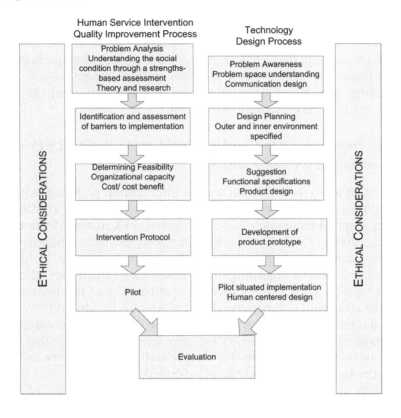

well-defined criteria for increasing and decreasing intensity over the course of involvement. The early development of a trusting, open, and constructive relationship between the parent and the home visitor is considered critical to engagement and retention, delivery of the intervention, and the attainment of desired outcomes. The home visitors are a mix of paraprofessional and entry-level professionals. The home visitor role is to provide emotional support, teach, model, screen, and assess risk and protective factors, and motivate change in knowledge, attitudes, and behavior. The home visitor is not intended to be a clinician or a counselor. When the need for professional therapeutic services is indicated, the home visitor's role is a referral one.

Grolleman, van Dijk, Nijholt, and van Emst (2006) have used scenario building as an approach to illustrate the combination of evidence-based practice approaches and persuasive technologies in a situation similar to that faced by HFA. We have adopted their illustrative scenario approach here. In this scenario, we propose design ideas for persuasive technology applications that are intended to increase the effectiveness of the physical home visitor. The technology enhancements are intended to more fully meet the goals of the existing home visitation program.

Design Imperative #1: Combine Problem Analysis with Problem Awareness and Design Planning

Problem analysis is the first step in intervention planning, whether designing a new program or engaging in a process of continuous quality improvement such as in our scenario (Kettner, Moroney, & Martin, 2008). Critical to a well-designed problem analysis is a thorough understanding of the social condition of concern, including, for example, facts regarding how many individuals are affected, demographic characteristics of who is affected, and information on how the condition is experienced and managed. In addition to examining data on the social condition, the problem analysis should be informed by theory related to the problem. It is critical that both the examination of data on the social condition and theory reflect a strengths-based as opposed to deficit-based approach.

Figure 5 provides a visual representation of a theory of child maltreatment used in the present HFA program. In Figure 5 the context of the problem that both the human service professional and the technology designer must understand is organized into a framework of four principal systems: (1) the individual parent and child, (2) the family, (3) the community, and (4) the larger societal system (Fraser, 2004). In this representation, multilevel forces transact to influence both parent and child, affecting how they respond, and in turn how they are responded to (Fraser, 2004). Each item under the headings in Figure 5 represents a potential risk or resilience factor to target for prevention. The goals of the HFA program include efforts to influence the parents' knowledge and behavior in terms of how he or she relates to the child and to others around these issues. Similarly, in the prenatal environment, HFA prevention efforts target access to prenatal care, improved nutrition, decreased

FIGURE 5. The Ecological Transactional Model of Child Abuse and Neglect

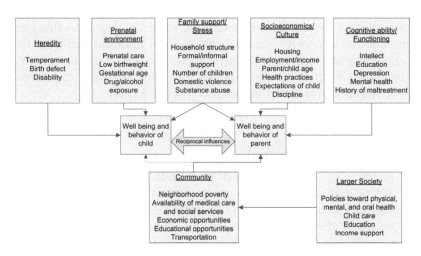

stress, and the avoidance of tobacco, drugs, and alcohol. Culture is viewed broadly in the program. For instance, it is recognized that considerable child maltreatment occurs through parental discipline (Regaldo, Harvinder, Inkelas, Wissow, & Halfon, 2004; Straus & Dinnelly, 1994). Discipline is affected by cultural practices related to ethnicity as well as to education level and the socioeconomic status of the parent (Pinderhughes, Bates, Dodge, Pettit, & Zelli, 2000). In the area of violent discipline, the HFA program is challenged to reach out beyond the mother, who is typically the focus of the home visit to other caregivers in the child's life. Failure to understand the systemic nature of the condition may lead to an exclusive focus on the mother or a failure to acknowledge protective factors already in existence in the family network.

Eric Dishman, Director of the Intel Proactive Health Lab, a lab that designs technologies for elderly persons, recommends that an ideal design model would start with the designer initiating needs assessment activities such as stakeholder and expert interviews, observations, and focus groups with consumers and service providers (Dishman, 2003). The technology designer may also decide to do abbreviated forms of ethnographic study to understand the cultural practices involved in the target population (Laurel, 2003). These activities indicate that wide-ranging human service knowledge is required to understand the problem. We would suggest that human service professionals be involved in the design consideration of the problem from the outset. For example, since the design in this paper is intended to deal with the problem of child maltreatment, the technology designer must be educated to understand the four principle systems and their interrelationships and how they are experienced by the home visitor and the members of the family.

Design Imperative #2: Combine, Identify, and Assess Barriers to Implementation with Suggestion

A second step in the process of continuous quality improvement is to examine existing barriers to program implementation. It is important not only to identify barriers to problem implementation but also to assess why the barriers exist. In our scenario, a barrier of significance to HFA is program fidelity. It is used here as an example that could benefit from the captological approach advocated in this paper. Program fidelity, the consistency between practices in the field and the program model, has been increasingly recognized as a critical factor in examinations of program effectiveness (Blakely et al., 1987; Dane & Schneider, 1998). In HFA, a lack of program fidelity has been implicated for null findings in two randomized control trials (Duggan et al., 2004; Duggan et al., 2000). In a review of evaluation studies on home visitation, Gomby, Culross, and Behrman (1999) stated, "Ultimately, better-implemented programs may produce stronger effects" (p. 24).

One method of systematically assessing program fidelity is to examine each phase of the HFA intervention, that is, the service tasks. On paper, service tasks follow a chronological order and are represented by a client flowchart that depicts the intervention process from entry to exit. In a typical intervention the service tasks emerge in the situation and include some variation of recruitment, screening and assessment, case planning, implementation of the case plan, monitoring of service provision, measurement of outcomes, revised case planning and monitoring, termination, and follow-up. An examination of program evaluation data related to process and outcome can assist in identifying barriers to program fidelity. For instance, in our scenario, these data will answer questions related to the percentage of HFA participants that have been screened for substance abuse at set intervals, the percentage of screens that were positive, and the proportion of those who screened positive that is receiving treatment. If the percentages associated with any of these process indicators are low, then a barrier to program fidelity has been identified. Once barriers are identified, research that includes both the service recipient and the service provider can assist with the assessment of why the barrier exists.

If the design problem resides in the service tasks, the human service intervention designer may be examining barriers to fidelity at the same time as the technology designer is trying to understand service task concepts. *Suggestion* is a phase of the design process in which the technology designer focuses on finding the key concepts needed to solve the design problem (Tankeda et al., 1990). At this point, the design development approach is usefully informed by key concepts from the intervention theory. A designer needs to know the key concepts of the suggested protocol before observing the home visit. Human service practice is messy—in our example we draw on Suchman (1987) and the concept of situated action. *Situated action* relates people's behavior to context and argues that context is very important in understanding how people act in a given situation. The designer will observe three things about context: (1) what takes place during the home visit has no "best" structure or sequence—it emerges from the interactions between participants in performance, (2) the performance changes from visit to visit, and (3) information requirements will not be obvious to the technology designer and involve knowledge of human service practices as well as intervention goals (Markus, Majchrzak, & Gasser, 2002). Here the design process needs to take into account key concepts that involve the *situation* of the client and the service provider and how the participants act during the intervention.

To illustrate, there can be a mixed affiliation experienced by the home visitor, particularly the paraprofessional, who is ostensibly in this case acting as a parent mentor. In one face-to-face HFA program, questions related to the discipline of the child were removed from the periodic parenting assessment instrument because the home visitors were reluctant to administer them. The home visitors possibly saw the disciplinary assessment questions as culturally inappropriate or a violation of their *understood* role. Whatever the reason, not only can paraprofessional and entry-level professionals be constrained by a lack of clinical skills in addressing client difficulties, but they may also lack experience and must resolve personal conflicts related to their professional role. The consequences of misalignment are likely to include expressed value conflicts, subversion of program components that do not fit the internalized parenting values of the home visitor, and ultimately lower retention rates of home visitors and participants. The human service professional will view dissonance between practitioner action and program goals in the performance of the service task and understand that misalignment is taking place. But such misalignment would likely be invisible to the technology designer until they are *prepared* to see it (Suchman, 1987). In this design imperative, we argue that a human service professional involved in design could contribute the knowledge that misalignment was a key concept as a barrier to implementation. This would prepare the designer to see it in the suggestion phase of the design. In that case, the initial design could address the need to support the authentic realignment of the program model and the parenting model of the home visitor.

In response to this issue, the technology designer could suggest that the technology enhancements include the creation of a set of cell-phone-delivered service tasks. The cell-phone-delivered service tasks could vary. For example, it could be an audio or text message, a video of the home visitor, or even a video of an animated character delivering the message. For example, the designer could suggest that all participants be queried on a regular basis, via cell phone, to complete a brief disciplinary practices assessment. These results could be sent directly to a supervisor rather than the home visitor. The HFA supervisor could decide to become directly involved when there is an indication of harm to the child. Parents could receive reminders periodically about discipline that are tailored based on their responses to the automated discipline assessment. The reminder messages could be both educational and supportive. For example, there may be a message encouraging the parent to continue progress, that is, an example of conditioning as presented in Table 1. The analysis of the periodic discipline assessments could lead to designing the assessments so that the participant's responses trigger changes in her or his assessment, which is an example of tailoring. A participant whose responses indicated difficulty could be led directly to a sequence that allows her or him to request immediate assistance— and to be connected directly to a counselor, that is, tunneling. The analysis of the responses to the assessment could also lead to an understanding of how the role of the home visitor could be used to increase the participant's capacity for change. Home visitors could be asked to participate in the analysis of the assessment and make suggestions, another persuasive tool. They could also be asked to participate in constructing the messages that would be sent to participants; for example, via text or video, thereby engaging the participant in learning constructive and nonviolent discipline strategies.

Design Imperative #3: Determine Feasibility

In a 20-year NIDA study of technology transfer by Simpson (2002), organizational elements related to the feasibility of technology adoption were highlighted. These included decisions at the leadership level including motivation as well as resources, staff exposure and training, and institutional support for implementation including the stages of exploratory and routine use. While these elements need to be considered, they also represent what Simpson (2002, p. 176) called "targets for organizational intervention."

Knudsen and Roman (2004), commenting on the widespread concern of the slow rate of adoption of technological innovations, suggest that an organization's absorptive capacity, defined as the ability of an organization to access and effectively use information, may be positively associated with its use of innovative practices. As organizations increase their information processing and application capabilities, they become more likely to use technology based innovations. A thoughtful design that is based on a thorough problem analysis will be wasted if it is not feasible within the context of the organization.

Cost is also a major consideration in assessing design feasibility. In a recent description of a cell phone intervention with young mothers, it was suggested that the cost of the technology would prevent its widespread use in large intervention programs (Robert Wood Johnson Foundation, 2004). As the cost of technology decreases, feasibility for use with large numbers improves. Included in any discussion of cost should be the consideration of cost benefit by the design team. For example, in HFA, the cost of one missed home visit by a home visitor to a family in a rural area is high in terms of lost productivity and travel cost. One less visit per month would more than cover the cost of providing a family with a cell phone and a service contract that could be used to avoid missed home visits as well as assist to achieve other outcome-oriented goals of the program, such as improved health maintenance, safety, social support, and employment.

The cell phone can offer advantages in states where HFA serves a transient, largely Latino group. For example, recent research that examined Latino perceptions of cell phones and the impact those perceptions have on use, found that Latino/a focus group participants discussed how cell phones provide an effective way to make interpersonal contact, while computers and the Internet were viewed as damaging to the communication necessary for good social relations (Leonardi, 2003). Pertierra (2002, 2005) has examined the effect of cell phone use on the user's perception of identity and claims that cell phones allow absent subjects to exercise a daily presence in their communities of origin. For Pertierra, cell phones have a role in helping people to construct and live the "story" of their lives while involving others who are absent in mutually supportive ways. In this design imperative example, we are indicating that feasibility in the human services always involves the cultural distinctiveness of the target population. In this example, the most obvious feasibility issue is the selection of the delivery vehicle, in this case a cell phone rather than the Internet and computer. What would not necessarily be obvious to the design scientist as a feasibility issue is the importance of the delivery vehicle to achieve social support in a collectivist culture.

Design Imperative #4: Combine Intervention Protocol with Development

Design imperative #4 deals with the issue that the development of the computing product prototype cannot be successful in behavioral science terms unless it conforms to the practice demands of the intervention protocol. The example that follows uses an intervention protocol based on the transtheoretical model of change. In this design imperative, imagine that a persuasive technology application is under development to increase the recovery rate from substance abuse. The application is intended to persuade the parent to use e-mail communications with a home visitor to support her or his recovery from substance abuse. The human service intervention protocol in this example is informed by the transtheoretical model of change (TTM)

(Prochaska, DiClemente, & Norcross, 1992). The persuasive technology tool that applies is tailoring a computer application to the individual. The TTM includes three primary components: stages of change, processes of change, and levels of change. As we have indicated earlier, tailoring is one of the persuasive technology tools that the designer will be able to use. In this case, the example of combining TTM and persuasive technologies is drawn from long-term investigations by Alemi and colleagues (2007). Their protocol for therapeutic e-mail would be studied at this stage of the design process by all of the disciplines involved in the design plan. The design plan for HFA at this point would recognize that substance-abusing mothers and fathers enter the program in varying states of recognition of the need and desire for change. The design team would then tailor the technology application to respond to the individual's change stage and use that knowledge in the therapeutic e-mail protocol to engage and support the parent at the appropriate stage.

Design Imperative #5: Combine, Pilot, and Evaluate

One way to address piloting and evaluation is to identify subgroups of the population and focus persuasive technologies on these groups. In our example, one approach would be to target subpopulations with one or more risk factors predictive of substantiated reports of child abuse and neglect. Research on the major risk factors associated with substantiated Child Protective Services (CPS) reports in a HFA population revealed nine factors that were significant in predicting substantiated child abuse and neglect. These included: young maternal age, Caucasian mother, substance abuse, a childhood history of abuse and neglect, multiple children, social isolation, attitudes in favor of violent discipline, difficulty in bonding and attachment with the child, and elevated potential for violence in the home (LeCroy & Milligan Associates, 2005). Using this human service research, important design foci for the combined pilot and evaluation would be the selection of the persuasive strategies used to address specific risk factors of the target subpopulation and whether or not the resulting applications will be adopted by the organization and used by the target population.

Technology designers and human service professionals need to work closely in staging this design imperative, as their interests will differ. In technology design, the process of prototyping and evaluating is iterative and evolutionary (Tankeda et al., 1990). There is the expectation that the technology designer will evaluate user experiences as the basis for judging whether or not the design is effective. Those evaluations become the basis for the next iteration, and for moving forward with progressively broader-scale implementation plans. The primary technology design question is: how well does the design work now? For the human service professional, the evaluation can be a theoretical assessment, where the primary question might be: when using this persuasive technology application, how well does the intervention work in producing the desired outcome? There is always the possibility that even a well-executed technology design will not produce the desired outcome. In the case of intervention research involving the HFA program, this might imply a comparative evaluation of the face-to-face condition compared to the approach with persuasive technology enhancements. Where more than one persuasive technology enhancement has been made, for instance, our scenario included an automated assessment process for discipline practices and a virtual coach for substance abuse, a multigroup evaluation design that is capable of testing several conditions in order to disentangle the effects of the multicomponent intervention is preferred. Technology can be used in evaluation by designing the technology-enhanced interventions to collect data on process and outcome as they are being used. For example, technology can deliver the cell phone administered assessment when deemed appropriate and collect information such as connect time, so that evaluative data can be continuously collected. Also, data mining techniques can be combined with post implementation program evaluation to allow practitioners to take an evidence-based practice approach to their work.

Design Imperative #6: Assess Ethical Considerations

Ethical considerations permeate the entire design process, from problem analysis to implementation and evaluation. In their Bill of Rights, Glastonbury and LaMendola (1992) suggested that the overarching principle of human rights, as declared in the Universal Declaration of Human Rights, is a reasonable and prudent starting point in all processes of Internet, web and wireless services development and use for the human services. This thinking emerges in grounded fashion in later work (Altschuller, 2004; Berdichevsky, Fogg, Sethi, & Kumar, 2005; Berdichevsky & Neuenschwander, 1999; Fogg, 2003). Similarly to Glastonbury and LaMendola, Berdichevsky and colleagues argue that if an act is considered unethical, it is also unethical in the context of computing technologies. Both advise respecting privacy, practicing full disclosure, and holding the creators of the intervention responsible for all reasonably predictable outcomes.

The expectation is that the human service and technology designers will not lie, will not hide important information, provoke emotions in an unwarranted fashion, or hide intentions. What the designer must consider is the interest of the service recipient and the service provider, and the designer must be responsible to organize technology-enhanced human services in a manner that he or she believes will not take advantage or act against the users' interests. Based on work by Berdichevsky and colleagues (2005), the ethical principles that have emerged in previous persuasive technology discussions could be summarized as including:

1. *Equivalency*: the creators of a persuasive technology realize that motivations, methods, and outcomes that are unethical in non-technical applications of human persuasion are also unethical when used in persuasive technology.
2. *Reciprocation*: the creators of a persuasive technology must never try to persuade a user of something if they themselves would not consent to be persuaded of it.
3. *Privacy*: the creators of a persuasive technology must regard the privacy of users with as much respect as they regard their own.
4. *Personal protection*: the creators of a persuasive technology must not relay personal information about a user without their knowledge to a third party.
5. *Disclosure*: the creators of a persuasive technology must disclose their motivations, methods, and intended outcomes.
6. *Outcomes*: the creators of a persuasive technology must assume responsibility for all reasonably predictable outcomes of its use.

We find that these ethical principles are often mixed in practice. For example, it would be unethical to make the results of the self-administered disciplinary assessments mentioned earlier available to the HFA supervisor without participant knowledge and consent. This could be an example of honoring the principles of privacy, disclosure, and personal protection. This example is also intended to indicate that the examination of potential ethical dilemmas involved in captology undertakings, though at an early stage, can be involved in each design imperative we have identified.

Other ethical issues are unique to the technology enhancements. For instance, we know that individuals tend to reveal more criminal and personally sensitive information to a computer than to another human. In our scenario, this may result in more reports to child protective services. Persuasive technology ethics have been recognized as one of the most important directions for further research (Ijsselsteijn et al., 2006). The ethical principles also infer that the involvement of human service professionals as advocates is essential to address ethical concerns throughout the design process. In the meantime, a more comprehensive assessment of the utility of existing ethical frameworks is needed.

CONCLUSION

Persuasive technology will increasingly be utilized to enhance existing evidence-based interventions—the question is how to go about it. This paper presents a first look at how captology might approach an answer. Our framework included evidence-based intervention design in the human services and design science approaches and illustrated how they might be collaboratively mixed despite their differences in purpose and method. Our approach is one that is human service based, considering not only the service recipient in a holistic manner, but also the service provider, and the organizational culture. Ethics is not a step in the framework or an afterthought, but permeates the entire design process. The framework marries the theory of the problem and the intervention with theory and research related to persuasive technologies and the process of design research. It is a first step toward understanding how the new science of captology can serve the development of therapeutic interventions in the human services.

REFERENCES

Alemi, F., Haack, M. R., Nemes, S., Aughburns, R., Sinkule, J., & Neuhauser, D. (2007). Therapeutic e-mails. *Substance Abuse Treatment, Prevention, and Policy*, 2(7). doi:10.1186/1747-597X-2-7.

Altschuller, S. (2004). *Developing an IT view-based framework for IS ethics research.* CIS Working Paper Series. New York: Baruch College.

Arbib, M. A. (Ed.). (2006). *Action to language via the mirror neuron system.* New York: Cambridge University Press.

Berdichevsky, D., Fogg, B. J., Sethi, R., & Kumar, M. (2005). Analyzing the ethics of persuasive technology. Retrieved May 7, 2007, from http://credibility.stanford .edu/captology/notebook/archives.new/2006/06/ethics_of_persu.html.

Berdichevsky, D., & Neuenschwander, E. (1999). Toward an ethics of persuasive technology. *Communications of the ACM Archive, 42,* 51–58.

Blakely, C. H., Mayer, J. P., Gottschalk, R. G., Schmitt, N., Davidson, W. S., & Roitjman, D. B., et al. (1987). The fidelity-adaptation debate: Implications for the implementation of public sector social programs. *American Journal of Community Psychology, 15,* 253–268.

Dane, A. V., & Schneider, B. H. (1998). Program integrity in primary and early secondary prevention: Are implementation effects out of control? *Clinical Psychology Review, 9,* 27–43.

Dillard, J. P., & Pfau, M. (2002). *The persuasion handbook: Developments in theory and practice.* Thousand Oaks, CA: Sage.

Dishman, E. (2003) *Designing for the new old.* In B. Laurel (Ed.), *Design research: Methods and perspectives* (pp. 41–48). Cambridge, MA: MIT Press.

Duggan, A., McFarlane, E., Fuddy, L., Burrell, L., Higman, S. M., Windham, A., et al. (2004). Randomized trial of a statewide home visiting program: Impact in preventing child abuse and neglect. *Child Abuse and Neglect, 28,* 597–622.

Duggan, A., Windham, A., McFarlane, E., Fuddy, L., Rohde, C., & Buchbinder, S., et al. (2000). Hawaii's Health Start program of home visiting for at-risk families: Evaluation of family identification, family engagement, and service delivery. *Pediatrics, 105,* 250–259.

Fogg, B. J. (2003). *Persuasive technology: Using computers to change what we think and do.* San Francisco, CA: Morgan Kaufmann Publishers.

Fraser, M. (Ed.). (2004). *Risk and resilience in childhood: An ecological perspective.* Washington, DC: NASW Press.

Glastonbury, B., & LaMendola, W. (1992). *The integrity of intelligence: A bill of rights for the information age.* London: St. Martin's Press.

Gomby, D., Culross, P., & Behrman, R. (1999). Home visiting: Recent program evaluations, analyses and recommendations. *The Future of Children, 9,* 4–26.

Grolleman, J., van Dijk, E. M. A. G., Nijholt, A., & van Emst, A. (2006). Break the habit! Designing an etherapy intervention using a virtual coach in aid of smoking cessation. In *Proceedings Persuasive 2006. First International Conference on Persuasive Technology for Human Well-Being* (pp. 133–141). Lecture Notes in Computer Science 3962. Heidelberg: Springer Verlag.

Ijsselsteijn, W., de Kort, Y., Midden, C., Eggen, B., & van den Hoven, E. (Eds.). (2006). Proceedings Persuasive 2006 First International Conference on Persuasive Technology for Human Well-Being, May 18–19, 2006, Eindhoven, The Netherlands. Lecture Notes in Computer Science Series 3962. Germany: Springer Verlag.

Kettner, P. M., Moroney, R. M., & Martin, L. L. (2008). *Designing and managing programs: An effectiveness-based approach* (3rd edition). Thousand Oaks, CA: Sage.

Knudsen, H. K., & Roman, P. M. (2004). Modeling the use of innovations in private treatment organizations: The role of absorptive capacity. *Journal of Substance Abuse Treatment, 26,* 353–361.

Laurel, B. (Ed.). (2003). Design research: Methods and perspectives. Cambridge, MA: MIT Press.

LeCroy & Milligan Associates. (2005). *Healthy families Arizona longitudinal evaluation—1st annual report.* Tucson, AZ: Author.

Leonardi, P. M. (2003). Problematizing "new media": Culturally based perceptions of mobile phones, computers and the Internet among United States Latinos. *Critical Studies in Mass Communications, 20,* 160–179.

Markus, M. L., Majchrzak, A., & Gasser, L. (2002). A design theory for systems that support emergent knowledge processes, *MIS Quarterly, 26,* 179–213.

Nass, C., & Brave, S. (2005). *Wired for speech: How voice activates and advances the human–computer relationship.* Cambridge, MA: MIT Press.

Owen, C. L. (1998). Design research: Building the knowledge base. *Design Studies, 19,* 9–20.

Parker-Oliver, D., & Demiris, G. (2006). Social work informatics: A new specialty. *Social Work, 51*(2), 127–134.

Pertierra, R. (2002). *The work of culture.* Manila, Philipines: DeLa Salle University Press.

Pertierra, R. (2005). Mobile phones, identity and discursive intimacy. *Human Technology, 1,* 23–44.

Pinderhughes, E. E., Bates, J. E., Dodge, K. A., Pettit, G. S., & Zelli, A., (2000). Discipline responses: Influences of parents' socioeconomic status, ethnicity, beliefs about parenting, stress, and cognitive-emotional processes. *Journal of Family Psychology, 14*(3), 380–400.

Prochaska, J. O., DiClemente, C. C., & Norcross, J. (1992). Stages and processes of self change of smoking: Toward an integrative model of change. *Journal of Consulting and Clinical Psychology, 51,* 390–395.

Reeves, B., & Nass, C.. (1996). *The media equation: How people treat computers, television, and new media like real people and places.* New York: Cambridge University Press.

Regalado, M., Harvinder, S., Inkelas, M., Wissow, L. S., & Halfon, N. (2004). Parents' discipline of young children: Results from the National Survey of Early Childhood Health. *Pediatrics, 113,* 1952–1958.

Ritterband, L. M., Andersson, G., Christensen, H. M., Carlbring, P., & Cuijpers, P. (2006). Viewpoint: Directions for the International Society for Research on Internet Interventions (ISRII). *J Med Internet Res,* 8(3):e23. Published online 2006 September 29. doi:10.2196/jmir.8.3.e23 Available: http://www.jmir.org/2006/3/e23/.

Robert Wood Johnson Foundation. (2004, December). *Cell phones give researchers a window on young mothers' parenting practices—Leads to NIH funded study.* Retrieved May 21, 2007, from http://www.rwjf.org/reports/grr/037224.htm.

Simon, H. (1996). *The sciences of the artificial* (3rd edition). Cambridge: MIT Press.

Simpson, D. D. (2002). A conceptual framework for transferring research to practice. *Journal of Substance Abuse Treatment, 22,* 171–182.

Straus, M. A., & Dinnelly, D. A. (Eds.) (1994). *Beating the devil out of them.* New York: Lexington Books.

Suchman, L. (1987). *Plans and situated actions: The problem of human-machine communication.* New York: Cambridge University Press.

Tankeda, H., Veerkamp, P., Tomiyama, T., & Yoshikawa, H. (1990). Modeling design processes. *AI Magazine,* 37–48.

Wantland, D. J., Potillo, C. J., Holzemer, W. L., Slaughter, R., & McGhee, E. M. (2004). The effectiveness of web-based vs. non-web-based interventions: A meta-analysis of behavioral change outcomes. *J. Med. Internet Res.* 6(4): e40. Published online 2004 November 10. doi: 10.2196/jmir.6.4.e40.

White, W. (2006). *Sponsor, recovery coach, addiction counselor: The importance of role clarity and role integrity.* Philadelphia, PA: Philadelphia Department of Behavioral Health and Mental Retardation Services.

Therapeutic Applications of Online Gaming

Paul P. Freddolino
Christina M. Blaschke

When readers think of "etherapy" or online treatment, most will assume the reference is to mental health services provided through the Internet, probably involving some combination of e-mail, chat rooms or instant messaging, threaded discussions, and/or live audio or video conferencing (Gingerich, 2007). Each of these exemplifies ways to meet the National Association of Social Workers (NASW) standard to "remain knowledgeable about ... the ways in which technology-based social work practice can be safely and appropriately conducted" (NASW & Association of Social Work Boards [ASWB], 2005, p. 18).

Online gaming is a medium for etherapy that uses emerging Internet-based technology for therapeutic purposes. In this article we will review some consequences of online gaming and examine some contemporary examples of online gaming used for therapeutic activities. We will conclude with a discussion of implications for research, practice, and social work education. To begin, however, we will provide background information on the evolution of online games, demographics of online gamers, and an overview of the online gaming environment and why it appeals to its wide audience.

EVOLUTION OF ONLINE GAMES

Etherapy games are a subset of a broader genre of games that have evolved on computers, stand-alone consoles, and, more recently, on the Internet. Nearly 50 years ago the first electronic video game was introduced to the public. In 1958 Tennis for Two used a simplified tennis court with an oscilloscope and a gravity-controlled ball that had to be played over the "net." Tennis for Two was quickly followed by the first multiuser game, Pong, a coin-operated table tennis arcade game that also became popular for video game consoles. Many advances occurred during the 1970s, and the arcade game industry entered its "Golden Age" in 1978 with the release of Space Invaders, Asteroids, and Pac-Man, which became common fixtures in shopping malls, restaurants, and convenience stores throughout the country. Another important development in the gaming world was the successful transition from limited-use university mainframe computer games to more widely used personal computer games like Zork in the 1980s ("History of Video Games," 2007).

Video game consoles are now in their seventh generation. Microsoft's Xbox 360 (2005) was the first to have wireless controllers and an Xbox Live service that allowed players to connect with other players worldwide through a built-in Ethernet port or wireless accessory. The Xbox 360 console was quickly followed in 2006 by Sony's PlayStation 3 with advanced graphics, and the Nintendo Wii, which allows players to physically participate with a wireless controller (e.g., throwing a ball) ("History of Video Games," 2007). All of these enhancements increase the appeal of the gaming environment.

Single-player etherapy games emerged while video game consoles and computer game genres were developing. They have evolved from the interest of game designers in using some of the perceived potential of games for educating clients to understand problems, make better choices, examine the consequences of their behavior, etc. Games have been designed to help people relax, learn about proper nutrition, and cope with or overcome phobias (Kharif, 2004). Examples of this class of etherapy games include substance abuse prevention and intervention games from the National Institute for Drug Abuse (http://www.teens.drugabuse.gov/havefun/index.asp), stress relief games from MindHabits (http://www.mindhabits.com/english/index.php), and a variety of substance abuse prevention and related games from the University of Texas at Arlington (http://www3.uta.edu/sswtech/sapvc/games/).

Faster progress in the online gaming world occurred in other areas. The first text-based multiplayer adventure game called Multi-User Dungeon (MUD) was launched in England in 1979 (Mulligan, 1999), and within a few years, various versions of MUD appeared in academia, gaining interest and participants. The first commercial version of a MUD, Islands of Kesmai, came onto the public market in 1984. By the late 1980s and early 1990s commercial massively multiplayer online role-playing games (MMORPGs) gained acceptance in mainstream gaming culture ("History of Video Games," 2007).

By the early 1990s, between four and six million households had active subscriptions to online services, paving the way for personal and commercial applications of games (Mulligan, 1999). Coupled with the ever improving computational power and graphics technologies, multiplayer games moved toward a three-dimensional (3D) virtual environment. Here, people take on alternative characters in 3D virtual spaces, collecting and constructing virtual items, communicating, and trading with one another. Today, the growth of online services for video game consoles has allowed gamers around the world to turn on their television, plug in their remote control, and battle fictitious enemies with one another.

The year 1997 marked a leap forward for MMORPGs with Origin Systems release of Ultima Online for home computers. Ultima Online is a strictly online game deploying numerous game servers to host thousands of online players simultaneously. The popularity of Ultima Online opened the door for MMORPGs like EverQuest (http://everquest.station.sony.com/), World of Warcraft (http://www.worldofwarcraft.com/), and RuneScape (http://www.runescape.com/), which currently boast millions of subscribers worldwide. Reynolds (2006) estimates that MMORPGs are played by more than 100 million people worldwide.

The most recent evolution of the computer-based simulated environments is no longer just a fantasy-based world but a virtual world with advanced social networking communities. One of the best known and widely used is Second Life by Linden Labs (http://secondlife.com/). This type of social virtual world is based on real-time, real-world environments with human characters, and not based on game objectives and plot lines. Second Life is a user-defined exploratory virtual environment in which people interact with one another, socialize, attend events, create virtual goods, and buy and sell them using virtual currency, Linden Dollars, which are exchangeable for U.S. currency. Other examples of social virtual worlds include The Sims Online (http://thesims.ea.com/), There (http://www.there.com/), Coke Studios (http://www.mycoke.com/), and Teen Second Life (http://teen.secondlife.com/).

In less than 40 years, online gaming has evolved from a two-person game played on one university campus to millions of people interacting in 3D virtual worlds, becoming a significant part of future socialization, business, and education for millions of people. One indicator of the perceived potential for gaming is the fact that more than 200 colleges and universities have partnered through the New Media Consortium (NMC) in creating a Virtual University in Second Life, where credit and noncredit courses are already offered (http://www.nmc.org/proj). Current offerings include mock trials for law students (Harvard University), an experiential opportunity to learn about hallucinations (University of California, Davis), and opportunities for faculty to learn how to teach in Second Life (Bowling Green State University). There are also numerous examples of courses that include a component of a regular course in the Second Life environment. Based on the number of colleges and universities becoming involved in NMC's activities, we predict it will not be long before human service courses are available.

CHARACTERISTICS OF ONLINE GAMERS

Obtaining accurate, up-to-date data to answer the question "Who's playing online games?" in the United States is challenging due to both definitional issues and the reality that the number of players increases daily. Even less information is known about users of online etherapy games. With these as caveats, however, a general sense of the potential "audience" can be drawn from a variety of sources.

The targeted age range for online gaming, exploration, and social networking sites covers preteens through senior citizens. One example of an online game for preteens is Club Penguin (www.clubpenguin. com), reported to have had four million unique visitors in January 2007 (Hawn, 2007). Among teenagers, Teen Second Life (http:// teen.secondlife.com/) claims to have members from thirteen countries, with the United States having the most. Exact numbers could not be located, but a corporate spokesperson noted that about 75 percent of the users are male, and most users are 15 years of age (Goodstein, 2005). At the opposite end of the age scale, the increased interest in and use of gaming sites and "brain games" by senior citizens points to an emerging market (Cohen, 2006). In between preteens and senior citizens are the mass of online gamers at sites such as Second Life with more than six million "residents" (with individual accounts of varying longevity), and World of Warcraft, with more than eight million paying members.

Gender is an important dimension in gaming as well. According to the Entertainment Software Association (2007), 58 percent of online gamers are male, and 42 percent are female. Female players are considerably older than male players in MMOGs (massively multiplayer online games): 44 percent of male players are 22 years of age or younger, compared with 20 percent of female players (Yee, 2006). According to Taylor (2003b), games such as EverQuest are "offering venues for the interesting exploration of activities typically bounded off from each other—sociability and power, mastery and cooperation—and women are finding dynamic ways to inhabit these mass virtual worlds" (p. 41).

While no specific data related to online gaming use by ethnic and language groups could be located, ethnicity and language are clearly related to access to the Internet in the United States for all purposes—including gaming. A report from the Pew Internet and American Life Project (Rainie, 2007) notes that among the "digital gaps" remaining in the United States, English speakers have the highest Internet use, while it is lower among those who speak a language other than English. Internet use is also higher among whites and Asian Americans, but lower among African Americans.

Online gamers can be divided into eight categories: newcomers, time killers, stress relievers, social players, enthusiasts, professionals, devotees, and addicts (Game Research, 2002). The first four are considered casual players. "The casual gamer is characterized by the fact that gaming is not a primary activity or something that he or she is willing to sacrifice other things for" (Game Research, 2002, p. 41). The remaining four categories of online gamers (enthusiasts, professionals, devotees, and addicts) are considered hard-core players, players that are very engaged in gaming and are prone to playing too much. According to Greenfield (1999), as many as 6 percent of Internet users could be classified as addicts. In June 2007 the American Medical Association (AMA) decided there was not enough evidence to add video game addiction to a list of formal disorders and called for more research into the public health risks of video and Internet games. The discussion was triggered by an AMA report from the group's Council on Social and Public Health that not only wanted to label excessive use of video games an addiction, but also pushed the AMA to pressure the American Psychiatric Association to include Internet/video game addiction in the next edition of the *Diagnostic and Statistical Manual of Mental Disorders* that will be published in 2011 (Mundell, 2007; Steenhuysen, 2007).

THE ONLINE GAMING ENVIRONMENT AND WHAT MAKES IT ATTRACTIVE

Why do so many people find the online gaming environment so attractive? What motivates gamers to spend multiple hours in virtual worlds? The answers to these questions differ from person to person.

322   *Paul P. Freddolino and Christina M. Blaschke*

The most common motivations behind online game playing are fun (BBC News, 2003a; Game Research, 2002; Oser, 2004), relaxation (Oser, 2004), leisure (BBC News, 2003a; Wan & Chiou, 2006), intellectual stimulation (Oser, 2004), competition (Game Research, 2002), and socialization (BBC News, 2003a; Game Research, 2002; Oser, 2004; Wan & Chiou, 2006). Etherapy games seem to draw players interested in improving their emotional, psychological, and physical health (Kharif, 2004).

For many players, online gaming is a social activity in which they meet new friends or play with friends they already had outside the online world (BBC News, 2003a; Game Research, 2002). Gamers create social communities revolving around the games they play, and they often play online games while they are physically together with someone who is also playing. Fifty percent of gamers extend their social network by meeting friends in real life that they first met online, a number that increases to 80 percent when female gamers are isolated (Game Research, 2002). Examining online game players from the United States, United Kingdom, and the Nordic countries, the majority of online gamers play with random people they met online or friends they know only online (60.1 percent); an additional 36.7 percent of online gamers play with friends they know from "real life" or from school (Game Research, 2002). Similar features appeal to young players as well. For example, Club Penguin is a kid-friendly virtual world designed for 8- to 14-year-olds where children can play games and interact with one another all while earning virtual coins that they can use to buy clothing for their penguin or furniture for their penguin's igloo (www.clubpenguin.com).

Engagement is another motivator for online game players. Games that keep the players working for weeks or months at a time are usually very difficult and complex. Players are constantly challenged with increasingly advanced goals, and they build close-knit communities to discuss and resolve their problems. The new generation of education/serious games attempt to emphasize the constructive components from commercial games, in terms of experiential environments, choice and consequences, peer-to-peer teaching, team collaboration, and complex decision making. Online games bring together challenges and interaction. Players treat a game as both a challenge and a place for creation and recreation. A game provides a story, puzzles to solve, and often tools to build and customize the environment. Talking to one another is just an instinctive human need for social interaction (Freddolino et al., 2007).

Other discussions of the online gaming environment have highlighted the transformative nature of the online experience, such as the feelings of mastery felt by young players in sports games, where they can accomplish feats unattainable on a real playing field (Turkle, 1995). By their very nature avatars facilitate players' capacity for transformative experiences, for being and doing what you cannot be or do in the real world (Levine, 2007). Children can be sports heroes, and people with disabilities can walk, run, and even dance (Bennett & Beith, 2007). These are powerful attractions of the online environment.

These characteristics of the online gaming environment have been shown to lead to some negative consequences as well as therapeutic opportunities, and we turn to these experiences in the next sections.

NEGATIVE ASPECTS OF ONLINE GAMING

The number of people becoming part of the virtual online gaming world is growing exponentially. With millions of people, young and old, logging on every day, the concern for any possible consequences has also grown among human services professionals, parents, employers, and educators. These concerns span across a broad range including technological, psychology/social, medical/health, and academic issues.

At the present time there is very limited research specifically focused on the negative aspects and consequences of online gaming. Most of the attention has been directed to the broader topic of Internet addiction, which is just developing as a field of research. While addiction to the Internet or online gaming is not listed specifically as a DSM-IV diagnosis, some studies have suggested that as many as 6 percent of Internet users could be considered addicts (Greenfield, 1999).

The Internet is neutral and not a source of addiction in and of itself. However, certain types and styles of applications, such as online gaming, appear to lend themselves to the development of the pathology that can lead to addiction (Young, 1998). Traditional addiction has centered on the use and abuse of a substance such as heroin or alcohol. Young (1998) in describing Internet addiction referred to it as "an impulse-control disorder which does not involve an intoxicant." Nonsubstance addictions, such as gambling and shopping, are considered to be process addictions (Soule, Shell, & Kleen, 2003) and have been magnified by the use of the Internet. Online gaming would fall into this subcategory of process Internet addiction, with some considering it to be the most addictive (Young, 1998). Two-way communication, personal interaction, and socialization may be the reasons why the Internet and online gaming in particular are so addicting (Grohol, 2003).

Virtual gaming environments are created and hosted on networks of computers, exposing users to certain technological risks such as network intrusion, computer viruses and worms, and identity theft. Of particular concern regarding younger gamers is the potential sharing of personal identifying information while playing the game that could provide online predators with enough details to locate someone. Another growing threat comes from cyberbullying (Center for Safe and Responsible Internet Use [CSRIU], n.d.).

Research on negative consequences has focused on psychological-social areas. Among these have been studies of the impact on personal relationships, anxiety, loneliness, depression, suicide ideation, and violence (Lo, Wang, & Fang, 2005; Wan & Chiou, 2006; Young, 2004). A recent study reported that the greater amount of time spent playing online games by college-aged students increased social anxiety and decreased interpersonal relationships (Lo et al., 2005). Reynolds (2006) describes a new class of video game widows who have even started an online support group (www.gamerwidow.com). One of the overlooked health concerns regarding online gaming is game-induced seizures. While infrequently measured, a recent study (Chuang, 2006) described the clinical presentation of 10 patients who experienced epileptic seizures during their participation in a MMORPG.

Players in other countries have demonstrated some of the extreme negative outcomes of gaming. In South Korea, online gaming has seeped into every societal and cultural crevice of the country and provides a glimpse of what the future of online gaming might look like throughout the world. According to BBC News (2005), more than 15 million people in South Korea are registered online gamers, equivalent to 30 percent of the total population. According to Farrand (2006), "online role playing has a strong appeal to Koreans who live in a tightly woven and hierarchical Confucian society" (p. 30). But some gamers take it too far and actually play themselves to death. In 2005, the deaths of at least seven South Koreans were attributed to excessive game playing. In response, private telephone emergency services have been created that can "dispatch ambulances for children who collapse while gaming, or refuse to come out of their rooms, glued to online games" (Farrand, 2006, p. 31). In Thailand, concern about rising levels of gaming addiction has led to imposed curfews (BBC News, 2003b). In China, the government has taken action to stop the "grave social problem" of teenage Internet addiction by funding inpatient rehabilitation clinics across the country (Cha, 2007).

POSITIVE ASPECTS OF ONLINE GAMING

The problems summarized previously tend to be what first come to mind when practitioners who are not gamers themselves are introduced to the concept of online gaming. Many have read about gaming addictions or spoken with a colleague who has treated an adolescent for whom an addiction to online gaming is one of several symptoms or problem areas. Schott and Hodgetts (2006) note, however, that this negative perception has been a common reaction over time to new media technologies by health and human service professionals; for example, television addiction. We used to talk about television addiction, now we talk about the television as a babysitter for the poor who work two jobs and cannot afford child care. Rather than simply dismissing all digital games as risks, Schott and Hodgetts (2006) suggest that consideration be given to "the social practices within which gaming is situated" (p. 310). This will bring us to consideration of some of the "social" dimensions of online gaming.

Health and human service professionals, working with skilled game designers, have harnessed aspects of the online gaming environment described previously to develop new therapeutic applications across a wide range of health and social problem areas. From our review of numerous games we have identified five features that characterize these online therapeutic games:

1. The content is controlled by the creators of the game. For example, the creators of Full Spectrum Warrior developed the content that permits users to "relive" the traumatic events that caused their post-traumatic stress disorder (PTSD) (http://kotaku.com/gaming/military/games-used-to-treat-ptsd

-191088.php). In the case of continuous virtual environments, the framework in which users will develop content is controlled by the creators. Linden Labs, creators of Second Life, make widely available the tools for users to develop content for the environment.

2. The games are designed to incorporate high levels of fun based on available evidence concerning what gamers seek. Some games incorporate continuous suggestions and feedback from target users in the development process. The National Institute on Drug Abuse (NIDA) enlisted the help of teens when developing its prevention and intervention games to make sure that the content is appropriate and addresses issues affecting teens.

3. The games are designed to be appealing to users in terms of color, graphics, sounds and music, speed, and other characteristics known to generate satisfaction, repeat visits, and positive comments to peers (also known as buzz). Reach Out Central argues that "the program appeals through its colorful aesthetic, use of popular music, ease of use, and overall fun of gameplay." They also note that 80 percent of the site is developed collaboratively with Youth Ambassadors who help write content and ensure that the site is relevant to the needs of youth (http://www.reachout.com.au).

4. Gaming sites have been and will continue to be developed in numerous countries, using multiple languages, reflecting many cultures; within gaming sites it is common to see information and conversations in multiple languages, reflecting the diversity and global residence of the players. For example, Re-Mission is available in English, Spanish, and French. Ben's Game is available in nine languages: English, Dutch, French, German, Greek, Italian, Japanese, Russian, and Spanish. The international appeal of online virtual environments such as Second Life is reflected in the emerging Chinese version of a similar gaming space (Adams, 2007).

5. Games that involve only one player frequently also provide collateral opportunities for players to exchange commentary, evaluations, strategy tips, etc. When not provided by the designers—and even when they are provided—users will establish their own chat rooms, forums, blogs, and other new interactive media as communal activities. The game's "community" *will* be established. Re-Mission designers have created community forums in which players can discuss the game, their experiences with

cancer, and general news (http://www.re-mission.net/forums/ index.php?act=idx). World of Warcraft has both official forums (http://forums.worldofwarcraft.com) and "unofficial" forums (http://wow.incgamers.com/forums/) for players.

There are many suggestions in the literature that time spent in gaming activities brings some positive benefits. In addition to the most obvious outcomes of entertainment, leisure, and fun (Wan & Chiou, 2006), one of the most important outcomes appears to be the extension of the players' social networks (Albuquerque & Velho, 2003; Axelsson & Regan, 2002; Chou, 2001; Farrand, 2006). That these networks now reach around the globe is illustrated by the reaction to the death of a well-known online personality (Banks, 2006). Steinkuehler and Williams (2006) describe the process of expanding networks in terms of building social capital.

Because the very nature of virtual worlds permits players to purposefully substitute virtual relationships for real-world social contacts (Lo et al., 2005), virtual worlds provide additional and potentially therapeutic venues for people with physical and/or other disabilities for whom real-world contacts are accompanied by anxiety or stigma or are even physically impossible (Bennett & Beith, 2007).

Other commentators and reviewers have identified more specific outcomes. The opportunities to learn social, group, and decision-making skills have attracted the eye of audiences from the corporate (Dignan, 2006; Fox, 2006) to the military (Riddell, 1997). The potential richness of virtual worlds epitomizes the creative value provided by some gaming and exploration environments (Taylor, 2003a). Bers (2001) describes the creation of "identity construction environments (ICEs)" that provide opportunities for teens—and potentially other age groups—to learn about their own identity, particularly in regard to personal and moral values. These outcomes are possible because of the almost limitless creative potential of online environments. One example of an ICE designed for teens is Reach Out Central, an interactive single-player game designed to help teens explore important aspects of their identity (i.e., thoughts, feelings, and behavior).

There are many examples of games intentionally designed to have a positive impact across a wide range of problems and/or desired goals. One game type focuses on individual player goals; a lengthy list is available at: http://www.socialimpactgames.com/. There are games for language issues (http://www.quia.com/pages/havefun.html), special education (http://www.parentpals.com/gossamer/pages/Special_Education_Games/index.html), and color therapy (http://www.magicmnemonic.com/pair/color01.html). Other games already mentioned include: NIDA for Teens (http://www.teens.drugabuse.gov/havefun/index.asp), MindHabits (http://www.mindhabits.com/english/index.php), and Games at SubstanceAbusePrevention.org (http://www3.uta.edu/sswtech/sapvc/games/).

An interesting example of the individual player genre is Personal Investigator (Coyle & Matthews, 2004), which implements a version of brief solution-focused therapy in a mental health intervention for teens. The game was one of the first to use an online game to "build stronger therapeutic relationships between therapists and adolescents" (Coyle, Matthews, Sharry, Nisbet, & Doherty, 2005, p. 73). In Personal Investigator, teens are trainee detectives for the Detective Academy, hunting for clues to resolve personal problems. With the assistance of master detectives, trainees learn about solution-focused therapy in order to move forward in the investigation. While playing the games, teens also learn about how other young people have been able to use techniques of solution-focused therapy to overcome personal problems (Coyle, 2007). Personal Investigator is available as a 3D computer game, but only to mental health professionals participating in the PlayWrite games study (www.cs.tcd.ie/~coyledt/index.htm).

The models provided by Personal Investigator and the other games mentioned previously can be used in designing other online games and activities for teens. One online therapeutic game aimed at teens uses many of the game features noted previously to construct an experience both appealing to teens and potentially able to impact areas in which teens frequently struggle (see Vignette 1). The game is one of many online tools, resources, and social networking opportunities provided by an agency focusing on teens (http://www.reachout.com.au/home.asp). Data related to outcomes or effectiveness of the site could not be found.

Children with cancer have benefited from several games available online. One of the best known is Ben's Game, distributed in multiple languages by the Make-a-Wish Foundation. The object of the game is for the player to destroy all mutated cells and collect seven shields that protect against common side effects of chemotherapy. Ben's Game is available for free download on the game's website

VIGNETTE 1. Reach Out Central

(http://www.reachout.com.au)

Reach Out Central (ROC) is an interactive environment designed for teens and young adults in which a player examines the interplay between the way he or she thinks, feels, and behaves. A player chooses a character and sets his or her mood (happy, sad, stressed, confident, scared, etc.). The player then goes through a series of real-life situations and must choose one of two reactions, such as whether to apply for a job or how to respond to an embarrassing situation. After each decision is made, the player is given the "Big Picture" about being nervous, seeing the positive side of things, anger control, stress, dealing with bullies, or accepting that no one is perfect. ROC incorporates a backdrop of current alternative rock music, hip fashion, and modern popular culture into every scene.

(http://www.makewish.org/site/pp.asp?c=bdJLITMAE & b=81924) (Greater Bay Area Make-a-Wish Foundation, 2005). Another example of a targeted individual player online game is Re-Mission, a game for adolescents and young adults with cancer (http://www.re-mission. net/) coupled, as is frequently the case, with several online tools to support networking among the patient-users, including message boards and blogs. What is somewhat unique about this game is the randomized clinical trial research that showed increases in users' quality of life, knowledge of cancer, and self-efficacy. Significantly, the data also showed that Re-Mission players "maintained higher blood levels of chemotherapy and showed higher rates of antibiotic utilization," both suggesting better adherence to cancer therapy regimens (Cole, 2006). Anyone can download or order Re-Mission from the game's website. HopeLab, a nonprofit organization that developed the game, requests a $20 donation in order to offset the cost of providing the game free of charge to young people who have cancer. Since the game was first introduced in April 2006, HopeLab has delivered 76,000 copies on disc or through downloads on the game's website (Baertlein, 2007). This game and its multiple ancillary tools reflect a sizable development effort requiring considerable resources. According to Ryan and Warhol (2006), the cost to develop Re-Mission was more than $2.5 million, not including internal costs incurred by HopeLab. Obesity is the next major health issue affecting young adults that HopeLab will target (HopeLab, 2007, http://www.hopelab.org/aboutus.html).

Military, first responder, and other categories of clients with intense symptoms related to PTSD now may be able to benefit from an online gaming approach that has great promise for significant results in reducing symptoms (Rizzo, 2006). Rizzo and Hollander (2006) and their colleagues have used game-based technologies to create an environment where victims of terrorist bus bomb attacks relive aspects of their experience in a controlled setting. Similar approaches are being developed for treating a wide range of anxiety disorders and phobias such as fear of flying (Bergfield, 2006; Virtual Reality Medical Center, n.d.).

One emerging arena for online gaming involves what are referred to as "persistent worlds" (International Game Developers Association, 2004) or "virtual worlds" (Freddolino et al., 2007). Unlike the linear play experienced in traditional online games, in nonlinear games such as Grand Theft Auto, Oblivion, or World of Warcraft, the worlds are freely explorable and what gamers do with their time is up to them. In these situations, gamers are free to choose how their characters perform and behave in this environment. Elements of story and narrative are available, but only if the gamer chooses to interact with this functionality. An interesting aspect of these types of games is how they enable the users to imagine or role-play their own narrative by developing a character with a unique personality and set of behaviors. For example, bullying victims can be encouraged to create an avatar with a more assertive personality and then engage other players in a virtual playground (Stutzky, personal communication, May 2, 2007).

In a recent article Parris (2007) describes examples of simulations in Second Life that allow players to engage in environments as diverse as schizophrenia and oil drilling. The former is used to teach an understanding of the disease and how to treat it; the latter is a prototype to see how this environment can be used for education. The Centers for Disease Control and Prevention have also established virtual clinics for training emergency workers. Parris notes that environments such as Second Life touch two very important human needs and preferences: social contact and visual stimulation. How far things may go in environments such as Second Life are related to the "business" dimension of the site. Already in Second Life major universities (Parris, 2007) and corporations (Cain, 2007) have made their

VIGNETTE 2. Second Life's Support for Healing

(http://secondlife.com/)

Support for Healing is a virtual island in Second Life where avatars can go for relief from life's problems. Island resources are free to any avatar in Second Life and are available around the clock. Looking for a support group for depression; anxiety; gay, lesbian, bisexual, and transgender issues; psychosis; chronic pain and illness; women's issues; or weight loss? Support for Healing provides a meeting place for all of these support groups. Meeting schedules are updated regularly and can be picked up when an avatar "teleports" to the island. Aside from support groups, the Support for Healing island also provides avatars with quiet areas for meditation and relaxation. The landscape has been beautifully crafted, with running streams, blue skies, and colorful flowers.

presence known. It should come as no surprise then that individuals are offering therapeutic services in Second Life. Anyone can now locate—in the Second Life environment—many examples of e-counseling or etherapy ranging from fee-for-service sessions or activities to free support groups. In some cases etherapy is provided in Second Life in exchange for Linden Dollars. One such e-therapist charges avatars 1,000 Linden Dollars for 10 minutes of therapy, equivalent to four U.S. dollars. Other e-therapists use the Second Life environment to advertise services provided outside of the virtual game. One example of a site in Second Life that provides free support groups for avatars is captured in Vignette 2. Of course, all of it is virtual . . . . or is it?

FUTURE DIRECTIONS

The NASW Technology Standards (NASW & ASWB, 2005) clearly require that practitioners keep current with best practices utilizing technology. This in turn requires research related to emerging applications and solutions, and the development of courses and continuing/professional education opportunities to aid in their dissemination. In this section we present an overview of possible efforts in these three arenas.

Research

The research agenda related to therapeutic uses of online gaming has two complementary tracks. One area should focus on improving our understanding of the gaming process—what happens within various types of games such as role-playing games and virtual environments—as well as the social networking activities that seem inevitably to evolve from gaming activities. Some of the research questions that develop along these lines will require the strategies and approaches typical of qualitative analysis. In this work, the methodological toolkit developed by Consalvo and Dutton (2006) will be useful. They describe approaches that focus on features such as the "object inventory" built by players, studies of the game interface itself, analyzing the interactions that occur within the game, and studies of the game log. Researchers can add more traditional analyses of the discussion boards, blogs, and other interactive tools associated with the games. These research efforts will increase knowledge of the games themselves that can parallel studies of the impacts and outcomes of playing these games.

To develop the types of research most supportive of the concepts of "best practice" and "evidence-based practice" the research in this field must move more toward experimental designs used in real-world settings. A good example is provided by the randomized field trials employed in the study of outcomes of the Re-Mission game (Cole, 2006). To deal with the myriad challenges of validity, representativeness, and generalizability, several different designs will have to be utilized. For example, to test for the "do no harm" issue some experimental designs will have to include a "no intervention" condition. Other studies will have to compare the online game condition with conditions in which some recipients receive "standard practice" as defined in the arena of service (e.g., substance abuse) while others receive a more realistic "minimal practice." Comparisons with the best face-to-face evidence-based practice would reflect the gold standard, but would not necessarily provide the most realistic comparison. Another approach would be to compare any of these levels of current practice with the same level *plus* the online gaming tool under study.

The field needs evaluations of the impacts and outcomes of online games, and the challenge is to make the forthcoming studies both rigorous in design and realistic in the nature of the comparisons. At the same time, researchers venturing into this field must confront some serious ethical challenges. For example, there is no consensus on whether the content of open, public virtual environments and games is public or private relative to researchers. Thus a valid informed consent prior to capture and analysis of content from a game environment may be required. The adult status of online subjects is difficult to validate, and researchers must provide adequate grounds for accepting the procedures of private companies and websites that claim to keep minors out. It may be difficult to ensure the respondent's comprehension of the risks involved in a particular study. These and similar concerns must be acknowledged and addressed by researchers wishing to study these environments. To increase their ability to control some of the factors that create ethical dilemmas, researchers may opt to collaborate with game designers and develop their own gaming worlds within which their research can be conducted.

Practice

There is almost always a wide gap between any new set of standards and the actual adherence to the standards in the field. Furthermore, the significant lag time between publication of findings of effective interventions and their actual utilization in agencies is well known (Cournoyer, 2004). It is not likely that "gaming" interventions will be high on clinicians' priority lists given what are perceived as more important or promising evidence-based approaches; however, these approaches are promising in their potential for therapeutic change and social support, warranting further investigation by the practice community. In addition, practitioners cannot help consumers with issues related to gaming addiction if they do not have an understanding of what is involved in this activity. At the very least, practitioners need to screen clients about their involvement in the online world as part of any thorough assessment process.

At the same time, we would submit that advances can and should be made in fairly simple ways by both individual practitioners and the agencies and programs in which they practice. This approach would be consistent with the Standards for Technology (NASW & ASWB, 2005), which address responsibilities of agencies in terms of providing access to appropriate technology (Standard 2, p. 8), including support for client access to technology. Practitioners are expected to seek "appropriate training and consultation to stay current with emerging technologies" (Standard 4, p. 10).

One way to encourage movement in this direction is for agencies to have available on site at least one Internet-enabled computer where staff can demonstrate to clients websites that provide useful information; games with effective, evidence-based skill-building opportunities; and other tools. This would also permit the information flow to be reversed, where clients can demonstrate to their practitioners where they go for information, relaxation, gaming sites for skill-building, etc.

Another strategy would be to connect with social workers and other practitioners already using gaming interventions effectively and learning how they have dealt with the threats implicit in online gaming. This can be done by the associations that sponsor practitioner conferences, or through online community-building efforts sponsored by NASW, CSWE, and other organizations.

These may be only small steps, but moves in these directions could initiate an increase in interest on the part of both practitioners and clients—something completely consistent with the Technology Standards.

Education

In order for some of these changes to occur, faculty in social work degree programs and managers of social work continuing education programs must become much more active in learning about the role of technology in social work practice. They also have a responsibility to incorporate such knowledge in the social work curriculum and professional development offerings (Freddolino, 2002).

Although the Standards for Technology are addressed primarily to practitioners, our educational and professional development programs are in some ways responsible for the knowledge, skills, and values with which their students enter practice. It is hoped that someone in each academic and continuing education program learns more about the use of gaming and then develops modules or short courses on therapeutic uses of gaming. Numerous blogs, wikis, lists, and other interactive networking tools are being developed to support efforts of educators and practitioners in using Second Life. One example for those in the health field is the Second Life list "Health Care Support and Education" (https://lists.secondlife.com/cgi-bin/mailman/listinfo/healthcare). More positive outcomes are likely where educators utilize some of these new technology tools directly in their courses, especially when the tools are used in connection with social work problems and solutions (Delwiche, 2006).

CONCLUSION

The NASW Standards for Technology and Social Work Practice requires practitioners to "remain knowledgeable about" new technology-supported interventions and how they can be used safely and effectively. This review has demonstrated both some of the risks and the possibilities of online games and creative online environments. Among the characteristics of these environments that attract players are the lively interactive social support networks and the potential for transformative and therapeutic change. The appeal of such environments for average people—including those who could be our clients— argue strongly for the need for practitioners to inquire about clients' involvement in online worlds just as they might ask about participation in neighborhood and other social groups. It is also clear that human service professionals must explore the ways in which they can become more active in designing online games to meet the needs of the clients we serve. Certainly much more research is needed to determine who plays online and what outcomes and impacts result from their participation.

It will probably be quite some time before online gaming interventions have become one of the standard approaches used by even a significant minority of practitioners. In fact, it may well be the case that various game developers market online gaming options in which people find fun, peace, growth, and other rewards directly to the people who will become our clients. For all we know, our clients may already be engaged in interactive play in virtual worlds like Second Life. They may already be interacting there...with some of our peers who have joined for many of the same reasons.

REFERENCES

Adams, J. (2007, July 30). Roam un-free. *Newsweek, International Edition.* Retrieved July 31, 2007, from http://www.msnbc.msn.com/id/19887681/site/newsweek/.
Albuquerque, A. L. P., & Velho, L. (2002). Togetherness through virtual worlds: How real can be that presence? In Universidade Fernando Pessoa (Ed), Fifth

Annual Workshop Presence 2002 (pp. 435–447). Porto, Portugal: Universidade Fernando Pessoa.

Axelsson, A. S., & Regan, T. (2002). *How belonging to an online group affects social behavior—A case study of Asheron's Call.* Redmond, WA: Microsoft Research.

Baertlein, L. (2007, May 30). Video game maker target teens with cancer. Retrieved July 24, 2007, from http://www.reuters.com.

Banks, G. (2006, March 5). Reality of a death saddens the virtual world. *Pittsburgh Post-Gazette.* Retrieved May 14, 2007, from http://www.post-gazette.com.pg/06064/665353=sl.stm.

BBC News. (2003a, July 8). Gaming "part of student life." Retrieved May 14, 2007, from http://news.bbc.co.uk/2/hi/technology/3052482.stm.

BBC News. (2003b, July 8). Thailand restricts online gamers. Retrieved May 14, 2007, from http://news.bbc.co.uk/2/hi/asia-pacific/3054590.stm.

BBC News. (2005, August 10). S Korean dies after games session. Retrieved May 14, 2007, from http://news.bbc.co.uk/2/hi/technology/4137782.stm.

Bennett, J., & Beith, M. (2007, July 30). Alternate universe. *Newsweek, International Edition.* Retrieved July 31, 2007, from http://www.msnbc.msn.com/id/19876812/site/newsweek/.

Bergfield, C. (2006, July 26). War vets get a dose of virtual reality. Retrieved July 31, 2007, from http://www.msnbc.msn.com/id/14048170.

Bers, M. U. (2001). Identity construction environments: Developing personal and moral values through the design of a virtual city. *The Journal of the Learning Sciences, 10*(4), 365–415.

Cain, P. (2007, February 21). Companies are finding Second Life. *Investor's Business Daily.* Retrieved May 14, 2007, from http://www.investors.com/editorial/IBDArticles.asp?artsec=17 &issue=20070221.

Center for Safe and Responsible Internet Use. (n.d.). Cyberbullying. Retrieved May 15, 2007, from http://www.cyberbully.org/.

Cha, A. E. (2007, February 22). China treats Internet "addicts" sternly. *Washington Post.* Retrieved February 22, 2007, from http://www.msnbc.com/id/17251571/.

Chou, C. (2001). Internet heavy use and addiction among Taiwanese college students: An online interview study. *Cyber Psychology & Behavior, 4*(5), 573–585.

Chuang, Y. (2006). Massively multiplayer online role-playing game-induced seizures: A neglected health problem in internet addiction. *CyberPsychology & Behavior, 9*(4), 451–456.

Cohen, A. (2006, December 7). Digital culture: Video-game players discover a new, older, market. National Public Radio.Retrieved May 14, 2007, from http://www.npr.org/templates/story/story.php?storyId=6589941.

Cole, S. (2006). Hopelab: Research results for helping kids with cancer using a videogame. Games for Health Day Expo. Retrieved May 14, 2007, from http://www.hopelab.org/docs/HopeLab%20-%20Re-Mission%20Outcomes%20Study.pdf.

Consalvo, M., & Dutton, N. (2006, December). Game analysis: Developing a methodological toolkit for the qualitative study of games. *The International Journal of*

Computer Game Research, 6(1). Available: http://gamestudies.org/0601/articles/ consalvo_dutton.

Cournoyer, B. R. (2004). *The evidence-based social work skills book*. Boston, MA: Allyn and Bacon.

Coyle, D. (2007). PlayWrite games.Retrieved August 1, 2007, from https:// www.cs.tcd.ie/~coyledt/playWriteGames.htm.

Coyle, D., & Matthews. M. (2004, April). Personal investigator: A therapeutic 3D game for teenagers. Presented at Social Learning Through Gaming Workshop, Vienna, Austria.

Coyle, D., Matthews, M., Sharry, J., Nisbet, A., & Doherty, G. (2005). Personal investigator: A therapeutic game for adolescent psychotherapy. *Journal of Interactive Technology & Smart Education*, 2(2), 73–88.

Delwiche, A. (2006). Massively multiplayer online games (MMOs) in the new media classroom. *Educational Technology & Society*, 9(3), 160–172.

Dignan, L. (2006). Second Life: Virtual world training wheels for corporate America. Retrieved May 14, 2007, from http://blogs.zdnet.com/BTL/?p=4039.

Entertainment Software Association. (2007). Facts & research: Game player data. Retrieved May 14, 2007, from http://www.theesa.com/facts/gamer_data.php.

Farrand, T. (2006, November 6). Gaming: All the world's a stage. *Brand Strategy*, 30–31.

Fox, S. (2006, October). The great escape. *Associations Now*, 2(11), 41–43.

Freddolino, P. (2002). Thinking "outside the box" in social work distance education: Not just for distance anymore. Originally published online in the *Electronic Journal of Social Work*, 1(1), 1–13.

Freddolino, P., Heeter, C., Stutzky, G., Detskas, A., Blaschke, C., Chen, J. (2007). Using virtual environments and multi-player games to support teens at risk, their families, and the professionals who work with them. White paper prepared for the Family Research Initiative, Michigan State University, East Lansing, Michigan.

Game Research. (2002). Online gaming habits.Retrieved May 14, 2007, from http:// game-research.com/2/wp-content/uploads/2006/05/Online%20Gaming%20Habits%20Standard%20Version.pdf.

Gingerich, W. J. (2007). eTherapy.Retrieved May 14, 2007, from http://www. gingerich.net/etherapy.htm.

Goodstein, A. (2005, December 22). Virtual teen entrepreneurs. *Ypulse*. Retrieved May 14, 2007, from http://ypulse.com/archives/2005/12/virtual_teen_en.php.

Greater Bay Area Make-A-Wish Foundation. (2005). Ben's game.Retrieved May 14, 2007, from http://www.makewish.org/site/pp.asp?c=bdJLITMAE & b=81924.

Greenfield, D. (1999) *Virtual addiction: Help for netheads, cyberfreaks, and those who love them*. Oakland, CA: New Harbinger.

Grohol, J. (2003). Internet addiction guide. Retrieved May 14, 2007, from http:// www.psychcentral.com/netaddiction.

Hawn, C. (2007, March 23). Time to play, money to spend. CNN Money.Retrieved May 15, 2007, from http://money.cnn.com/magazines/business2/business2_archive/2007/04/01/8403359/index.htm.

History of video games. (2007). *Wikipedia*. Retrieved from http://www.answers. com/topic/history-of-video-games.

HopeLab. (2007). About HopeLab. Retrieved July 24, 2007, from http://www. hopelab.org/aboutus/html.

International Game Developers Association. (2004). 2004 persistent worlds whitepaper. Retrieved May 14, 2007, from http://www.igda.org/online/IGDA_PSW_- Whitepaper_2004.pdf.

Kharif, O. (2004, June 14). My therapist is a joystick. *Business Week*. Retrieved July 30, 2007, from http://www.businessweek.com/magazine/content/04_24/ b3887088_mz063.htm.

Levine, K. (2007, July 31). Alter egos in a virtual world. National Public Radio. Retrieved July 31, 2007, from http://www.npr.org/templates/story/story. php?storyId=12263532.

Lo, S., Wang, C., & Fang, W. (2005). Physical interpersonal relationships and social anxiety among online game players. *CyberPsychology & Behavior*, *8*(1), 15–20.

Mulligan, J. (1999). Online game timeline. Retrieved May 14, 2007, from http:// www.skotos.net/articles/bth.html.

Mundell, E. J. (2007, June 27). Video games' addictive nature unclear: AMA. Retrieved July 24, 2007, from http://abcnews.go.com/Health/Healthday/Story?- id=4507723&page=1.

National Association of Social Workers & Association of Social Work Boards. (2005). Standards for technology and social work practice.Retrieved May 14, 2007, from https://www.socialworkers.org/practice/standards/NASWTechnologyStandards. pdf.

Oser, K. (2004). Moms are unsung players in gaming world. *Advertising Age*, *7*(22), 56–57.

Parris, C. (2007, May 1). Viewpoint: Do better business in 3D. *Business Week*. Retrieved from http://www.businessweek.com/technology/content/may2007/ tc20070501_526224.htm?chan=top+news_top+news+index_technology.

Rainie, L. (2007). The new digital ecology: The growth and impact of the Internet (and related technologies). Washington, DC: Pew Internet & American Life Project. Available: http://www.pewinternet.org/presentation_display.asp?r=86.

Reynolds, C. (2006, January). Videogame widows. *Macleans*, *119*(3), 42.

Riddell, R. (1997, April). Doom goes to war: The Marines are looking for a few good games. *Wired*, *5*(4). Available: http://www.wired.com/wired/archive/5.04/ ff_doom_pr.html.

Rizzo, A. (2006). Expose, distract, motivate and measure: Virtual reality games for health. *Nuevas Ideas en Informatico Educativa*, *2*, 1–4.

Rizzo, A., & Hollander, A. (2006). Game environments and post traumatic stress disorder. Presented at the Game Developers Conference 2006, March 20–26, San Jose, California.Retrieved May 14, 2007, from https://www.cmpevents.com/ gd06/a.asp?option=C & V=11 & SessID=2501.

Ryan, T. & Warhol, D. (2006, September 29). The making of Re-Mission: A case study on the integration of entertainment software and games for health. Presented at Games for Health Conference, September 28–29, Baltimore, Maryland.

Retrieved July 24, 2007, from http://www.gamesforhealth.org/presentations/the-making-of-remission.ppt#279,28,CostImplications.

Schott, G., & Hodgetts, D. (2006). Health and digital gaming: The benefits of a community of practice. *Journal of Health Psychology*, *11*(2), 309–316.

Soule, L. C., Shell, L. W., & Kleen, B. A. (2003). Exploring Internet addiction: Demographic characteristics and stereotypes of heavy Internet users. *The Journal of Computer Information Systems*, *44*(1), 64–73.

Steenhuysen, J. (2007, June 27). Doctors want more study on overuse of video games. Retrieved July 24, 2007, from http://www.alertnet.org/thenews/newsdesk/N27312681.htm.

Steinkuehler, C. A., & Williams, D. (2006). Where everybody knows your (screen) name: Online games as "third places." *Journal of Computer-Mediated Communication*, *11*,885–909.

Taylor, T. L. (2003a). Intentional bodies: Virtual environments and the designers who shape them. *International Journal of Engineering Education*, *19*(10), 25–34.

Taylor, T. L. (2003b). Multiple pleasures: Women and online gaming. *Convergence*, *9*(1), 21–46.

Turkle, S. (1995). *Life on the screen: Identity in the age of the Internet*. New York: Simon and Schuster.

Virtual Reality Medical Center. (n.d.). Virtual reality therapy. Retrieved May 14, 2007, from http://www.vrphobia.com/therapy.htm.

Wan, C., & Chiou, W. (2006). Why are adolescents addicted to online gaming? An interview study in Taiwan. *CyberPsychology & Behavior*, *9*(6), 762–766.

Yee, N. (2006). The demographics, motivations, and derived experiences of users of massively multi-user online graphical environments. *Presence: Teleoperators and Virtual Environments*, *15*, 309–329.

Young, K. (1998). *Caught in the net: How to recognize the signs of Internet addiction and a winning strategy for recovery*. New York: John Wiley & Sons.

Young, K. S. (2004). Internet addiction: A new clinical phenomenon and its consequences. *The American Behavioral Sciences*, *48*(4), 402–415.

Cybercounseling Online: The Development of a University-Based Training Program for E-mail Counseling

Lawrence Murphy
Robert MacFadden
Dan Mitchell

The majority of training programs in psychotherapy employ a traditional face-to-face (FTF) method of delivery. Even though web-based education and Internet blended approaches are becoming more popular in human service fields, many educators question whether this type of virtual education is appropriate for the clinical area, which requires development of FTF skills and relationship building. In a national study of social work educators in the United States, Moore (2005) found that faculty perceived FTF education to be more effective than web-based education in all curriculum areas, but particularly for less "content-based" based areas such as practice. These perceptions stand in contrast to much of the research comparing FTF and web-based education that generally reports "no significant difference" (Namsook, Krug, & Zhang, 2007). There is a great need for description and research about the effectiveness of specialized online training directed at developing clinical skills for counseling to be delivered exclusively over the web.

This article describes the development of a university-based cyber-counseling certificate program that is situated within a continuing education program in a graduate faculty of social work. Some of the issues, challenges, and accomplishments of the program over three years of operation are explored along with important lessons learned.

The term *cybercounseling* has been used along with others such as online counseling, etherapy, web-based therapy, and Internet therapy to denote some type of technology-enhanced form of counseling or therapy. The cybercounseling program discussed in this article refers specifically to the asynchronous type of counseling that occurs through e-mail. This type of counseling has been identified currently as the most prevalent type of web-based intervention (Chester & Glass, 2006). This article describes the inception and structure of the training program followed by a description of how the training is delivered through PrivacEmail Professional, the software system used to deliver both the training and the cybercounseling. Learner demographics and evaluation data are presented, concluding with a section on lessons learned.

BACKGROUND AND NEED

The delivery of clinical intervention via technology has been occurring for decades. Telephone counseling has been discussed in the literature for more than 30 years (Mallen, Rochlen, & Day, 2005), and in one sample of 600 doctoral level American Psychological Association members, 98 percent reported delivering some service over the telephone (VandenBos & Williams, 2000). Two of the authors of this article (DM and LM) have been delivering e-mail counseling since 1995 and have written some of the early publications in this area (Murphy & Mitchell, 1998; Collie, Mitchell, & Murphy, 2000; Mitchell & Murphy, 2004).

INCEPTION AND STRUCTURE OF THE CYBERCOUNSELING PROGRAM

The Director of the Continuing Education Program at the graduate faculty of social work became familiar with one of the other two authors who had been a regular guest presenter on cybercounseling at a credit course on IT in social work at the master's level. Impressed by Murphy's and Mitchell's pioneering work with its heavy emphasis on ethics and security, the director invited the two cybercounselors to deliver a cybercounseling certificate program that would be be a collaboration of the cyber-counselors' company, Worldwide Therapy Online Inc., and the Continuing Education department of the faculty. Continuing education would conduct the advertising, and Therapy Online would look after registration and delivery of content. The two organizations agreed on a cost-sharing format. An FTF workshop called "Cybercounselling: Doing Therapy Online" was delivered at the university each year to introduce the area broadly to learners and to increase registration within the larger certificate program. The director also connected the cybercounselors with groups within the community who were either delivering cybercounseling or who were interested in exploring the possibility. The first cybercounsel-ing certificate program commenced in the fall of 2004.

Continuing education departments cannot depend solely on faculty resources for innovative programing. Indeed, much inno-vation occurs within the field, and continuing education offers an opportunity to provide field-based innovations to our professional community. Some advantages are that collaboration with field collea-gues broadens the offerings, provides increased revenues, and brings additional practice experience and wisdom into the faculty. As an example, Therapy Online is assisting the faculty pro bono in designing a pilot training program to introduce cybercounseling skills to supervised graduate social work students who are volunteering for an online-posting-based distress center. Disadvantages of this type of partnership include the need for heightened quality assurance reviews of outside programs, concerns about collaboration with "for profit" organizations, and the validity of new approaches.

Given the newness of the field of online counseling, this training is available only to those who have a strong base of professional qualifications. The program requires membership in an accredited organization or association, with an associated professional code of ethics or code of practice. Through this affiliation there must be a mechanism in place for clients to lodge complaints. Educationally, a graduate degree in the human services field and three years experience in FTF counseling or an equivalent combination of education and experience is required for admission to the program. We set these minimums because we believe that much of online counseling is qualitatively different from FTF work. Online counseling is not simply a set of new techniques; it is a challenging and uniquely different way of working and as such requires that counselors already have experience with ethical decision making, the counseling process, and the range and severity of client experiences.

THE PROGRAM

The program presently consists of two levels of training. Level 1 provides qualified learners with the knowledge and skills necessary to do e-mail-based counseling. Level 2 was created at the behest of learners who had completed the first training level and who were interested in a deeper understanding of the therapeutic aspects of the online work and some ideas about the business and marketing aspects of operating an online practice. Some concepts and features of the training in the brief descriptions that follow will appear familiar to readers (e.g., ethics). Descriptions of the components unique to this training appear in subsequent sections.

Level 1

Level 1 is composed of three modules that focus on building the learning community of students within the program and introduces them to the cornerstones of cybercounseling: theory, skills, technology, and ethics. The first module in Level 1 is intended to serve as an introduction to the field of cybercounseling and to help learners decide whether to continue with the certificate program. All modules are four weeks in duration. Each week requires between five and seven hours of work on the part of the learner.

Module 1 provides a welcome, personal introductions, and a cybercounseling overview: theory, ethics, skills, and technology; Module 2 presents theoretical issues and beginning practice ideas; and Module 3 offers additional practice, text-enhancing techniques, and personal clinical consultation.

Level 2

Level 2, which also consists of three modules, emphasizes the practical application of cybercounseling skills and techniques for effective intervention. The prerequisite is completion of Level 1. All modules are four weeks in duration, and each week requires between five and seven hours of work on the part of the learner.

Module 1 emphasizes role plays between learners; Module 2 discusses online business, marketing, and related cybercounseling issues; and Module 3 offers advanced clinical consultation and guided self-reflection, including opportunities for learners to review and analyze, in a structured way, their experience, progress, and future in cybercounseling.

A Certified Cybercounselor Certificate is issued to each graduate at the successful completion of each level. The certificate signifies that the learner has successfully completed the tasks that are incorporated into each module within the level. In addition, completion of each level entitles graduates to a discount on the development of a 25-page cybercounseling website, including use of the PrivacEmail system.

Because Therapy Online also delivers online counseling and sells software and services, including the PrivacEmail system, some students go on to become affiliates with Therapy Online or to purchase the software for their own use. Others already have systems in place or are taking the training as employees of other agencies. Recognizing the potential for a conflict of interest here, or indeed even the appearance of such a conflict, we include a number of specific components in the training to address this. These include telling trainees that our objective is not to promote the PrivacEmail system although we do sell it through another arm of the company; PrivacEmail is used as illustrative because it has the components that we believe are critical to the delivery of ethical online counseling and because the students get firsthand experience using it; PrivacEmail is not the only system out there that delivers encryption and security; students are in no way required to use the system once they've completed their training; and no negative consequences would arise for a student who decided to go with another software approach and wanted to maintain a relationship with Therapy Online (e.g., take Level 2).

ETHICAL ISSUES OF INTEREST

There are many ethical issues unique to the online modality, and the program discusses these in detail, with specific attention paid to those issues raised in the literature (e.g., Mallen, Vogel, Rochlen, & Day, 2005; Mitchell & Murphy, 2004). Trainees are exposed to ethical issues and considerations throughout the training. The sessions that focus specifically on ethics include assigned readings, discussion and debate, and an online scavenger hunt in which trainees must search the web for online counseling sites and then return to the group with comment on, and critique of, those sites. The scavenger hunt is also used as a way to expose trainees to other options for e-mail encryption.

This section reviews a number of the more frequently asked-about ethical issues in cybercounseling.

Cross-jurisdictional concerns have been an issue in the United States for some time. Many American licensing bodies require counselors to practice only in states where they are licensed (Mallen, Vogel, & Rochlen, 2005). Generally these bodies have decided that cybercounseling occurs in the state where the client resides. From our perspective this belief is debatable. Counseling does not happen in a particular place since cyberspace is not a single place in the legal sense. It could easily be argued that the counseling happens where the counselor resides. Regardless, jurisdiction is a concern in the United States. It also may soon be an issue in Canada, where a number of provinces are in the process of licensing counselors and psychotherapists.

Reporting in cases of threat of harm to self or other or in cases of child abuse and neglect is also a concern. Learners are taught to collect adequate information to enable them to report wherever the client may reside. Such information includes name, location, and telephone number as examples. We take the position that we must adhere to the rules and regulations of our place of residence: Canada. To this end, all clients are required to consent to counseling by reading a consent form online and clicking a box acknowledging this. This has led to peculiar situations where we have contacted authorities in other countries with reports of what Canadian authorities would deem child abuse only to be told that the behavior is perfectly acceptable in the country where the child lives.

This issue of collecting information about clients also relates to knowing the identity of one's client. Our experience is that people are not willing to pay for online counseling in order to pretend that they are someone they are not. That said, clients are required to provide passwords at two levels to enter the system in order to protect their information. The passwords and encryption together provide protection that is equivalent to the protection that their banking information receives online. The passwords and encryption together provide enhanced protection.

More subtly there are situations in which a client might lie about some aspect of their past or personality. In addition, there is no lack of FTF clients who may hide, lie about, or distort some part of their past or personality. One of the more interesting aspects of the online modality is that clients disclose more quickly and more completely online than face to face. The phenomenon of "swift trust" that is developed in online relationships has been noted elsewhere (MacFadden, 2005).

Insurance is a consideration for any professional, and coverage for cybercounseling should be considered specifically. Not all insurers and not all policies cover cybercounseling. Indeed, professionals using e-mail to connect with clients in any way should be speaking to their insurer about their policy.

E-mail security and confidentiality must be assured. Even though the counselor may simply be asking the client via e-mail about changing an appointment, the request reveals the client's involvement in counseling. Should this message be inadvertently sent to the wrong address or the information stolen from the computer or in transit (Mitchell & Murphy, 2004), it seems reasonable to assume that an insurer would ask whether the counselor had malpractice coverage for working online.

Finally, there are a number of issues that we discourage learners from addressing online. These include: serious mental health problems that involve distortions of reality, crisis situations requiring quick responses, and suicidal situations that may require a physical presence. Our approach has been to encourage clients who are experiencing problems that may require a speedy crisis response to seek FTF counseling. For those clients who begin working online and then experience severe crisis there is material on the website that they can access for assistance. And in extreme cases, clients are encouraged to contact their counselor by phone.

CLINICAL ISSUES OF INTEREST

In many respects, cybercounseling is qualitatively different from FTF work and in our experience, being an outstanding FTF counselor is not enough to ensure competent online clinical work (Murphy & Mitchell, 1998). Building a therapeutic alliance is essential in any helping endeavor. Clients want to be connected and believe that we have their best interests at heart. What is necessary is to find ways to join with clients and to create the substance of a helping relationship.

This essential work is done using our *presence* techniques. Clients do not need another explanation of their behavior, the origins of their problems, and the solutions they ought to pursue. Instead, clients need a therapeutic experience. One of our concerns is that the way some professionals use e-mail does not create such an experience for the client. Although it may provide interesting advice and information, it does not create a "therapeutic space"; that is, a supportive, safe, and empathic relationship in which a client can explore issues, feelings, and alternatives related to their concerns (Corcoran, 1981). The presence techniques (Murphy & Mitchell, 1998) appropriately used, accomplish this.

For example, *emotional bracketing* is a technique that is used with clients to convey nonverbal elements of a therapist's written communication such as thoughts and feelings of the counselor. In counseling emotional bracketing is used primarily in joining with clients, in conveying warmth, and in tempering and highlighting other elements in the text. It can be used in training as well, as in the following example:

A warm hello to all of you as we approach the finish line of Module 1 [for me it feels like we've been in a marathon this past month!] w-h-e-w!!!

All month the work that each of you have done has been exemplary. A pleasure to review. And this session is perhaps the most challenging. I hope for more great work.

So [looking about the class suddenly serious]. Don't let me down now! [eyebrows raised with a playful smile]

Okay, okay. Let's get right to Session 4 [a more business-like tone pervades].

Descriptive immediacy is another technique frequently employed in cybercounseling. This involves the description of the counselor, scene, and setting and is used to intensify the experience of the client and the counselor being in the presence of each other. It is also used in strengthening the connection between client and counselor and to convey importance and depth. It is equally effective in training as the following example illustrates:

> I am sitting in my office in the early evening. The weather outside continues to be cold here in Southern Ontario. And, despite spring's alleged arrival, I still have that warm feeling one has inside when it's wintery outdoors. My office is a decent size, and if you were all here with me we would be sitting comfortably on the couches and various overstuffed chairs that abound. My office has the feel of an old library, with books and wood . . . and wood and books. It's a friendly place of learning and sharing and I welcome each of you, grateful for your presence and participation.

Another concern is the lack of control counselors have over the process the client engages in once the counselor has sent an e-mail. Clients may read through the material too quickly, failing to engage with the text in a meaningful way. FTF counselors can be taught ways to exert control over the pace of counseling. Similarly, learners are taught the use of spacing and pacing techniques in an online environment that allows the counselor to exercise a higher measure of control over the process.

Sentence construction and spacing, for example, can be modified to alter the reader's pace. A sentence such as, "Okay, so let's stop and review this material" can be changed as illustrated to slow down the process:

> Okay.
> So.
> Let's stop.
> And review this material.

The *presence* and the *spacing and pacing* techniques can be used by counselors working from virtually any theoretical perspective. This is also true of the other practical material that trainees are taught. And although the authors operate from a combined solution-focused and narrative perspective, our trainees come to us working with a range of counseling models and are encouraged to integrate the techniques into the approach with which they are already familiar.

THE DELIVERY SYSTEM: PRIVACEMAIL PROFESSIONAL

PrivacEmail Professional is the name of our integrated software system that incorporates secure e-mail, registration information, and access to the Online Learning Community for the course. This area provides course outlines, calendars, readings, and assignments. PrivacEmail Professional is also used for lectures and communication between instructors, students, and peers.

The Course Process

In order to participate in the courses, learners are provided a secure PrivacEmail e-mail address and password protected access to the Online Learning Community: the course website. To get started, learners are provided a link to an extensive course orientation web page that describes the technology used as well as the online learning process. Technical assistance is available by e-mail and telephone.

When the course begins, instructors use regular e-mail to prompt learners to login to the training site at https://learning.privacemail. com. Since learners' accounts are set up in advance, their passwords are provided by Therapy Online. They can, however, change their passwords at any time. Once logged in, learners click on an e-mail link and provide a second password to access their secure Privac-Email in-box and retrieve their first lecture, which has been sent to all course registrants. Accessing their in-box is, metaphorically, the means to "take their seat" in the virtual classroom. Learners must use the PrivacEmail system and cannot engage in the course through any other e-mail system.

Each week a new lecture is e-mailed to learners. After reading a given lecture, learners access the Online Learning Community website by clicking a link and entering their username and password. The site is loaded with readings and proprietary information for general study and to complete assignments. It contains the details of assignments for each session of the course as well as calendars with assignment deadlines. Learners then complete the assignments within the deadlines identified and engage and interact with their colleagues as required. All lectures and training conversations take place within the confines of the PrivacEmail secure e-mail system. A sense of "classroom" is created by use of a distribution list within the Privac-Email system. The instructor sets up the distribution list to include all registrants.

Every lecture is written in conversational style, and descriptive imagery, along with all of the other presence techniques, is modeled to learners, so learners have the experience of sitting in a real classroom. The standard features of e-mail, such as reading, printing, composing, and sending messages are the primary features used by learners. While the PrivacEmail system is capable of much more (e.g., sending encrypted file attachments), simplicity is important in the early stages of training (or cybercounseling for that matter). A single Level 1 course can include anywhere from 6 to 16 learners. The Level 2 cybercounseling courses tend to be smaller and more intimate with as few as 4 learners involved.

System Security

The PrivacEmail Professional system was designed to serve clients online. It was not originally designed for online education. Because of its original clinical application, the system uses several technically distinct approaches to data security. Nevertheless, from a learner or client perspective, the system functions as a seamless integrated unit.

When learners go to https://learning.privacemail.com, their browsers automatically engage the secure sockets layer (SSL) 128 bit encryption. In layperson's terms, this means that every bit of information traversing the Internet between the learner and the server is randomized. This layer of encryption is maintained throughout navigation of all parts of the cybercounseling courses. SSL encryption secures en route data from unauthorized interception.

Data storage security is required for passwords and registration data (such as names, telephone numbers, and so on) as well as the contents of e-mail messages. When engaged in the course, learners are actually accessing three firewall protected servers—two in Ontario (one that runs the software and another for data storage), and one in British Columbia (for encrypted e-mail). The data stored on the server in Ontario uses three different security methods, depending on the type of data. The data on the e-mail server in British Columbia is stored using 2048-bit encryption. So for example, when learners login to https://learning.privacemail.com, they are accessing the data stored on the server in Ontario; when they access their PrivacEmail in-box they are logging in to the secure e-mail server in British Columbia. In addition to SSL encryption, the PrivacEmail system offers users the option of enabling an unparalleled 2048-bit end-to-end encryption. In essence, e-mail messages are double encrypted—they are encrypted on learners' local computers before they are sent and they are also encrypted en route via the SSL protocol.

The PrivacEmail Professional system is a hacker's nightmare. In the unlikely case of a successful break-in, the information that is exposed will be limited and meaningless. To make sense of the information, the hacker would need to break through another locked door, so to speak, and then another, and another. The more sensitive the information, the more vaultlike the doors become.

In the unlikely case of a server failure clients can be contacted either by phone or regular e-mail as both pieces of information are provided by clients during registration. Any e-mails sent by regular e-mail simply refer to the system shutdown and note that they will receive another e-mail when the system is up and running again. So all e-mail between client and counselor is via the trainer/author's servers.

UNIQUE ELEMENTS OF THE TRAINING

The training has a number of unique elements that distinguish it from traditional university-based courses. First, weekly e-lectures, or content with instructions and comments are sent out to learners. It would be simpler, and less intensive for the facilitator, to have learners read material from the Online Learning Community website each week, complete the assignments, and do a quiz at week's end. However, the weekly e-lectures encourage ongoing contact between learners and facilitator, model the skills and techniques necessary for professional e-counseling, deepen their relationship, and add to the sense of community.

Second, facilitators use the cybercounseling techniques developed by the authors (Murphy & Mitchell, 1996 in their delivery of e-lectures and additional course materials. Presence and pacing techniques, collectively known as SITCOMs (skills in text-based **communication**) are used as part of the teaching process. This models the use of the techniques for learners and helps to ease them into their use. Equally important, the techniques do in the teaching environment what they do in the counseling setting: establish a connection, deepen the bond between facilitator and learner, allow the facilitator control over the flow of the process, and draw participants into the presence of one another creating a genuine learning experience.

Third, the courses are small. Online courses through Canadian universities regularly have 100 or more students. The cybercounseling courses are kept small so that e-mail may be used for communication within the course rather than a bulletin board or some other solution. The purpose here is to ensure that the process, as much as possible, mirrors what counselors will experience with clients. A class too large would overwhelm even the most diligent student with e-mails. Keeping class sizes small also allows more personal interaction between the facilitator and each learner.

LEARNER DEMOGRAPHICS

This training program is conducted entirely online, and learners come from around the world. Of the 66 learners who have taken these courses to date, 53 (80 percent) have been Canadian, 4 (6 percent) were American, 4 (6 percent) from the United Kingdom, 2 (3 percent) were Australian, 2 (3 percent) were from Singapore, and 1 (1.5 percent) was Malaysian.

Of the various organizations to which learners have been members, 7 belonged to the Canadian Counseling Association, 3 were members of the Ontario Association of Counselors Clinicians Psychotherapists and Psychometrists, and 22 have been members of social work associations. The rest were members of individual associations or organizations in their respective countries.

We also require a graduate degree in a field related to counseling and 3 years of FTF experience or an equivalent combination of education and practice. All learners must also have significant experience with computers, the Internet, and e-mail. Any professional who is planning on doing online work must be able to resolve problems that their clients have with hardware and software as easily as they are able to assist their FTF clients with the use of the parking garage or bathroom door key. The course website registration page outlines these requirements. In the case of association membership we require a member number to confirm membership. In the case of all other requirements, the learners are trusted to be honest about their experience and qualifications.

Only 9 (14 percent) of the 66 learners hold bachelor's degrees. Each of these has significant FTF experience or other training that allowed them to participate in the course. Of the rest, 6 (9 percent) hold PhDs in fields ranging from counseling to social work to marital and family therapy. The remaining 51 (77 percent) are trained to a master's level. This group of 51 includes 26 (51 percent) MSWs, 3 (6 percent) clinical psychologists, and 14 (28 percent) master's in counseling psychology. The remaining 8 (16 percent) learners were from a host of other individual disciplines (e.g., divinity).

Also of interest to us is the work experience and present employment situation of each learner. The average number of years FTF experience is 12, with a range of 3 to 25 years. The average number of years of experience interacting with clients via e-mail (for whatever reason) is 3 with a range of 0 to 12 years. Twenty learners had no experience interacting with clients via e-mail.

Interestingly, almost exactly half of our learners work as employees in a counseling center or clinic. The other half are in private practice. After completing the training those learners who meet Therapy Online's standards are invited to join Therapy Online as affiliates. The company delivers counseling and also subcontracts with other agencies. Other learners return to their agencies to practice while some add the service to their existing private practices. In these latter situations learners and their agencies may purchase the PrivacEmail system for their cybercounseling work. This is another advantage of using the system for the training: learners who move on to do their own cybercounseling are already intimately familiar with the system when they begin cybercounseling.

The picture that emerges is one of a group of well-educated and highly trained professionals. These are experienced, capable individuals who know their profession, the ethics of counseling, and the skills and techniques that contribute to client change. Despite this, the online text-based modality is a challenging one for even these individuals. As evidenced by the evaluative data in the following section, doing online therapy is a qualitatively different experience for both counselor and client. A solid educational background and significant FTF experience is a prerequisite for cybercounseling training, not a replacement.

EVALUATION SURVEY RESULTS

Following completion of the cybercounseling training, learners are asked to complete an evaluation form. This form was revised in 2005 and as a result this section will review only the results of this revised evaluation. In addition, trainings were ongoing at the time of publication, and so some data was not yet available for inclusion. Finally, all learners are asked for permission to use their results for purposes such as this article. Some declined, and so their responses are not included. Thus, content of 25 of the 66 individual feedback forms makes up the data here reviewed.

The form itself is a qualitative survey consisting of 22 questions. The survey is split into four sections: (1) questions about the instructors, (2) questions about the PrivacEmail technology, (3) questions about the content and process of the course, and (4) a narrative section that asks about goals and allows learners to write anything additional they choose to about their experience.

Instructor Questions

The course is conducted on the premise that the process should reflect the content. That is, the instructors use techniques and approaches drawn from the actual online counseling methods to join with learners, create an atmosphere of trust, and engage both intellectually and emotionally within the virtual classroom. When asked about teaching styles, learners comment that our instructors "walk the walk," "set the tone," and "display the techniques as well as teaching them."

Another consequence of this approach is that learners experience the instructors as real people. Learners in turn become more real themselves. That is, their own personalities and unique approaches show through in the text. Rather than their work being a repetition of the facilitator's work, it becomes their own. They use words such as *warm, compassionate, supportive*, and *humane*. They also tell us that it is "easy to take risks" because of our approach. By this learners mean that they feel safe in trying out the techniques and using novel approaches confident that they will be supported and encouraged rather than criticized in their efforts by the instructors.

When the authors initially proposed the idea of doing online therapy they were met with significant resistance from virtually all members of the counseling community to whom they reported their new ideas and approaches. Many of the comments pointed to the coldness of the modality, the absence of tone and nonverbal communication in the text-based medium and the lack of anything "personal" in the experience. Such comments and the concerns underlying them informed our training approach and led to a training experience that is both intellectually stimulating and highly experiential.

Technology Questions

There are two components to the online training experience. First is the PrivacEmail system that is in essence a secure encrypted e-mail system. The second is the Online Learning Community, a website that learners gain access to when they begin their training. The site contains all of the information about each session, including links to relevant articles, technical FAQs, and a calendar with due dates for assignments.

As discussed earlier, Therapy Online uses its PrivacEmail system for both counseling and training. However, the system is designed to be used for counseling. As such, there is a trade off between providing learners with experience using the system prior to working with it as counselors and using a system with them that does not have the robust teaching features that another system tailored for online learning would have. The decision was made to weigh the former consideration more heavily.

Learners were asked directly if they felt that the system would be a good one to use for counseling clients. All concurred although one felt that a minimum level of computer expertise was necessary to navigate the system, and we agree. The majority (66 percent) also felt that it was a great system for use in the training, although the authors suspect that part of this is due to the low student-facilitator ratio. The volume of e-mails would be overwhelming with 20 learners or more.

The Online Learning Community website was seen as a very valuable adjunct to the weekly lectures and the ongoing input from the facilitator and other learners. Specific elements that learners identified as being helpful were the layout broken down session by session, including links to articles that were required reading, and having a calendar with specific assignment deadlines.

Not all comments have been wholly positive. We regularly revise and rewrite the content when learners identify complicated or confusing elements of the site. In addition, a number of learners in each course always suggest that we have an hours estimate for each session, which is difficult given learners progress at different rates.

Course Content and Process Questions

Learners are asked a variety of questions about the content and process of the course. Two questions ask about the time commitment and the workload. Fifty-seven percent felt that the course load was just right, 14 percent felt it was too heavy, 7 percent found it too light, and 21 percent felt that it varied from week to week.

We estimate for students that they will average 5 to 7 hours of work a week. Seventy-one percent felt this was accurate. However, 19 percent spent anywhere from 10 to 15 hours a week working on the course. The remaining 10 percent said that they were able to get away with 3 or 4 hours a week.

Learners are asked what they hoped to learn but did not. Two-thirds replied that their "expectations had been met." Of those that identified material they wished had been covered, one in Level 1 identified "setting up a cybercounseling practice" as an unmet need. This is dealt with more in Level 2. Another wanted to have more personal clinical feedback and earlier in the process.

This issue of personal feedback also arose in responses to our questions about improving the course. There are at least one or two learners every course who identify a need for earlier direct one-to-one feedback from the facilitators. We have responded to this in the spring 2007 courses by integrating an individualized segment into the second session of the training. Following the second session, the facilitator provides feedback via e-mail to each learner on their initial use of the text-based techniques. On the positive side, this responds to an issue identified by a handful of learners over the years. It remains to be seen if personal clinical feedback at a time when learners are only just getting their feet wet will produce the benefits intended.

Another challenge handed down from past learners concerns partner work. Partnered up into cybercounselor and cyberclient dyads for role-playing, learners have wonderful opportunities to practice the online counseling techniques, receive feedback, and engage in a dialogue that allows them to teach and learn from one another. It also reduces the burden on the facilitator. He or she can observe and comment as appropriate, which is far less demanding than providing each learner with continuous personal feedback.

Understandably, learners identify the dyad work as some of the most valuable they experience during the course; that is, if they have a partner who sticks to the schedule, sends their messages, replies when they are supposed to, and generally holds up their end of the bargain. As positive as learners generally are about the dyad work, the handful of learners who add comments to our question about improving the process always mention the frustration of late and irresponsible partners.

One final element worth noting is the reading assignments. Learners were asked for their opinions, and all thought that they were an outstanding addition. About 25 percent of learners ask for additional readings. Our solution has been to include readings as optional assignments so as to keep to the five to seven hour weekly commitment. The one additional recommendation that has been made is for case studies. Some have been added to the Learning Community, although permission for real cases is often difficult to secure given what cybercounseling clients feel is the "public" nature of a website.

Narrative Section

Contributions in this section from learners range from a few brief words to many pages. This material is of course rich and varied. For the purposes of this paper, only themes that were evident in a majority of responses will be reported.

A good portion of the course focuses on the text-based skills and techniques necessary to turn a simple e-mail into a therapeutic experience for the client. The first theme that found majority support was the feeling that cybercounseling could indeed work when done well. One learner said "not only was I amazed at what I was able to bring forth in terms of enhanced counseling but I was blown away by what the rest of the class was able to accomplish (WOW)." Another wrote that "one of the most important things I have learned is how to adapt my words to the client in text which can be read and re-read easier by the client than the client having to 'remember' what was said in session." A third wrote: "when I look back at my counseling career I wonder if the more V-o-l-a-t-i-l-e clients would have done better with the Cooling influence of e-mail exchanges."

A second theme that emerged was the importance of reviewing the ethical and legal issues associated with online work. Too many professionals imagine that a small expansion of their ethics will accommodate what for them is a small change of including cyber-counseling in their repertoire. One learner shared that "like many others, I have been enlivened to ethical and legal issues. And here in particular I might want supervision." Another wrote, "there are still many questions that require further clarification such as confi-dentiality, legal aspects, acceptance by the mainstream counseling community, immediacy of response, enhancement of the human aspect and others."

What brought all of these comments together was not simply their breadth; it was the depth of thinking and reflection that this new approach evoked for them. The fact that cybercounseling can work, can be therapeutic, and can engage others in a process of change is evident from the training. Consequently, the learners themselves were left not to wonder "if," but rather, "what now?"

LESSONS LEARNED

Since these cybercounseling courses began changes have been made to the process and the content of the courses based on learner feedback.

Process Developments

A number of the sessions are quite complex with a variety of parts to the week's process. In these cases an assignment summary, simply a numbered list of required tasks for the week, was always included at the end of the e-lecture. This turned out to be a component that was much appreciated by learners and so in present versions of the course an assignment summary is included at the end of every e-lecture.

As noted in the evaluation section, learners consistently rate the dyad work one of the best parts of the course. This, however, can be a negative experience for some learners when their partners are late with their assignment. We have attempted to deal with this by asking learners to be honest about their assignment completion style (e.g., always-ahead-of-the-game or classic procrastinator) and then matching learners. This has proved successful.

Also noted in the evaluation section is the meaningfulness, for learners, of personal clinical feedback. For the first time this semester we are providing feedback early in the course on learners' use of the presence techniques before they have developed any expertise in the techniques or approaches. It remains to be seen the degree to which this is perceived as a positive addition.

Content Developments

Internal reviews of counseling work done by the authors and affiliate counselors working with Therapy Online regularly leads to additions in content. Examples of this are new pacing and presence techniques. Changes in law, regulation, and the like also lead to revisions in content. For example, if and when the term *psychotherapist* is regulated in Ontario the ethics component of the training will be revised to reflect this change.

We also respond to learner feedback in reviewing content changes. Graduates from Level 2 have recently suggested that more be included in Level 2 about business and integrating cybercounseling into private practice. We are reviewing this idea and may integrate a more in-depth business focus into the module that covers marketing.

Finally, there has been much discussion of adding a Level 3 course. Graduates report that they would like clinical consultations once they have begun doing cybercounseling for real. Practical considerations for integrating a third level into the training are ongoing and we anticipate that select graduates will be offered clinical consultations beginning in the fall of 2008.

OTHER TRAINING PROGRAMS

It is difficult to know the number of other cybercounseling training resources available on the Internet. As a point of comparison, two UK-based training programs (www.onlinecounsellors.co.uk and www.onlinetrainingforcounsellors.co.uk "Onlinetraining") offer similar training. Both programs are offered completely online. All information was obtained from the respective websites on August 1, 2007.

www.onlinecounsellors.co.uk stipulates eligibility requirements which include a recognized counseling or cybercounseling qualification, adherence to a code of ethics, membership in a professional body, and supervised, postqualification experience. This one-level, six-module program has no start date and learners can enroll anytime. The cost is approximately $1,215 USD and learners who complete the program receive a certificate from onlinecounsellors.co.uk that acknowledges this professional development and a verification logo for their websites. The training uses a discussion board and forum extensively with threads in areas such as technical, network, and course issues. There appears to be less emphasis on role-playing than other programs and on opportunity to explore both e-mail and IRC chat approaches to cybercounseling. The website identifies one person as the provider and emphasizes the use of the BACP (British Association of Counselling and Psychotherapy) Code of Ethics.

www.onlinetrainingforcounsellors.co.uk offers another UK-based training program for online counseling involving several professionals called the Counselling Online Ltd Directorate. Although no specific experience requirement is cited, applicants need to have a recognized counseling or psychotherapy qualification at the diploma level or equivalent. The program offers two levels—basic and advanced. The cost is approximately $848 USD for the basic and $970 USD for the advanced. A General Certificate in Online Counselling Skills is awarded to those who successfully complete required work submitted to a tutor as part of a learning portfolio. Much of the training in this eight-week general level program is group-based with a heavy emphasis on role-playing. Both synchronous and asynchronous approaches to training are employed, and each learner is assigned a tutor. In the advanced program there is an emphasis on the development of a personal practice model for online counseling and an opportunity to experience online supervision.

FUTURE DIRECTIONS

One direction we are taking is in conducting outcome evaluations of our work with e-clients to better inform both our practice and our training. In addition to providing training, Worldwide Therapy Online Inc. also provides subcontracted e-counseling, in collaboration with its trained affiliate counsellors, to agencies looking to provide such services to their clients. Initial evaluations of these clients' experiences, using simple online questionnaires modeled on agency paper and pencil questionnaires has been very positive.

Much of the research literature has also been finding a variety of positive outcomes related to cybercounseling, but this research is still very preliminary (Mallen, Vogel, Rochlen, & Day, 2005). For instance, there is minimal knowledge about the differences among the various cybercounseling technologies (e.g., e-mail, videoconferencing, chat) regarding quality of care.

While text-based asynchronous cybercounseling is the focus of our training program, the potential does exist to move into other forms of cybercounseling. However, the availability and simplicity of e-mail, along with the distinct advantages and challenges of text-based work, will form the main focus of our work for many years to come.

Questions arise about the possibility of doing video-conferencing style cybercounseling. We might assume that because client and counselor can see each other there should be virtually no difference between the work one would do in this format and the work one does face to face. However, it may be premature to draw such conclusions. It is likely that subtle but important distinctions exist and that training may be beneficial.

The cybercounseling courses discussed previously form the basis of what is required to do ethical, clinically impactful text-based online counseling. Professionals without training are not delivering the best that they can. It has been our experience in training and in doing cybercounseling since 1995 that specific techniques are required to create a therapeutic space, join with clients, and create change in a text modality that lacks nonverbal communication and tone of voice. In summary, the training discussed here is designed to prepare qualified professionals to do counseling that performs in the same way that all good counseling does: it engenders change.

*The terms PrivacEmail, PrivacEmail Professional, Descriptive Immediacy, Emotional Bracketing, Presence Techniques, SITCOMS, are Trademark terms belonging to Worldwide Therapy Online Inc.

REFERENCES

Chester, A., & Glass, C. (2006, May). Online counseling: A descriptive analysis of therapy services on the Internet. *British Journal of Guidance and Counselling, 34*(2), 145–160.

Collie, K., Mitchell, D., & Murphy, L. (2000). Skills for online counseling: Maximum impact at minimum bandwidth. In J. Bloom, & G. Walz (Eds.), *Cybercounseling and cyberlearning* (219–236). Alexandria, VA: American Counseling Association.

Corcoran, K.J. (1981). Experiential empathy: A theory of a felt-level experience. Journal of *Humanistic Psychology, 21*(1), 29–38.

MacFadden, R. (2005). Souls on ice: Incorporating emotion in web-Based education. In R. MacFadden, B. Moore, M. Herie, & D. Schoech (Eds.), *Web-based education in the human services* (79–98). Binghamton, NY: The Haworth Press.

Mallen, M., Vogel, D., & Rochlen, A. (2005, November). The practical aspects of online counseling: Ethics, training, technology, and Competency. *The Counseling Psychologist, 33*(6), 776–818.

Mallen, M., Vogel, D., Rochlen, A., & Day, S. (2005, November). Online counseling: Reviewing the literature from a counseling psychology framework. *The Counseling Psychologist, 33*(6), 819–871.

Mitchell, D. L., & Murphy, L. J. (2004). Email rules! Organizations and individuals creating ethical excellence in telemental-health. In J. Bloom & G. Walz (Eds.), Cybercounseling and cyberlearning: An ENCORE (203–217). Alexandria, VA: CAPS Press and American Counseling Association.

Moore, B. (2005). Faculty perceptions of the effectiveness of web-based instruction in social work education. In R. MacFadden, B. Moore, M. Herie, & D. Schoech. Web-based education in the human services (53–66). Binghamton, NY: The Haworth Press.

Murphy, L., & Mitchell, D. (1998). When writing helps to heal: Email as therapy. *British Journal of Guidance and Counselling, 26*, 21–31.

Namsook, J., Krug, D., & Zhang, Z. (2007). Student achievement in online distance education compared to face-to-face education. *European Journal of Open, Distance and E-Learning*. Retrieved July 8, 2007, from http://www.eurodl.org/materials/contrib/2007/Jahng_Krug_Zhang.htm.

VandenBos, G., & Williams, S. (2000). The Internet versus the telephone: What is telehealth anyway? *Professional Psychology: Research and Practice, 31*, 490–492.

Etherapy: A Training Program for Development of Clinical Skills in Distance Psychotherapy

Georgina Cárdenas
Berenice Serrano
Lorena Alejandra Flores
Anabel De la Rosa

The evolution of information and communication technologies (ICT) and particularly the growth of the Internet have changed the way in which we communicate and relate to one another. In recent years, there has been considerable emphasis on the use of ICT in various fields such as education and health. In the mental health field, there are several concepts that refer to therapy services provided through the Internet. In the area of psychology, online psychotherapy is a concept that emerged from the term *behavioral telehealth* proposed by Nickelson in 1998, which implies the application of telecommunications and technological information to provide behavioral health services. Thus, online psychotherapy is defined as the application of psychological health procedures and principles of human development through cognitive, affective, and behavioral techniques with systematic intervention strategies focused on a person's welfare, personal growth, and personal development (National Board Certified Counselors, 2007). Another often used concept is Internet therapy (IT), which describes a number of ways to deliver treatment over the Internet. By definition, IT is "any type of professional therapeutic interaction that makes use of the Internet to connect qualified mental health professionals and their clients" (Rochlen, Zack, & Speyer, 2004, p. 270). Other terms for IT, which are mostly interchangeable with one another, include cybercounseling, online therapy, Internet-based treatment, etherapy and interapy (Lange et al., 2000).

The use of online therapy is increasing, and IT is considered a powerful tool when it is used in addition to, or is adequately integrated with, the presence of a therapist. In addition, it can replace face-to-face therapy in the following cases: (1) when there is no access to psychological services, (2) when people prefer to keep their anonymity in the beginning of the therapeutic process, and (3) when people have problems identifying the therapeutic benefits that they can obtain and therefore have the first contact with professionals through the Internet (Bermejo, 1999).

Research into computer-aided psychotherapy has generated diverse ways of assisting with a variety of psychological disorders, such as anxiety, depression, phobia, substance misuse, and eating problems. Effective computer-based systems are coming online for a growing range of mental health difficulties (Marks, Cavanagh, & Gega, 2007). In 2006, England's National Institute for Health and Clinical Excellence (NICE, 2006) recommended two computer-aided systems for mild and moderate depression and phobia/panic as a routine care option. This may be the first recommendation of such systems by a government regulatory institution worldwide.

Schneider (1999) evaluated the effectiveness of three modes of psychological treatment (face-to-face, two-way audio, and two-way video). The study was carried out with 80 clients divided into 3 treatment groups and a control group on a waiting list. Each treatment group had five sessions of a brief cognitive-behavioral treatment. There were no significant differences between the three treatment groups. The results suggest that therapy with technological support can be as effective as a face-to-face therapy.

From an educational perspective, mental health professionals who provide Internet therapy base their treatment on professional competencies acquired during their professional formation (Oravec, 2000). This suggests that in order to provide psychotherapy through the Internet, it is necessary to learn how to transfer professional knowledge and skills previously acquired in a face-to-face way into practices carried out through an ICT. Colon (1996) and Murphy and Mitchell (1998) suggest that online psychotherapists have to develop more specific competencies—for instance, therapeutic reading and writing, or bibliotherapy techniques.

In Mexico, professional training in psychology is carried out at the undergraduate level of studying. This level is responsible for endowing students with the basic knowledge and professional competency that will allow them to apply the discipline in an appropriate and effective way. One of the main aspects in the students' training is the development of professional competencies that will allow them to generate and propose solutions to problems in their future work. The current psychocological studies, however, are focused on more theoretical knowledge than professional practice. In order to provide more opportunities for direct practice and to teach newly developing online practice skills, the psychology program developed the Virtual Teaching and Cyberpsychology Laboratory, which is a teaching program to train clinical psychology students in providing psychotherapy via the Internet to treat anxiety and depressive disorders. The purpose of this paper is to present a description and the preliminary evaluation of this teaching program. The program allows students to (1) have access to innovative courses that teach techniques and procedures for diagnosis, intervention, and psychological assessment via the Internet; (2) practice their clinical skills via the Internet; and (3) provide psychological services to the university community.

METHOD

The teaching program was set up for the clinical psychology students' final three semesters. It was designed to contribute toward forming clinical skills and training in the use of Internet-based clinical practice in mental health. A pilot study of the first generation of participating students was conducted in order to obtain general indicators to improve the teaching program.

Participants

In the first semester of training we had 17 students participating (15 female, 2 male) with an average age of 22 years. For the next 2 semesters we had just 6 students (4 female, 2 male) choosing to continue the professional training. Their average age was 22.5 years. In order to be selected, participants must have had an educational background in the field of clinical psychology, indicated by their attendance of the following courses: Introduction to Psychotherapy, Psychometric Diagnosis, Integration of Psychological Tests, Behavioral Rehabilitation, Psychodynamics of Groups, and Clinical Interviews. In addition, the students had to be familiar with the use of information technologies.

Setting

The training was carried out in a multimedia classroom equipped with 27 personal computers, Internet access, microphones, headsets, and video conference cameras. The room had an X-Class monitoring system through which real-time supervision could be accomplished (Sun-Teach International Group Ltd., 2004).

TEACHING PROGRAM

The teaching program lasted three semesters. The first part was an introduction to etherapy, in which the particular characteristics of this mode of therapy were examined. Students were encouraged during this time to reflect on the ways that using the Internet or other information technologies and software could be used to provide mental health services. After this introduction, various intervention programs were examined, taking into account the characteristics, symptoms, evaluations, and diagnosis of specific cases. Once the students knew what their program of treatment consisted of, they were trained in the specific cognitive-behavioral techniques for treating disorders. This allowed them to formulate a specific method of treatment and put the relevant clinical processes into practice when offering psychological services online. Students were required to strictly adhere to scientific and ethical codes; for example, the APA Ethical Principles of Psychologists and Code of Conduct and the APA statement on services by phone, teleconferencing, and Internet (American Psychological Association Ethics Committee, 1998), as well as the professional attitude of a psychologist.

During the first semester, the students attended a 16-week intensive training (12 hours per week), divided in five units:

Unit 1. Etherapy: Participants have their first contact with this new therapy mode through an introductory course, supported by a training manual developed for this aim (Cárdenas, Moreyra, et al., 2005), which was based on professional competencies, antecedents of the new therapy modality, applications, types of communication, and tools used in online psychotherapy. The structure of therapeutic intervention via Internet, ethical principles, and recommendations for this modality were also included during the course.

Unit 2. Programs of intervention: Participants learn the characteristics and symptoms of anxiety and depression disorders and how to provide treatment through the Internet, adapting techniques they already know with the aid of new technologies.

Unit 3. Cognitive-behavioral techniques for the Internet: Participants are trained in the application of cognitive-behavioral treatments and treatment protocols supported by multimedia elements and the Internet.

Unit 4. Treatment formulation (based on a problem solving model): Participants elaborate the design of their treatment and they test it in a simulated practice before initiating practice with patients. This treatment formulation is based on the model of problem solving proposed by Nezu, Nezu, Peacock, and Girdwood (2003), as well as a case study.

Unit 5. Training in the use of support software for etherapy: Participants are trained in the use of software developed for the support of the therapist during the sessions with the patient. Psychological services are provided in two ways. The first is *synchronous* or simultaneous manner. This allows the therapist to interact in real time via text, audio, and video with the patient, using commercial text-based instant messenger programs (e.g., Skype or Microsoft Messenger). The second is *asynchronous* or delayed manner. This refers to messages and tasks that are sent by the therapist via e-mail and are read at a different time by the receiver. The etherapy software was designed to work simultaneously with commercial "chatting" software (Messenger, Skype, etc.), which further facilitates communication between the service provider and the user.

Unit 6. Supervised practice: During second and third semesters, some clinical sessions are carried out to supervise participants and give them feedback by the supervisor and the group. To reinforce supervision, individual sessions are carried out. A clinical session is carried out weekly with the student-therapist, so they may ask questions as well as review excerpts of texts produced during the interactions between therapist and patient. The therapy room has a monitoring system that allows supervising the therapist's work with his or her patient in real-time from a different computer. This is more comfortable for the supervisor and less stressful for the therapist.

Before students are allowed to provide any kind of psychological service, they carry out three practice sessions with simulated clients in which their knowledge, skills, setting-up of goals, and carrying out of the session are evaluated by the supervisor during the interview; afterward, they are given feedback by the supervisor. Students are constantly evaluated throughout their training by means of formative evaluations of their progress and performance as therapists. Instructors also give continual feedback as a way to improve students' clinical skills.

Student-therapist clinical activities begin when the student makes telephone contact with the patient, explaining the mode of therapy and providing the patient with a website address where he or she can find information about etherapy. In order to be helpful in evaluating nonverbal cues and to solve his or her doubts with regard to the mode of therapy, a face-to-face appointment is arranged with the patient. The reason for requesting services is dealt with in this appointment.

Session texts for three months were saved with the patient's consent in order to aid in the therapist's training. Patients were also informed about the safety measures taken to protect their data. Note that patients voluntarily requested psychological support from the Psychological Care Center of the Faculty of Psychology. Under the inclusion/exclusion criteria they were assigned to the etherapy program. The criteria used were: patients between 18 to 45 years old with specific anxiety and depression problems considered mild to moderate and basic notions of the use of computers and the Internet.

Materials Used in the Program

- *Etherapy Procedures Manual* (Cárdenas Serrano, Patoni, & Plata, 2005) includes outlines, procedures, service schedules, records, and use of software when providing psychological therapy via the Internet.
- Support software for etherapy (González & Tellez, 2005). This software was created in order to supervise the practice effectively as well as to administer the psychological services provided online. It is divided into the following modules: administration, initial assessment, personnel module, patient module, and intervention module. The modules process data from various psychological instruments. For supervision, the clinical administrator can enter notes to specific records, indicating instructions to the therapist working with the specific patients. The software allows participants to create an electronic record in which they can attach a general clinical history, the reason for requesting consultation, and an identification card. In addition, there is a module in which all psychological tests, along with the patient's answers, are stored. The software also has a scheduler that allows therapists to make their appointments in order to properly monitor their patients.

Assessment Instruments

- Questionnaires evaluate knowledge of concepts, definitions, diagnosis, and intervention techniques for anxiety and depression disorders. They are based on the general intermediate assessments found in the multimedia teaching tutorials regarding different anxiety disorders (Cárdenas, Moreyra, et al., 2005). They evaluate knowledge of definitions, diagnosis, and treatment techniques with a cognitive-behavioral approach through multiple choice items.

- Cognitive therapy scale (Young & Beck, 1980). The scale has two main sections: (1) evaluating general therapeutic skills and (2) evaluating conceptualization, strategies, and techniques. The first section is mainly concerned with the use of time, efficient scheduling, and the relationship between therapist and patient. The second focuses on identifying behaviors and cognitions as well as on applying cognitive behavioral techniques. The scale used was six points per item, where a zero represents poor ability and a six represents an excellent ability.

- Use of services and managing software questionnaire. This assessment instrument measures student's knowledge of the use of service software as well as the ability to use such software.

RESULTS

The results obtained in this research project are described in three sections. In the first section we show the percentages of the 17 students who started the training process as Internet therapists. In the second we describe the percentages only of therapist students officially qualified to provide mental health services under this modality. Finally, we show the qualitative results of the therapist students. Results obtained from the pilot study are based on students' conceptual knowledge, case formulation, and clinical skills evaluation, as well as the social validation responses.

Figure 1 shows the evaluation of conceptual and declarative knowledge before and after students completed the four months of intensive training. The evaluation includes knowledge of psychological disorders to be treated, cognitive-behavioral techniques, etherapy concepts and definitions, case formulation, and use of specialized software. The lowest score is 0 and the highest is 10. The minimum passing score is six. Overall, the 17 students improved their knowledge scores from 52 percent at pretest to 88 percent at posttest.

The evaluation of student's clinical skills using the cognitive therapy scale (Young & Beck, 1980) was carried out using the six students who were enrolled in the program. The cognitive therapy scale was

FIGURE 1. Pre- and Postevaluations of Students About Anxiety Disorders and Depression (N = 12)

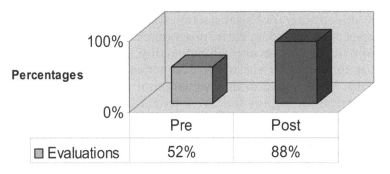

Pre and Post Evaluations of students about Anxiety Disorders and Depression N=17

given three times, at the beginning of the first semester and at the end of the second and third semesters. Figure 2 shows results indicating that students felt more confident at posttest when working with a patient. The six students' results from pre, post, and follow-up evaluations show increased therapeutic skills. Student therapists are considered competent if they score over 60.6 percent (blue line). The data shows an increase in clinical skills from the 15.8 percent in the initial evaluation to 84.7 percent and 83.8 percent at the end of the second and third semesters of supervised practice, respectively.

FIGURE 2. Therapeutic Skills Students Evaluation (N = 6)

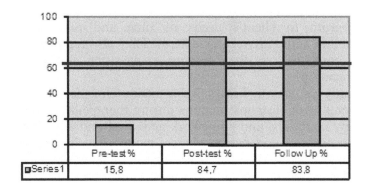

Students believed that they had enough knowledge to know what to do throughout treatment and that they could be advised should any doubt arise. They reported, through standardized questions in the previously mentioned scale, being able to carry out a more thorough functional analysis for treatment formulation and to better design psychological interventions as well as evaluate their effectiveness.

The student-therapist's satisfaction was evaluated from a qualitative perspective regarding costs, program characteristics, communication with the patient, scenario, functionality, system requirements, and whether or not he or she would recommend the modality to other clinicians. With regard to the evaluation of the therapeutic modality as a practical setting for the development of clinical skills, the students responded that objectives, instructions, and requirements to provide psychological services online were clear and comfortable. In addition, they reported that the therapy modality was well adapted to the counseling necessities of their patients and that time devoted to therapy was adequate. Finally, students indicated that it was easy to keep contact with the patient during sessions because the patients were highly motivated to receive psychological advice. Students pointed out that etherapy was easy to apply, generated interest from patients, and increased their own clinical competencies.

In connection with the evaluation of the training program, students reported that the use of technologies to provide psychotherapy via the Internet motivated them and made them feel confident. They reported that their patients told them that instant messaging programs make communication easier during the therapeutic process than asynchronous communication since synchronous communication allowed them to have sufficient interaction with their therapist. In addition, students reported that instant messaging makes collaboration with the patient easier and permits students to adapt the therapy program to client's needs of time and physical distance (webcam and audio are recommended). They also reported that their patients could express their feelings easily using text-based online communication.

Etherapy software makes a suitable medium for the patient, providing patients with clear instructions during therapeutic sessions, bibliotherapy materials, and homework activities, and allowing student therapists to send and receive clinical material such as records and psychological tests. All student-therapists concluded they would recommend this therapy modality as a means of training in clinical skills.

DISCUSSION

A teaching program training clinical psychology students to provide psychological services online seems to be promising for carrying out a teaching-learning process in order to teach clinical skills in an innovative manner. Initial data from the pilot study shows that clinical psychology students improved by 36 percent (52 percent to 88 percent) on declarative knowledge after the intensive first-semester training program. During this period, students learned the characteristics and symptoms of anxiety and depression and eventually how to evaluate the disorders and formulate diagnosis and treatment. In addition, they learned how to use the software to provide psychological services online. This confirms the Colon (1996) and Murphy and Mitchell (1998) findings that suggest that online psychotherapists need to develop more specific competencies in order to provide psychological services online.

The evaluation of students' clinical skills using the cognitive therapy scale (Young & Beck, 1980) was carried out using the six advanced students who were enrolled in the program. Results obtained in this group show an improvement of therapeutic skills, an increment from the initial assessment from 15.8 percent to 84.7 percent at the end of the second semester and to 83.8 percent at the end of the third semester. Thus, the majority of learning took place during the second semester and was maintained in the third semester. This data is satisfactory, considering that after the second evaluation the students had scored more than the 60.6 percent necessary to be considered competent according to the scales used in the assessment instrument. These results seem to confirm the Oravec (2000) study suggesting that mental health professionals who provide services online base their treatment on competencies acquired during their training in this treatment modality.

As far as the students themselves are concerned, it has been a novel experience. For instance, the program allows the student-therapists, who are still in the process of professional formation, to have a first online contact with the patient without it being a highly stressing event. Results generated by the qualitative student evaluation stress the utility and satisfaction obtained from the teaching-learning process. The positive evaluations include the satisfaction of using the application of an innovative treatment modality and support for the possibility of providing psychological treatment to a greater number of people (or locations) through low-cost modalities.

From an educational perspective, the program represents an alternative setting for professional formation; that is, a classroom provided with computers and Internet that allows continuous supervision. Due to the lack of enough settings to teach professional skills, there is a great need for a teaching environment different than institutions such as hospitals and research centers. We provided a classroom-based environment that offers a new modality of psychological services and an educational scenario to link theory with practice.

Students reported that their patients accepted the new online modality as an alternative mode of psychological support. In addition, patients were satisfied with the convenience of using the modality from any location (their house, work, or school) without the need of transportation. Furthermore, the patients indicated that they noticed better communication with their therapist by combining sessions through "chatting" programs with sessions through e-mail. With respect to the therapy time, we observed that if audio was not used during the Internet communication, therapy time was prolonged extensively. This was because the information that could be exchanged in written communication was less and took more time than the one possibly transmitted by an audio system.

Counseling and conducting therapy sessions can be wholly effective through e-mail. From the patient side, we had two patients reporting the effectiveness of sending an e-mail about a difficulty or emotional conflict right at the time they were experiencing it. Similarly, the therapists could send an appropriate reply or comment, accompanied with a list of tasks, exercises, or suggested bibliotherapy concerning the specific problem.

FUTURE DIRECTIONS

We expect to see future growth in online psychological practice in Mexico. This is due to the universality of the medium, the easy access to the World Wide Web, the expected technological advances that will improve the infrastructure of the communication between patient and therapist, and the low cost of the treatment. Services via Internet cost between 300 and 500 Mexican pesos (approximately $27 to $45 respectively) for each full treatment, whereas face-to-face treatment at the Psychological Care Center costs approximately 5,400 Mexican pesos ($490) for each full treatment. The previous paragraph highlights the importance of training students in this innovative therapeutic modality. It is also worth mentioning that this mode of teaching allows the educator to provide students with specialized knowledge, a knowledge that will fortify their competence level and modernize them as professionals in these newly developing specialties. The availability of teaching programs that strengthen the university students' integral formation—in particular the linking of theory and practice—represents a great contribution to the field of teaching in psychology.

One limitation of the present pilot study is that the results obtained represent the first assessment of the teaching program. As such, they can allow only tentative conclusions due to the small sample that is not sufficient to test the real efficacy of our training program. It is necessary to test the efficacy of this training program in larger samples using group designs, including control groups and other treatment groups. Moreover, further research is necessary to assess the patients' clinical results as well as the factors associated with successful treatments. Additional empirical studies are needed in order to establish ethical regulations for practicing psychology under this modality of service; to assess results, cost-effectiveness, technological development needs; and to investigate the limits of distance intervention. These would lead to better teaching of the emergent modalities in these times of change.

REFERENCES

American Psychological Association Ethics Committee. (1998). Services by telephone, teleconferencing, and Internet: A statement by the Ethics Committee of the American Psychological Association. *American Psychologist, 53*, 979. Retrieved from http://www.apa.org/ethics/stmnt01.html.

Bermejo, M. (1999). *Eficacia y Aplicación de la Terapia Cognitivo-Conductual Vía Internet*. Valencia: IV Congreso Internacional de Psicología Cognitiva/Conductual. Retrieved May 22, 2006, from http://www.cop.es/colegiados/pv04735.

Cárdenas, G., Moreyra, L., Serrano, B., Richards, C., Villafuerte, M., Ramírez, A., et al. (2005). *Tutoriales multimedia: Diagnóstico y tratamiento en trastornos de ansiedad*. México, DF:UNAM.

Cárdenas, G., Serrano, B., Patoni, R., & Plata, L. (2005). *Psicoterapia vía Internet: Manual de entrenamiento*. México, DF: UNAM.

Colon, Y. (1996). Chattering through the fingertips: Doing group therapy online. *Women & Perfomance*, *9*, 205–215.

Lange, A., Schrieken, B., Van de Ven, J., Bredeweg, B., Emmelkamp, P., Van der Kolk, J., et al. (2000). Interapy: The effects of a short protocolled treatment of posttraumatic stress and pathological grief through the Internet. *Behavioral and Cognitive Psychotherapy*, 28, 175–192.

Marks, I., Cavanagh, K., Gega, L. (2007). *Hands-on help. Computer-aided psychotherapy*. New York: Psychology Press.

Murphy, L., & Mitchell, D. (1998). When writing helps to heal: E-mail as therapy. *British journal of Guidance & Counselling*, *26*, 21–33.

National Board Certified Counselors (2007). The practice of Internet counseling. Retrieved from http://www.nbcc.org/webethics2.

National Institute for Health and Clinical Excellence (NICE) (2006). Annual report and accounts 2006/7. Washington, DC: TSO.

Nezu, A., Nezu, C., Peacock, A., & Girdwood, C. (2003). *Case formulation in cognitive-behavior therapy*. In *Behavioral Assessment* (Vol. 3), *Comprehensive Handbook of Psychological Assessment*. New York: Wiley.

Nickelson, W. (1998) Telehealth and the evolving health care system: Strategic opportunities for professional psychology. *Professional Psychology: Research and Practice*, *29*(6), 527–535.

Oravec, J. (2000) Online counseling and the Internet: Perspectives for mental health care supervision and education. *Journal of Mental Health*, *9*(2), 121–135.

Rochlen, A., Zack, J., & Speyer, C. (2004). Online therapy: Review of relevant definitions, debates, and current empirical support. *Journal of Clinical Psychology*, *60*(3), 269–283.

Schneider, P. (1999, August). Psychotherapy using distance technology a comparison of outcomes. Presented at the Annual Meeting of the American Psychological Association, Boston, Masssachussetts.

Sun-Teach International Group Ltd. (2004) X-Class One-click Teaching System. Retrieved from http://www.suntechgroup.com/classroomcontrol/index_es.htm.

Young, J. E., & Beck, A. T. (1980). *Manual de calificación de la escala de Terapia Cognitiva*. (E. See, Trad.) Philadelphia: University of Pennsylvania, Center for Psychotherapy Research.

Conclusion

Dick Schoech
Jerry Finn

Changing from an old to a new technology involves two distinct phases. The first is overlaying the existing technology with the new technology. For example, the first cars were called and literally were horseless carriages and the first planes were bicycles with wings. The second phase involves redesigning objects and processes based on the new technology; for example, current automobiles are fundamentally different from the horseless carriage because they are designed around the internal combustion engine and modern transportation systems. The articles in this issue suggest etherapy is at the first stage of using information technology (IT) with only a few articles containing concepts and ideas related to the second stage. Consequently, we have a long way to go to in fully using IT to deliver therapeutic interventions. While we have a long way to go, we have come a long way over the past 20 years. We can see how far we have come by examining the articles in *Using Computers in Clinical Practice* (Schwartz, 1984). Chapters in this book concerned selecting and using computers for education, accounting, word processing, testing, assessment, interviewing, diagnosis, and information management and reporting. Only a few articles in the book discussed what today we call etherapy.

The articles herein describe many etherapy approaches, discuss many issues, and raise many more issues. One consistent issue concerns nomenclature, classification, and definitions. The introduction to this special issue lists about 20 terms for describing online therapeutic interventions. We may not be at a place where terminology issues can be resolved, because etherapy is technology driven, and the Internet is rapidly evolving with new features such as targeted search (Google), social networking (MySpace), video sharing (YouTube), and user-developed resource repositories (Wikipedia). Technological developments are moving etherapy from therapist-dominated text and phone applications to applications that use interactive multimedia with therapist support. As the underlying technology of etherapy changes, additional terms and concepts will emerge. Definition and classification issues may be with us for some time in the future.

Another issue concerns training the workforce to practice in an online environment (see Abbot, Klein, & Ciechomski). Questions remain whether an online workforce can be trained in the traditional face-to-face classroom or whether this training must be online (Cárdenas, Serrano, Flores, & De la Rosa-Gómez; MacFadden, Murphy, & Mitchell). These articles also question whether existing therapeutic techniques are adequate or whether new techniques that are specific to online therapy need to be developed.

The fact that the articles on training online therapists are from other countries illustrates another issue, the role of legal liability and regulation. Various articles allude to the role of governments and professional associations to regulate and monitor Internet-delivered therapeutic interventions (Zack; Midkiff & Wyatt). One question is whether a stand-alone etherapy application should be considered a therapeutic device and thus be regulated by the U.S. Food and Drug Administration, as are other health devices. Alternatively, should regulation be by professional associations that currently are struggling to find their role and keep up with new technology? Courts will have to decide these and many other issues; for example, whether the client's or the clinician's locale has the legal authority to regulate online practice. Similar issues, such as the e-therapist being licensed in the state in which the client resides, may require legislation to be resolved on other than a state-by-state basis. Clients can be highly mobile, for example, a therapist in the UK stated that he treats a client who lives periodically in the United States, Europe, and Asia. Issues concerning etherapy and local juris-diction are more difficult in a global but interconnected workplace.

Another group of issues concerns the design and delivery of online interventions. Some issues concern the theoretical base of online practice (Peng & Schoech). Others concern viewing the application development process in ways that encourage computer scientists and human services professionals to communicate effectively (LaMendola & Krysik). Associated with this group of issues is how to evaluate online interventions, especially those experimenting with phase two applications that use interactive multimedia (Pahwa & Schoech). Games are an example of phase two applications that raise many issues (Freddolino & Blaschke). For example, with therapeutic games, no two players receive the same intervention, thus making it difficult to insure fidelity to the intervention for evaluation purposes.

Other issues emerge when delivering therapeutic interventions; for example, client suitability (Abbot, Klein, & Ciechomski). These issues are complicated by uneven broadband coverage. For example, while South Korea has about 90 percent broadband coverage, Africa has less than 1 percent broadband penetration ("Broadband Use Swells," 2007). Only 4.5 percent of the world's households have broadband connectivity that is necessary for some forms of etherapy. Etherapy is not value free but incorporates the philosophical value and world-views of researchers and developers who reside in modern wealthy economies. Consequently, etherapy interventions are typically designed for clients who are urban, mobile, and relatively isolated from their family and neighbors. However, these applications can easily be delivered to clients in countries where mental health interventions typically involve traditional healers, extended families, and tight-knit communities. This point was illustrated by a colleague's discussion about how some Native American students often "disappeared" for several weeks and explain on their return that they were addressing a family problem. Inquiring further, she found that when someone in a local Native American family had a problem, members of the extended family gathered around that person and processed through the problem for the number of days needed to reach a resolution. None of the etherapy techniques in this issue is able to support, structure, or deliver help to this extended family process for solving human problems. Developers must be careful that etherapy delivered outside the culture in which it was developed support rather than replace family and community networks and natural ways of healing.

Surprisingly, the issue of etherapy effectiveness seems to be resolved. Meta-analyses (Barak, Hen, Boniel-Nissim, & Shapira) and the research presented throughout this issue suggest that properly designed and implemented etherapy is effective. The range of problems addressed by etherapy range from panic, anxiety, depression (Andersson et al.), fear of public speaking (Botella et al.), sexual victimization (Finn & Hughes), and sex offender recovery (Kernsmith & Kernsmith). While potential effectiveness seems well established, delivery issues remain such as informed consent, confidentiality, privacy, identity verification, and data security

(Abbott, Klein, & Ciechomski). Another unresolved issue is the role of professionals in online intervention. Some articles describe the Internet as a tool to assist practitioners in delivering etherapy, while others suggest etherapy can be delivered independent of professional contact, although under professional supervision. While both roles may continue, how predominant a role the practitioner will play depends on effectiveness research, cost, client preference, and other factors that will surface in the future.

Future perspectives on Internet-delivered therapeutic interventions depend on how far in the future one looks. Clearly, the rapid development of online interventions is the result of positive outcomes along with client acceptance and demand (Lintvedt, Sørensen, Østvik, Verplanken, & Wang). We failed to receive an article discussing future approaches to online delivery, although this is an important topic. Some online therapeutic sites, such as www.live-counselor.com, take a marketplace approach where consumers rate therapists like any other online service, with 1 to 5 stars with customer comments (Finn & Bruce). However, receiving therapy is not the same as buying a television or renting a movie. During some stages of therapy, a client may experience discomfort or dissatisfaction as therapists challenge and address their destructive practices. Also, the concept of transference suggests that client satisfaction can be an unreliable measure of success. The consumer rating approach is in sharp contrast to the approach where human service professionals come together to in virtual office space to take advantages of etherapy IT infrastructure, specialized training, and support (MacFadden, Murphy, & Mitchell). These virtual offices can then market their services to individuals or obtain contracts from corporations that view etherapy as one tool in their employee assistance program. Still another approach is where a research teams designs, tests, and then moves proven interventions out to the public (Andersson et al.; Abbot, Klein, & Ciechomski). It will be interesting to watch which delivery approach—individual, group virtual office, or research team—will prove more viable. While client choice will be important, sadly we were not able to find an author to articulate the client perspective.

In conclusion, the Internet offers many alternatives for addressing client's problems in effective but nontraditional ways. Many issues remain concerning etherapy design, delivery, liability, and the role of the professional. Just as the authors in the 1984 Schwartz book could not have foreseen the development and importance of the

Internet platform for etherapy, future professionals will probably look back on this special issue as describing rather primitive approaches to online practice. It seems clear, however, that online practice will continue to grow and evolve, and become an important addition to human service delivery.

REFERENCES

Broadband use swells to 300 million worldwide. (2007). *The Inquirer*, June 14. Retrieved January 14, 2008, from http//www.theinquirer.net/en/inquirer/news/2007/06/14/broadband-use-swells-to-300-million-worldwide.

Schwartz, M. (Ed.). (1984). *Using computers in clinical practice: Psychotherapy and mental health applications*. Binghamton, NY: The Haworth Press.

Index

Page numbers in *Italic* are tables
Page numbers in **Bold** are figures

T - #0139 - 071024 - C0 - 234/156/22 - PB - 9780415845311 - Gloss Lamination